Quality of Life in Ireland

Social Indicators Research Series

Volume 32

This new series aims to provide a public forum for single treatises and collections of papers on social indicators research that are too long to be published in our journal *Social Indicators Research*. Like the journal, the book series deals with statistical assessments of the quality of life from a broad perspective. It welcomes the research on wide variety of substantive areas, including health, crime, housing, education, family life, leisure activities, transportation, mobility, economics, work, religion and environmental issues. These areas of research will focus on the impact of key issues such as health on the overall quality of life and vice versa. An international review board, consisting of Ruut Veenhoven, Joachim Vogel, Ed Diener, Torbjorn Moum, Mirjam A.G. Sprangers and Wolfgang Glatzer, will ensure the high quality of the series as a whole.

The titles published in this series are listed at the end of this volume.

Tony Fahey • Helen Russell
• Christopher T. Whelan
Editors

Quality of Life in Ireland

Social Impact of Economic Boom

Springer

Editors:
Tony Fahey
University College
Dublin
Ireland

Helen Russell
Economic and Social Research Institute
Dublin
Ireland

Christopher T. Whelan
Economic and Social Research Institute
Dublin
Ireland

The work has been previously published by IPA, Institute of Public Adminstration, Dublin, Ireland.
Original title: Best of Times? The Social Impact of the Celtic Tiger
Paperback published July 2007, ISBN 978-1-904541-58-5 (PB)

ISBN 978-1-4020-6980-2 (HB)
e-ISBN 978-1-4020-6981-9

Library of Congress Control Number: 2008928684

Printed on acid-free paper

9 8 7 6 5 4 3 2 1

springer.com

Contents

Contributors

Mary P. Corcoran is Senior Lecturer in the Department of Sociology, National University of Ireland at Maynooth

Merike Darmody is Research Analyst at the Economic and Social Research Institute, Dublin

David Duffy is Research Officer at the Economic and Social Research Institute, Dublin

Allison Dunne, until recently a research assistant at the Economic and Social Research Institute, is a PhD student in the European University Institute, Florence

Robert Erikson is Professor at the Swedish Institute for Social Research and a member of the Council of the Economic and Social Research Institute, Dublin

Tony Fahey, until recently a Research Professor at the Economic and Social Research Institute, is Professor of Social Policy at University College, Dublin

Jane Gray is Senior Lecturer in the Department of Sociology, National University of Ireland at Maynooth

Gerard Hughes is Research Professor (retired) at the Economic and Social Research Institute, Dublin

Richard Layte is Research Professor at the Economic and Social Research Institute, Dublin

Selina McCoy is Research Officer (Higher) at the Economic and Social Research Institute, Dublin

Frances McGinnity is Research Officer at the Economic and Social Research Institute, Dublin

Bertrand Maître is Research Officer at the Economic and Social Research Institute, Dublin

Anne Nolan is Research Officer at the Economic and Social Research Institute, Dublin

Brian Nolan, until recently a Research Professor at the Economic and Social Research Institute, is Professor of Public Policy at University College, Dublin

Philip J. O'Connell is Research Professor at the Economic and Social Research Institute, Dublin

Ian O'Donnell is Director of the Institute of Criminology at University College, Dublin

Michel Peillon is Associate Professor in the Department of Sociology, National University of Ireland at Maynooth

Emma Quinn is Research Analyst at the Economic and Social Research Institute, Dublin

Helen Russell is Senior Research Officer at the Economic and Social Research Institute, Dublin

Emer Smyth is Senior Research Officer at the Economic and Social Research Institute, Dublin

Christopher T. Whelan is Research Professor at the Economic and Social Research Institute, Dublin

Foreword

Frances Ruane, Director,
Economic and Social Research Institute

Irish and international scholars continue to be curious about Ireland's exceptional economic success since the early 1990s. While growth rates peaked at the turn of the millennium, they have since continued at levels that are high by any current international or historical Irish measures. Despite differences of view among Irish economists and policymakers on the relative importance of the factors that have driven growth, there is widespread agreement that the process of globalisation has contributed to Ireland's economic development. In this context, it is helpful to recognise that globalisation has created huge changes in most developed and developing countries and has been associated, *inter alia*, with reductions in global income disparity but increased income disparity within individual countries.

This book reflects on how, from a social perspective, Ireland has prospered over the past decade. In that period we have effectively moved from being a semi-developed to being a developed economy. While the book's main focus is on the social changes induced by economic growth, there is also recognition that social change has facilitated economic growth. Although many would regard the past decade as a period when economic and social elements have combined in a virtuous cycle, there is a lingering question as to the extent to which we have better lives now that we are economically 'better off'. In the context of economic change, there are always winners and losers, which gives rise to the issue of how we determine whether and to what extent we are better off as a society. Those who see the glass as being half-full point to increased employment opportunities, better housing, greater participation in education, reduced poverty and long-term unemployment, etc. Those who focus on the half-empty glass point to greater inequality at the top end of the wealth spectrum, greater commuting times, greater stress, longer waiting lists for health care, some increase in crime, etc.

However the glass is viewed, all agree that the change has generated new opportunities and created great challenges. If we are to realise the opportunities and face up to the challenges, we need to understand and appreciate the combined economic, social and environmental implications of the change. In effect, we need to understand in a more analytical way the issues which have been raised in the media by many commentators, perhaps most effectively by David McWilliams. Only with this type of analysis, can we be sure that our policy responses are strategic and evidence-based rather than reactive and anecdotally driven. We need to get a handle on the heterogeneity of people's experiences in the context of this massive social and economic change.

The chapters in this volume cover all of the main issues one would expect to see in a collection looking at the social changes induced by rapid economic growth. This coverage includes employment, health, education, housing, income inequality, immigration, social cohesion, work–life balance and quality of life. The chapters review the current state of knowledge and understanding about this social change, drawing on a range of recent research and data sources, most particularly within the ESRI and the CSO. In addition, the final chapter by the distinguished Swedish sociologist, Professor Robert Erikson, reflects on the overall picture created by the book and on the extent to which it meets its own objectives.

In essence, therefore, this volume brings together what we know from research about how Irish society has changed as it has become more prosperous. And while we know a lot, it is clear that there is more to be known. Some steps are already in place to begin to fill in some of the current gaps in our knowledge. For example, Ireland is finally about to undertake its first longitudinal study of children – this will inform us about what determines the outcomes for our children as they grow up in a very different context to that experienced by their parents and by the nation's policymakers. Steps are in motion to develop longitudinal studies of older people, which will help inform us about the health and care needs of a more numerous older population. It may also be timely to contemplate a longitudinal study of migrants so that we are better placed to evolve policy and avoid the huge social problems being encountered by some of our EU neighbours. And to understand life–work balance, should we now invest in collecting time-use data, which is key to understanding how economic and social factors operate at the household level? In a knowledge-driven society, it seems imprudent to under-invest in programmes whose objective is to gain a better understanding of ourselves, so that our policy interventions serve us well. For this understanding, we need more data to be collected and more research to be undertaken.

The breadth of this book reflects the very broad scholarship of researchers at the ESRI across a range of key social issues. It is enhanced by the addition of the aforementioned chapter by Robert Erikson, as well as by the chapter by Mary Corcoran, Jane Gray and Michel Peillon at NUIM on the quality of life in the new suburbs surrounding Dublin, and Ian O'Donnell of UCD on how crime and social cohesion have been impacted by growth. To these authors and to my colleagues at the ESRI, we are indebted for a collection of scholarly articles on how our society has changed in the face of rapid growth.

1

Quality of Life After the Boom

Tony Fahey, Helen Russell and Christopher T. Whelan

Best of times or worst of times?

Over the past decade the Irish economy has soared and has brought levels of average income to among the highest in the world. This economic 'miracle' has generated a great deal of congratulation both at home and abroad, not only because of stellar economic performance but also because, as some commentators believe, Ireland is a good society as well as a strong economy. In 2004, for example, the Economist Intelligence Unit (EIU) forecast that in 2005 Ireland would be the world's best country to live in – it scored the highest of 111 countries around the world on a quality-of-life index compiled on the basis of nine separate indicators, only one of which – Gross Domestic Product (GDP) per capita – was economic in the strict sense. Compared to other rich countries, according to the EIU's analysis, Ireland's quality-of-life advantage lay primarily in two key *social* factors: its higher than average level of stability in family life (measured by its low divorce rate) and its stronger community participation (measured by a combination of church attendance and trade union participation). These family and community factors together accounted for about three-quarters of Ireland's superiority on the quality-of-life index compared to the average for the EU-15 (Economist Intelligence Unit, 2004).

While one might query the details of the EIU's index and dispute its ranking of Ireland as the world's number one country, the key point to note is its view of Ireland as a socially as well as economically successful society. This point has evoked scorn in many quarters, and a chorus of commentators has portrayed the social side of the Celtic Tiger in darkly pessimistic terms. For example, in an address to a conference in Ennis, Co. Clare, on 3 November 2004, Emily O'Reilly, the current Ombudsman and Information Commissioner and formerly a high-profile journalist, excoriated Ireland's recent social and cultural record. She spoke of the 'vulgar fest' of modern Ireland – 'the rampant, unrestrained drunkenness, the brutal, random violence that infects the smallest of our townlands and

T. Fahey et al. (eds.), Quality of Life in Ireland, 1–10.

villages, the incontinent use of foul language with no thought to place or company, the obscene parading of obscene wealth, the debasement of our civic life, the growing disdain of the wealthy towards the poor, the fracturing of our community life' (O'Reilly, 2004). This unflattering portrait attracted a good deal of attention in the media, much of it sympathetic (*The Irish Times* printed an edited version of the address in a features page – 6 November 2004). A statement released by Céifin, the community development organisation that arranged the conference, reported a huge demand for copies of the speech and claimed that it 'articulated what the majority of people in Ireland feel about the direction Irish society is taking'.

Other observers have expressed similar sentiments. For example, in his introduction to a recent collection of sociological commentaries on the Celtic Tiger, Colin Coulter has written that '[t]he materialism that has overtaken the twenty-six counties in the era of the Celtic Tiger articulates a spiritual emptiness that invariably attends the process of modernisation'. He says that Ireland 'has become a place that elevates having over being' and criticises the 'rampant consumption', 'devotion to self' and 'arrogance and callousness' that has overtaken the country (Coulter, 2003, p. 25). Kieran Keohane and Carmen Kuhling, in a recent contribution with a similar tone, refer to the 'melancholy spirit of the Celtic Tiger' and catalogue a gloomy list of failings: '… urban growth that is squalid and blighted, a liberal culture that is shallow and vulgar, a new emancipated subjectivity that is aimless and listless, a promiscuous and indiscriminate "openness" to the new, … a derision of past beliefs and ideals, softened by a note of nostalgia and wistful romance for their passing ...' (Keohane and Kuhling, 2006, p. 40). Elizabeth Cullen, a public health specialist, has presented an equally negative judgement on a more empirical level, assembling a mass of statistical indicators to support her view that the economic boom 'has seriously damaged the nation's health and the bonds between its people' and 'has depleted our true wealth – our health, our society and our environment' (Cullen, 2004, pp. 9, 43).

Objectives

The negativity of this line of commentary is striking, and has been rejected by some as excessive (entertainingly so by David McWilliams who, in his recent bestseller on Ireland, lampoons it as the utterings of a 'confused commentariat' – McWilliams, 2006). Yet concern about the social effects of the economic boom is widespread enough for the underlying question to be taken seriously. Has the Celtic Tiger, on balance, been good for Irish society or has rapid economic growth come at too high a social cost? The purpose of this book – an edited collection of chapters written by specialists in their fields – is to bring to bear the latest research and empirical evidence to answer this question. It seeks to establish who has benefited from the economic boom and what it has done to Irish people's social and personal well-being and quality of life. There are some aspects of this question that are too elusive to come within the reach of conventional social science and so are passed over here – whether, for example, Ireland is becoming more 'vulgar' or 'shallow', or whether Irish people are less courteous or use more coarse language than before. The focus of the book on the *social* also rules out consideration of many important questions on other aspects of the Celtic Tiger's impact, such as its effects on the physical environment and its long-term sustainability even in economic terms.

Even with these restrictions, however, many questions remain for the book to grapple with. Some see Ireland's rising tide of prosperity as having lifted all boats, while others argue that the benefits have accrued mostly to those who were already well placed, leaving the disadvantaged further behind. Some highlight how economic growth has raised living standards, while others say that it has imposed strains on family life, eroded values and communities, and created problems in accessing adequate housing, health care and other services. Some see the 'Irish social model' as a template that the EU should learn from, while others criticise its failure to live up to European standards of social inclusion and solidarity. These issues arise against the backdrop of a larger debate in rich countries about current models of economic progress: do they bring real improvements in people's lives or do they increase the pressures we live under, over-emphasise work and competition for status, and encourage people to adopt selfish, materialistic values?

What can be said?

There are many reasons why this or indeed any other book cannot answer these questions on anything more than a partial and tentative basis. First of all, there is the *cultural relativity* problem. Conceptions of the good society, or of what constitutes social progress, are founded on ethical and philosophical worldviews that vary across cultures and even across social groups and cannot readily be determined as right or wrong (for a lucid and sophisticated discussion of this issue by a philosopher from University College Dublin, see Cooke, 2006). In Ireland in recent times, for example, whether one considers the declining social role of religion or the more liberal attitude to sexuality as progress or decline depends largely on one's philosophical standpoint. Second is the *apples and oranges* problem – how to weigh up different dimensions of social change and come to a judgement on the resulting balance. In most countries in recent decades, for example, crime has gone up (a bad thing) but so too have levels of education (a good thing). How can one add these two developments together in trying to decide whether social conditions have improved overall? Third is the *ambivalent good* problem: even those social changes that may be good in one sense may be bad in another. For example, more people in Ireland than ever before have a car, which greatly enhances personal mobility, but traffic congestion and environmental pollution have increased as a result, which restricts our mobility in some ways and makes our physical environment less pleasant. How can we decide whether the upside or the downside of any development be given more attention? Finally, there is the *ignorance* problem: we sometimes do not really know what has happened and therefore cannot begin to say whether change – if it has occurred at all – is progressive or not. Mental health, for example, is an important part of quality of life but is so difficult to measure that trends over time are difficult to track (as is outlined briefly in Chapter 2). Even areas of behaviour that would seem reasonably quantifiable in principle can have quite muddled data in practice (as is shown, for example, in connection with crime statistics in Chapter 14 of this volume).

Although these problems limit the judgements one can make about social change in Ireland, they do not place such judgement out of bounds altogether. There is cultural consensus on the valuation of many social trends – nobody disputes, for example, that unemployment or early death are socially undesirable – and even topics that are the subject of value dispute can be illuminated by good information. For example, it can help us to decide how much significance to attach to, say, an increase in marital breakdown if we know more about its precise extent and nature. Likewise, with the apples and oranges problem, factual details can help – it matters whether we are comparing five apples with five oranges or ten apples with one orange. The counterbalancing sides of an ambivalent good can similarly benefit from having factual light shone upon them. Even with the ignorance problem, it can help to point out where ignorance exists and thereby restrain us from jumping to ill-informed conclusions.

Starting from this somewhat cautious view of what it is possible to do in an exercise such as this, the book sought to encompass a fairly wide range of topics in assessing Ireland's present social situation – not an encyclopaedic list but enough to give some sense of an overall picture and to include core areas, such as living standards, health, family, education, and so on, that are widely assumed to be central to quality of life. The approach was guided in part by the Swedish 'level of living' concept of welfare measurement, which is concerned with people's access to resources in the form of money, possessions, knowledge, mental and physical energy and social relationships. It thus goes beyond economic resources to include, among other things, health, knowledge and skills. In addition, however, topics were included because of a mixture of their topicality in Irish public commentary and availability of research findings and expertise to write about them.

The analysis of these topics is mainly concerned with *outcomes*. It does not try to explain Irish economic performance nor assess its sustainability but focuses on the social consequences of the boom and their implications for people's well-being. The main time frame taken into account is the past ten years or so, that is, from the onset of the boom in 1993–94 to the present day, though longer periods are also considered where these are needed to set recent developments in context. Much attention is paid to relative and absolute change. Pre-boom Ireland was both more unequal and poorer than the norm for Western Europe. Today it continues to be unequal but in a context where even the less well-off have seen major absolute improvements in their circumstances. This combination of stasis and advance could be judged a success or failure, depending on one's point of view, but in any event it is important to keep both sides of the coin in mind and not simply focus on either relative or absolute change alone.

A further feature of the Irish case is the highly globalised nature of the Irish economy – it is exceptionally open to international trade and investment and to cross-border flows of labour. Some consider that such integration increases uncertainty, raises the risk of social marginalisation and reduces national autonomy, but others have stressed not only the positive potential of globalisation but also the continuing importance of domestic institutions, choices and values in mediating its impact (for an analysis of the European welfare state in these terms, see Ferrera and Rhodes, 2000). The Irish strategy, as Ó Riain and O'Connell (2000) argue, is far removed from the social democratic emphasis on equality and universalistic social services, though, equally, it is too wedded to such corporatist institutions as the national partnership agreements to be counted as a full-blooded instance of the Anglo-Saxon neo-liberal approach. The Irish social model, as Hardiman (2004) notes, involves a mix of market-oriented competitiveness, active labour market policy, an emphasis on incentives to work, sustained welfare provision, and a social partnership founded on a trade-off between pay and tax. In evaluating the consequences of this model, account must be taken not only of its distributional consequences but also the pre-boom starting point and the dramatic scale of absolute change.[1]

Outline of chapters

Doubts about the impact of the Celtic Tiger on our sense of well-being are a common source of the ambivalence sometimes expressed about the benefits, or lack of them, arising from the economic boom. While this theme recurs in a number of chapters, it is given primary attention in Chapter 2, which deals with the relationship between economic growth and happiness in Ireland in recent times. The claim that the rich are getting richer and the poor are getting poorer is another of the more commonly voiced criticism of the Celtic Tiger. Chapter 3 takes up this question by examining how rich and how unequal Ireland has become in income terms during the economic boom. It shows that Ireland's wealth has grown dramatically, though not as much as is suggested by some indicators, particularly GDP per capita. More meaningful measures of national income bring Ireland's relative position down more or less to the average for OECD countries. The chapter confirms that Ireland has a high degree of income inequality by rich country standards but disagrees that this problem has worsened in recent years: the Celtic Tiger may have failed to reduce income inequality but neither did it increase it.

Along with rising incomes, the jobs boom of the past decade has been one of the most striking products of the Celtic Tiger. Chapter 4 examines how widely spread and real its gains have been. It points to the decline in unemployment, including long-term unemployment, as a central transformation, and one that is broadly inclusive. Some groups, such as lone parents and those with low education, poor health or a disability, continue to have job problems, though less so than in the past. Trends in the nature of the jobs that are available contradict the sometimes expressed view that there has been a general decline in the quality of employment. Rather, the occupational structure has been upgraded and overall job quality has increased, with more job security, less involuntary part-time

---

[1] The need to do so is particularly well illustrated in Brady, Beckfield and Seeleib-Kaiser's (2005) comparative analysis of the consequences of globalisation for the welfare state, which encompasses the Irish case. They conclude that over the period 1975–2001 Ireland increased its trade, reduced its social welfare expenditure, in part due to an expanding GDP, while at the same time raising its level of 'decommodification' or insulation from market forces; as reflected in the combined effect of coverage, qualifying periods for eligibility and replacement rates for unemployment, sickness and pension welfare programmes.

work and temporary contracts, higher wages and a decline in long hours. These gains are tempered with a simultaneous growth in the lower-skilled service sector jobs but even these have a positive side since without them it would have been difficult to absorb the huge numbers of formerly unemployed. Furthermore, the Irish case has not been characterised by a polarisation into work-rich and work-poor households.

The contrast between intense growth and undiminished inequality has led many to argue that such growth has locked up social mobility and decreased equality of opportunity. Chapter 5 paints a picture that is a good deal more optimistic. There has been considerable intergenerational mobility in recent decades and the greater part of it has been upward. The rising tide has lifted many boats. However, the occupational playing field remained tilted in favour of children from more advantaged backgrounds even as the flow of children from working-class origins into middle-class positions increased dramatically.

Chapter 6 turns to those on the margins and assesses the recurring theme that social exclusion has increased amid the growing affluence. It identifies tiered levels of deprivation in Irish society, with the numbers affected decreasing as the intensity of the deprivation increases. However, it concludes that both levels and depth of such deprivation are less than in the past and are a good deal more modest than is suggested by the more extreme critics of the recent Irish experience.

Chapter 7 shows that there has been a considerable improvement in the health of the Irish population, though the advent of this improvement predates the economic boom. However, changing attitudes and expectations mean that very little of this improvement is reflected in people's assessments of their health. Despite the substantial increase in resources to the health system, the acute hospital sector remains under severe strain, primary care services have not expanded as intended and equity of access remains a major issue.

The booming housing market is often taken as emblematic of the social and economic transformation that has taken place since the mid-1990s. Chapter 8 looks at the social impact of the housing boom in Ireland in regard to issues such as affordability of housing, its implications for family/household formation, and significance for social inequality. The authors argue that the blockages and strains faced by new entrants to the housing market can be overstated. Young adults are more likely to form independent households now than ever before and problems of affordability are restricted to a minority of homebuyers, even among recent first-time buyers. The real losers in the current housing system are those in the private-rented sector and those who traditionally depended on social housing, where problems of affordability are much more common.

Inadequate provision of social housing has been a major factor behind this outcome. While this trend accentuated social inequalities, other groups who are income-poor, such as the elderly, are argued to have gained from the housing boom.

Chapter 9 examines an important part of children's experience – that represented by the education system, with particular reference to second-level schools. The authors argue that changes within Irish schools have not kept pace with changes in Irish society. Increased autonomy for young people within the family and in the spheres of work and leisure has not been matched by a greater involvement in school decision-making. Social relations in schools remain very hierarchical. While some positive steps have been taken to allow for the diversity of student needs and interests in terms of curriculum, the abiding picture of Irish secondary schools during a period of rapid social transformation is of continuity rather than change.

Chapter 10 looks at changes in attitudes and behaviour in relation to family and sexual relations in Ireland. It suggests that this area of life has been characterised by relative stability since the mid-1990s following a period of intense public debate over questions such as abortion, divorce and contraception. Attitudes have become gradually more liberal over the period, but there have been few radical changes in behaviour. The sometimes heralded collapse of the family is not backed up by statistics on marital breakdown or on family formation, which has stabilised at a level that is high by international standards. In contrast, economic growth is seen to have a relatively benign impact on family life. Changes in sexual behaviour have also been observed, but whether this should be interpreted as a sign of moral decline or a positive move away from a repressive sexual culture depends on one's moral standpoint.

The nature of wider social relationships within the community and neighbourhood are examined in Chapter 11, which considers the quality of life of those living in the expanding suburbs. In contrast with the negative view of the suburbs that infuses the popular and academic literature, the authors found a high level of satisfaction and social integration among the residents of four large suburbs. The majority of residents felt attached to their localities and sited positive reasons for the move to the suburbs. Young families, far from being isolated, had access to local social support, and embeddedness in the local community increased as children reached school-age. However, the demographic homogeneity of the suburbs may marginalise those at other stages in the life cycle. Involvement in more formal associations was also healthy, with between 31 and 48 per cent of residents in the four locations claiming membership of local voluntary associations.

Changing patterns of work, including the increased feminisation of the workforce, are the focus of Chapter 12. Burnt-out working parents, tensions between the demands of the workplace and the home, exhausted long-distance commuters, and children left in care for 12 hours a day are staple media symbols used to indicate all that is wrong with the Celtic Tiger (with the often implicit message that families would be far better off if women stayed at home). The chapter disputes many of these images. It finds high levels of work satisfaction and psychological well-being among those with paid jobs and a decline in the proportion reporting work–family tensions in recent years. There are some strains – some workers feel rushed and stressed and those who combine heavy workloads in the home and in the workplace feel less satisfied. But these factors do not cancel out the positive effect of employment on well-being. Rising female employment has not eliminated gender inequalities in earnings, training, occupational position and the division of unpaid work, though men's and women's attitudes in these areas are becoming less traditional.

Chapter 13 points out that the ending of mass emigration and the advent of net immigration are key indications of improvement in quality of life in Ireland in recent years – people now want to enter rather than leave the country. The economic impact of immigration has been favourable to date, with migrants making a positive contribution to GNP. Nevertheless, immigrant workers are often employed below their qualification levels and there have been a number of high-profile cases of exploitation, indicating the existence of some barriers to their proper integration into the labour market. Survey results show that the Irish population has a more favourable attitude to immigrants and immigration than many of our European neighbours, but a high proportion of asylum seekers and work-permit holders report experiencing harassment or have difficulty accessing jobs and services. The chapter concludes with a discussion of the need for a coherent policy for the integration of migrants into Irish society, for the sake of both migrants and the host community.

Chapter 14 assesses trends in crime and fear of crime since both can impact upon quality of life in society. Changes in recording practices and gaps in data make it difficult to compare crime rates across countries or over time. Official figures suggest no overall escalation in serious crime (including crimes against property, and violent crime) but there has been a rise in homicides. Victimisation surveys show a somewhat contradictory picture, with an increase in crimes against the person and no change in property crime. Public concern about crimes spiked after 1996 but has not led to public demands for harsher responses; this has prevented a shift in policy that has proved misguided in other countries. The chapter concludes that the crime problem remains manageable, despite periodic crises.

The overall picture

Taking all these chapters together, the conclusion they point to is that the Celtic Tiger, judged on the basis of its social as well as its economic impact, certainly deserves two cheers and perhaps even three. The authors have identified a fairly long list of social fundamentals that are stronger today than they were before the Celtic Tiger arrived. Subjective well-being and national morale are among the highest in Europe; living standards have risen and have done so more or less for everyone; jobs have become astonishingly abundant and have improved in quality; people are now flocking into rather than out of the country; young adults are forming couples and having children at an exemplary rate by rich country standards; and people are physically healthier and, as far as we can tell from the rather patchy evidence, generally feel good about their lives and the society around them. This is an impressive list of outcomes, and does not exhaust the positives identified in this book.

One could of course retort that problems still abound and point to the many warts that still mar Ireland's social face. Social inequalities are slow to narrow; the indignities of poverty and hopelessness, though less widespread than before, are still all too common; some public services are poor; traffic congestion frays the nerves; some types of crime have increased; and there is the niggling worry that the whole edifice of economic growth may come crashing down about our ears at some time in the future. There have always been and will always be problems, and they can hardly be said to be more abundant today than in the past. Utopia is not now and never has been available, though the struggle to do better must always go on. A curmudgeonly judgement might therefore be made that, at a minimum, Ireland now has the least worst of times – things may not be good everywhere, but on balance they are not as bad as they used to be. It would not be unreasonable, though, to go a little further than that. One might rather agree with President Mary McAleese when, in her address to the 'Re-Imagining Ireland' conference in Charlottesville, Virginia, in May 2003, she said that no generation had come as close to achieving a peaceful, prosperous, open, equal and opportunity-filled Ireland as this. As she imagined on that occasion, 'if the men and women of Ireland's past could chose a time to live, there would be a long queue for this one' (McAleese, 2003).

2

How Do We Feel? Economic Boom and Happiness

Tony Fahey

Much of the social science research on social progress has concentrated on things that can be measured, like income, housing conditions, educational levels, health, and so on. While all of these are important, the amount of attention they receive may lead to a feeling that some of the more crucial but less tangible aspects of the good life are being left out of the picture. This chapter deals with one of these: subjective well-being or, in plainer language, happiness. It addresses one of the big 'buts' that often arise in questions about the social impact of the Celtic Tiger: 'We are wealthier than ever but are we any happier?'

The aim of the chapter is in part to attempt to answer this question directly, since some factual information is available that enables us to go some way in responding to it in its own terms. In part also, however, the concern is to query the question itself, since the usefulness of happiness as a yardstick of social progress is by no means self-evident. The chapter, therefore, gives some attention to what social science research on happiness tells us in general terms, as well as to the specifics of the situation in Ireland. The thrust of the argument is sceptical: the idea that an across-the-board deficit in human happiness is a real problem in today's rich societies may be superficially compelling but seems doubtful on closer examination. Happiness may indeed be a vital human aspiration, and there are many afflicted people in the world today – mostly but not only in the poorer parts of the world – for whom a happier life is a real and urgently to-be-wished-for goal. It is a different matter whether the privileged majority in rich countries such as Ireland are, on the whole, seriously short-changed in happiness, whether there was a time in the past when they were substantially better off on this front than they are today, or whether a significantly higher plane of happiness is a real possibility for the future. At issue here are quite profound questions about the goals that the good society should be designed to pursue and, in the realm of human happiness, the limits of what is attainable within the constraints of the

T. Fahey et al. (eds.), Quality of Life in Ireland, 11–26.

human condition. This chapter cannot address these underlying questions, but it can present some thoughts and information that will throw light on the impact of the Celtic Tiger on the happiness of people in Ireland and what that tells us about the present condition of Irish society.

Happiness: issues and trends

Social science has recently discovered happiness, both as a subject of research and as a goal that human societies might be geared to pursue. Part of the impetus for this new interest is the accumulation of quantitative survey-based indicators which researchers in this area believe provide meaningful and reliable measures of subjective well-being in human populations (see the bibliography and databases on this issue in the *World Database of Happiness* at http://www.eur.nl/fsw/research/happiness). The two main dimensions of subjective well-being that are typically quantified in this way are *happiness*, which is viewed as the affective side of subjective well-being, and *life satisfaction*, which is thought to be based on cognitive evaluations of one's day-to-day situation. In practice, these measures are based on survey questions that ask people how happy they are or how satisfied they feel either with life in general or with particular domains of daily existence. The various measures that are available on these dimensions are often grouped together under a single label of 'happiness indicators'.

Based on a faith in the methodological soundness of these indicators, happiness has caught on as a research topic even in economics, the branch of the social sciences that traditionally was the least interested in human emotions (for a representative selection of work in this area, see Bruni and Porta, 2004). A recent prominent example is provided by Richard Layard's book, *Happiness: Lessons from a New Science* (2005). Layard, a leading British economist, sets out a now common view as to why happiness is important for social scientists and policymakers. He points to 'a paradox at the heart of our lives':

> Most people want more income and strive for it. Yet as Western societies have got richer, their people have become no happier. … [W]e have more food, more clothes, more cars, bigger houses, more central heating, more foreign holidays … and, above all, better health. Yet we are not happier. (Layard, 2005, p. 3)

This 'devastating fact', in Layard's view, should lead us to re-appraise our whole approach to how we try to improve our lot. Instead of continuous dedication to the 'joyless economy', to use Scitovsky's (1976) phrase, where people constantly pursue more wealth in the futile belief that it will make them happier, we should focus on the things that really matter, such as stronger social relationships, lower unemployment and poverty, less commercialism, and a stronger sense of moral values, and by that means strive for a real and meaningful increase in human happiness (Layard, 2005, pp. 233–235; for a similar view, see Diener and Seligman, 2004).

Economic growth and happiness

One part of the story that inspires Layard's views is not in doubt: economic output has multiplied manifold in recent decades in rich countries but the average level of human happiness, as measured by the standard instruments used for this purpose, has remained more or less unchanged. In the US since the 1950s, for example – the country with the longest time series on happiness indicators – economic output has grown almost fourfold but the trend in subjective well-being has been completely flat (Frey and Stutzer, 2002). The situation in Ireland is in keeping with this pattern. The longest data series we have on happiness in this country derives from Eurobarometer surveys which have been carried out a number of times per year since the early 1970s and which regularly include measures of life satisfaction, based on a four-point life satisfaction scale. Figure 2.1 compares the trend on these data for Ireland and two comparison countries that represent the extremes of variation found within the old EU–12, namely, the Netherlands, which consistently scores highest or nearly highest in the EU on various measures of subjective well-being, and Italy, which, among the original EU Member States, typically scores at, or close to, the bottom of the range on the same measures.

According to these measures, life satisfaction in Ireland was no higher in the late 1990s than in the 1970s, though it dipped for a time in the late 1980s. As the latter was a period marked by economic recession, high unemployment and the resurgence of high emigration, it is plausible to attribute the dip to the poor state of the economy, particularly since the sense of a crisis in the economy at that time was 'talked up' by the political parties in the context of the general election of 1987 (see Laver, Mair and Sinnott, 1987). However, following a recovery in the satisfaction level in the period 1987–1990, fluctuations around the longer-term flat trend resumed. The onset of an economic boom in 1994 brought no upward shift in the trend, and the much higher living standards that had emerged by the late 1990s merely left people with more or less the same level of life satisfaction that was present 25 years previously.

Figure 2.1: *Mean life satisfaction scores in Ireland, the Netherlands and Italy, 1973–1998*

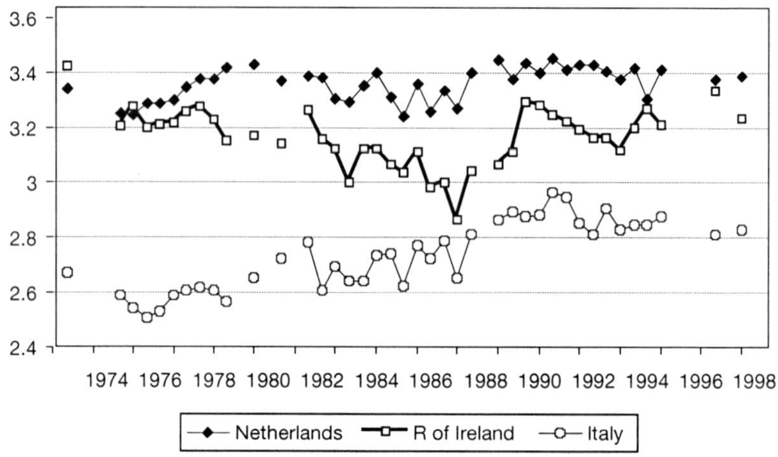

Note: Means are based on a four-point scale where 1 = not at all satisfied and 4 = very satisfied.
Source: Mannheim Eurobarometer Trend data file.

This more or less static level of happiness over long periods, despite economic growth, is replicated in many countries and has prompted Layard and those who write in a similar vein to question the benefits of rising prosperity for subjective well-being. It is this which leads Layard to ask, in one of the chapter titles in his book, 'If you're rich, why aren't you happy?' However, it is possible to view the static nature of happiness in rich countries in a more positive way than Layard does, since it matters a great deal for how we interpret this stasis whether happiness is stuck at a high or a low level and what further increases beyond present levels we think are attainable in normal human conditions. For many researchers in this field, the implicit view is that overall happiness levels are in an unacceptably low trough – especially in rich countries where one might have expected the abundance of resources to benefit people's sense of well-being – and can be significantly increased. The alternative possibility is that in the rich part of the world happiness is in fact on a reasonably high plateau, beyond which further increases are constrained by a ceiling effect: the upper limit of what is possible is so close to being reached that further large increases are more or less impossible.

The data assembled by happiness researchers seem to suggest that for most people in rich countries the high plateau rather than the low trough seems to apply – so much so that a concern for how unhappy people are, particularly rich people, would seem to be misplaced. The data report that the vast majority of people in rich countries, and especially the most affluent in those countries, have quite high levels of subjective well-being and indeed are so far up the scale of what happiness researchers usually measure in this area that further large increases seem hardly possible in their case. In the US, for example, according to data Layard cites, only 4 per cent of those in the upper quarter of the income distribution say they are 'not too happy'. All others – 96 per cent of this income bracket – are either 'very' or 'quite' happy. The situation in Britain is similar: here, 94 per cent of those in the upper income quarter are 'very' or 'quite' happy (Layard, 2005, p. 31). In these instances, in other words, it is the generally high level of happiness rather than of unhappiness that seems striking. This is not to say that the poor in these countries are unhappy: in the US and Britain, 85–90 per cent of those in the bottom quarter of the income range say they are very or quite happy – a slightly smaller share of happiness than for the better off but still very large. In the case of Ireland, surveys which posed a similar question (as was done in the European Values Surveys in 1981, 1990 and 1999–2000) revealed more or less the same result: the proportion of respondents who said they were 'not at all happy' was less than 1.5 per cent in all of these surveys, while in the region of 95 per cent said that they were either 'very happy' or 'quite happy' (Fahey, Hayes and Sinnott, 2006, p. 172).

These quite high levels of subjective well-being cannot be taken for granted, because when we look at poor countries we generally find that their populations score much lower on subjective well-being indicators (in Eastern Europe in particular, there are countries where over half the population say they are not happy – Halman, 2001, p. 17). Instances where people in these countries are 'poor but happy' do occur but they are the exception rather than the norm (Veenhoven, 1995). The positive link between national wealth and average national level of subjective well-being is particularly pronounced in Europe, as is shown in Figure 2.2, which is based on data for 28 EU Member States and candidate countries in 2003. Here the measure of subjective well-being employed is a ten-point life satisfaction scale, a standard indicator used for this purpose. National wealth is measured by means of GDP per capita, adjusted for differences in the cost of living (using purchasing power parities).

This graph shows that the higher the GDP per capita, the higher the level of satisfaction. Ireland, as a rich country, belongs to a group of countries with the highest satisfaction levels in Europe. Generally speaking, Northern Europe has higher levels of subjective well-being than Southern Europe, while Southern Europe is in turn happier than Eastern Europe. It should be said that a high level of economic development is itself strongly correlated with other societal characteristics that are known to affect

Figure 2.2: *Life satisfaction and GDP per capita in EU Member States and candidate countries*

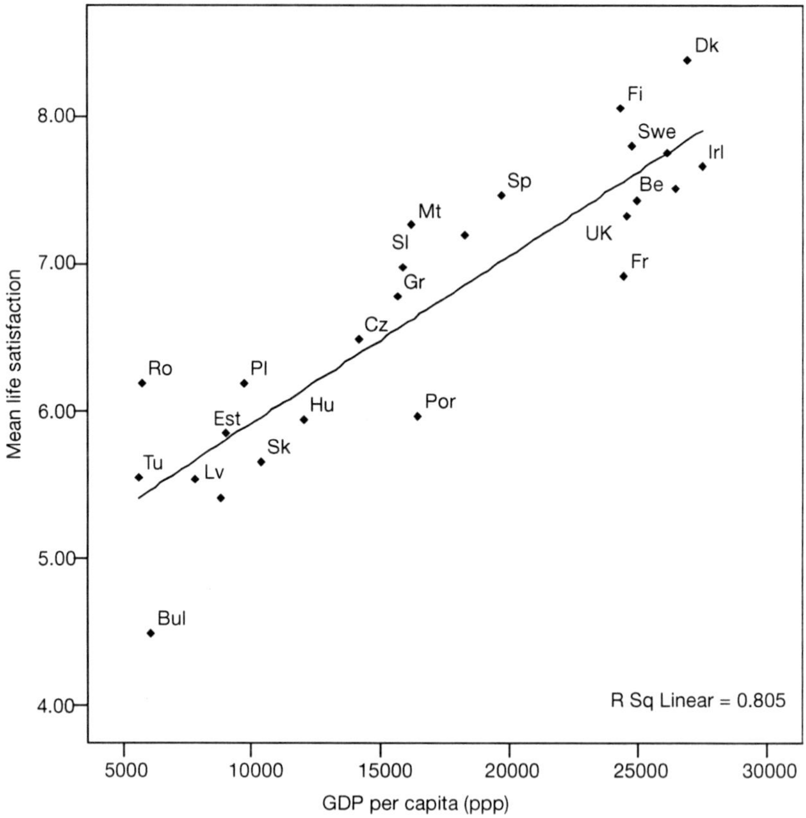

Source: European Quality of Life Survey (2003) micro data; see European Foundation (2004).

subjective well-being, such as long-established, well-functioning democratic political systems. Even in Western Europe, the countries with the most recent experience of non-democratic government – Greece, Spain and Portugal – may have the sunniest weather but nevertheless tend to have somewhat lower levels of subjective well-being. In Eastern Europe, the legacy of communism appears to have a strong depressing effect on subjective well-being. However, Turkey, which was never communist, is just as badly off in subjective well-being as most of the ex-communist states. Thus, we can say that while it is not necessarily national income on its own that supports national happiness, it is clear from Figure 2.2 that there is *something* about living in a rich country that tends to add to people's subjective well-being. These European patterns, therefore, give some grounds for believing that a high level of national prosperity is part of the package of advantages held by rich countries that help to sustain their happiness at reasonably high levels.

The second notable feature of Figure 2.2 is the corroboration it offers to the point made earlier about the ceiling effect on subjective well-being, arising from the closeness of happiness scores in some countries to the upper limit of the scale. In this instance, Ireland is one of a group of 5 countries with mean scores on the 10-point life satisfaction scale above 7.5, while a further seven countries have a mean between 7 and 7.5. Other surveys confirm that while the precise scores vary slightly, there are a number of Northern European countries (of which Ireland is one) that generally show average national scores on such 10-point scales in the region of 8 or slightly below, and few people in these countries rate themselves at less than 5 on the 10-point scales (Fahey and Smyth, 2004; Delhey, 2004; Böhnke, 2005).

Given how high these means are, the scope for further large increases among most of the population is limited, though the circumstances of the small minorities who fall further down the scale could be open to improvement. Even in the best of circumstances, there are always likely to be some people who are unhappy, either temporarily because of some upset in their lives (such as illness, bereavement or conflict with family members) or because of longer-term depressive tendencies, and these will pull population averages down from the top of the scale. It thus may be possible for national averages to rise just a little bit further, but the idea that there are large deficits in subjective well-being that can be made good in the future is not supported by these figures. In these countries, in other words, for the majority of the population who are already high up on these scales, it might well be said that as far as happiness is concerned, *this is as good as it gets*.

This finding could be dismissed as a measurement artefact, having to do with the bounded scales normally used to measure subjective well-being (such as the 10-point life-satisfaction scales just referred to). If the scales only go up to 10, how could measurement record increases beyond 10? However, this feature of the data, far from being a technical quirk, could reflect a profound truth. There is a real doubt as to whether human beings are psychologically hard-wired in such a way to enable them to sustain highly elevated levels of subjective well-being over a long time. The 'set-point' theory of happiness in psychology supports this view. It proposes that people have *set points* of subjective well-being that are largely determined by personality and that anchor our happiness to levels that are fairly stable over the long term, irrespective of changes in the social context (Argyle, 2001; Kahneman, 1999). The various negative shocks or bouts of good fortune that we experience in our lifetime affect our happiness only temporarily, either up or down, following which we return to our set point of subjective well-being. The upper bound on the happiness scales may thus reflect a limit of human nature, not a quirk of measurement.

Stated baldly, the set-point theory is excessively rigid: societal differences across countries, which cannot be attributed to personality factors, give rise to gaps in happiness levels between populations and, at the individual level, there seem to be certain factors (such as severe disability or unemployment on the negative side or a good marriage on the positive side) that produce a lasting downward or upward shift in people's levels of subjective well-being (Easterlin, 2005, pp. 31–41). However, the range of variation is not open-ended – positive or negative factors do not add together to produce ever-rising or ever-falling spirals of happiness. Furthermore, of the factors that are known to enhance people's happiness, most are already possessed in a large measure by people who live in the rich world – and indeed, as we have seen, living in a rich, stable democratic society is itself one of the main foundations of a high level of subjective well-being. Other important factors include not being unemployed, having supportive family and friends, not being seriously ill, having treatment available if one has mental health problems, and having meaningful goals in life (Diener and Seligman, 2004; Frey and Stutzer, 2002) – all of which, again, are commonplace in the developed world today and are lacking only as a minority rather than a majority experience.

The relationship between some of these factors and subjective well-being in Ireland is shown in Table 2.1, which sets out variations in the percentage who are 'very happy' and in mean life-satisfaction scores across a number of socio-demographic categories – gender, age, marital status, social class, and employment status. Looking at this table overall, it is clear that two factors stand out as having substantial links with happiness and life satisfaction. These are unemployment and marital status – and under the latter heading, the separated or divorced have the lower levels of subjective well-being. Among both the unemployed and the separated or divorced in Ireland, only around 20 per cent say they are 'very happy', which is less than half the percentages who are 'very happy' in the samples as a whole. Similarly, their life-satisfaction scores are the lowest – they are the only sub-groups to have means below 7.5 on the life-satisfaction scale. It might equally be said, however, that while these categories of people have lower subjective well-being than the rest of the population, in absolute terms their scores are still quite high. They are not so much unhappy as somewhat below the quite high levels of happiness of the population as a whole – in the case of life-satisfaction, for example, they are well into the upper rather than the lower half of the scale. This may be taken as confirming people's capacity to adapt to negative situations, even though adaptation may not be so complete as to bring people in these situations all the way up to the levels of subjective well-being found in the general population.

Table 2.1: *Happiness and life satisfaction by socio-demographic characteristics*

	% 'very happy'	Mean life-satisfaction score*
Gender:		
Males	39	8.13
Females	45	8.22
Age:		
18–34	40	8.13
35–49	46	8.18
50–64	42	8.17
65+	38	8.20
Marital status:		
Married	49	8.43
Widowed	33	7.98
Separated/divorced	19	7.32
Never married	33	7.73
Social class:		
Professional/managerial	49	8.49
Other non-manual	45	8.27
Manual	42	8.09
Farmers/agric. workers	41	7.92
Employment status:		
At work	44	8.23
Unemployed	22	7.18
Retired	39	8.45
Home duties	46	8.13
Other	33	8.02
Overall sample	42	8.20
[Base N]	[1,012]	[1,012]

* Means are based on a 10-point scale where 1 = dissatisfied and 10 = satisfied
Source: European Values Study, 1999–2000

What about mental disorders?

As mentioned earlier, happiness researchers base their work on a confident view of the validity of the subjective well-being indicators looked at in the previous section. One might wonder, however, whether that confidence is inflated and whether other kinds of indicators should be taken into account to get a rounded picture of people's psychological states. The most commonly cited such alternative indicators are those that relate to mental disorders. These are of particular interest because they are sometimes read as revealing a remarkable worsening of people's psychological health in rich countries over the past half century and so are at odds with the data just reviewed which show high and stable levels of happiness over time in those countries.

Diener and Seligman (2004), for example, present a particularly pessimistic view of mental health trends in their interpretation of survey data on mental disorders in the US. They speak of a 'huge increase in depression [in the US] over the past 50 years', and on the basis of their reading of one study, estimate that the risk of depression may have increased by as much as ten-fold over two generations (Diener and Seligman, 2004, p. 16). They point to these increases as evidence of a decline in psychological well-being in the midst of increasing wealth in the US and as an important part of the justification for shifting the focus of national development away from traditional economic goals towards improvements in subjective well-being.

There are, however, two general problems with arguments along these lines. One is the difficulty of reliably measuring trends in the mental health status of populations over time. Population-based measures of this kind have only recently begun to be developed and there are no consistent historical data sources that enable us to reliably measure trends for earlier decades. Thus, Diener and Seligman's (2004) dramatic conclusions on this issue for the US are not derived from actual trend data on mental health status but are based on comparisons between reported lifetime experience of depressive symptoms among older and younger age groups in point-in-time surveys carried out in the 1980s and 1990s. In effect, they use the recollections of previous occurrences of mental health symptoms among older people in the 1980s and 1990s to back-project estimated rates of depressive disorders for up to 50 years previously. They then compare these with more recent back-projections for younger people. Such means of measuring long-term trends in depression may have some value but clearly they are subject to so many possible sources of error that they have to be viewed with caution.

Apart from such data problems, the other difficulty with arguments about the significance of trends in the experience of depression for psychological well-being among human populations is that the connection between the specific problem of depressive symptoms and broader psychological well-being may not be as strong as might first appear. Layard (2005), for example, focuses on improvements in *therapies* for depression rather than on changes in the incidence of depression as the outstanding feature of developments in this area over the past half century. Effective chemical treatments began to emerge in the 1950s and 1960s, and these were complemented by developments in psychotherapy in the 1970s and 1980s. He therefore emphasises the new-found possibilities open to people who are prone to depressive disorders to live normal, happy lives as one of the major advances in quality of life in human populations in recent decades. This might help to explain a puzzling feature of the analyses in this area produced by Diener and Seligman (2004). Even though they point to a massive increase in the risk of depression and the experience of depressive symptoms in the US population over time, no knock-on effect on measured levels of happiness is evident – as we have seen, Americans today are as happy as they ever were. This could mean either that the supposed increase in depression is not real or that it is counter-balanced by other factors, such as better treatments for depression or improvements in other aspects of people's circumstances that off-set any increases that might have occurred in depression. Thus, even if people are increasingly likely to experience symptoms of depression at some point in their lives (and it is not at all clear whether or to what degree this is the case), it does not necessarily follow that overall psychological well-being is in decline.

In Ireland, long-term trend data on mental health are no more available than in other countries and so it is not possible to decide with any certainty whether mental disorders are becoming more or less common. Some relevant population-based data are available for shorter, recent periods. For example, a standardised indicator of psychological stress was collected in large population samples in Ireland in 1987, 1994 and 2002. These data are referred to by Layte, Nolan and Nolan in Chapter 7 of this volume and show that psychological stress *declined* substantially in Ireland over this period, thus countering the notion of a general worsening of people's mental health.

The most abundant data on mental health in Ireland are based on treatment statistics rather than measures of underlying psychological morbidity in the population, and these are available only for treatment in institutionalised settings (mainly psychiatric hospitals) rather than in community care (that is, through GPs and other non-institutional providers). Thus, it is not known how many people are being treated for depression in Ireland at any given time, though a new system of data collection on community care for mental health sufferers, now being instituted by the Health Research Board, means that such data will become available in the future (Daly et al., 2006, p. 17). However, even with the limitations of existing data, one striking feature of the evolution of mental health in Ireland is evident. This is the massive long-term decline in treatment for schizophrenia and the possibility this raises that the incidence of this extreme form of mental disorder in the population has also decreased (the account of this issue here is based on Daly and Walsh, 2004). In the 1950s and 1960s, Ireland had the highest rate of hospitalisation for schizophrenia in the world: in 1958, the year in which the number of schizophrenic patients reached its peak, there were 21,000 such patients in Irish mental hospitals, amounting to 0.7 per cent of the Irish population (Daly and Walsh, 2004, p. 83). It is not clear whether or to what extent the hospitalisation rate for this illness in Ireland overstated its true incidence in the population compared to other countries. For example, families in Ireland may have made more widespread use of committals to mental hospitals as a way of ridding themselves of troublesome or unwanted relatives, and diagnostic and treatment practices in the Irish medical profession may also have had an influence in inflating hospitalisation rates compared to other countries.

In any event, by 2001, despite population increase, the number of hospital patients with schizophrenia had declined by 80 per cent, to 4,000. This decline was due in part to the de-institutionalisation of mental health care, resulting in a large shift in services from hospital to community settings, and may also have been influenced by changes in diagnostic practice that would classify those formerly regarded as schizophrenic under other headings. However, Daly and Walsh consider that possible compensatory increases in non-institutional treatment and other categories of mental illness were not large enough to balance out the large decline in hospitalised cases of schizophrenia (Daly and Walsh, 2004, p. 85). They hesitate to conclude that the overall decline in the treatment of schizophrenia indicates a corresponding decrease in the incidence of schizophrenic-type mental health problems in the population, given the unreliability of treatment rates as a guide to population incidence. However, their judgement is that the evidence provides strong hints in that direction – and certainly, it might be added, provides no support for the view that extreme forms of mental ill-health have been on the *increase* in Ireland over time. This again should caution us against assuming that the Ireland of the Celtic Tiger era is a high-stress environment which is more damaging to our mental well-being than the supposedly more relaxed and humane world that has gone before.

National morale

As a final means of judging trends in subjective well-being in Ireland, we can move away from people's sense of their personal situation and look briefly at their perception of Irish society more generally. It is possible that people may be able to preserve a protected space of personal well-being, while feeling that the broader public sphere outside that space is in decline. The issue here is the level of morale evoked by the collective sense of Ireland as an entity rather than by the individual's experience of his or her own personal life.

A relevant indicator for this purpose is provided by a question on pride in national identity that was asked in a number of Eurobarometer surveys from 1982 to 2003. Figure 2.3 shows for selected age groups the percentages of Irish respondents in four of these surveys who stated that they were 'very proud' of their national identity. The striking feature of the results is the large increase in pride in national identity found among the younger age groups between 1982 and 2003. In 1982, 48 per cent of 18 to 24-year-olds in Ireland were very proud of their Irish identity. By 1997, that had risen to 70 per cent and it continued more or less at the same high level in 2003. A similar upward movement, though from a somewhat higher initial base, was recorded among 35 to 44-year-olds. The pronounced gap in levels of pride in identity between the young and the old which was present in 1982 – with the old more proud than the young – had largely disappeared by 2003 as younger people increasingly matched the levels of pride of older people. Data not shown here also indicate that Irish attitudes on this count were highly positive compared to the European average. In the Eurobarometer data in 2003 on this question, for example, the proportion of all Europeans who said they were 'very proud' of their national identity was 47 per cent, compared to 71 per cent in Ireland.

Fahey, Hayes and Sinnott (2006) asked whether the revelations of corruption in Irish public life that emerged during the 1990s and caused the setting up of a number of tribunals of investigation had a negative effect on people's perception of the Irish political system. Examining a range of indicators from successive rounds of the European Values Study, they found that Irish people's ratings in this area had, if anything, risen rather than fallen during the 1990s and by the end of the decade could be counted as almost enthusiastic compared to the glummer attitudes then found in much of the rest of Europe. In 1999–2000, for example, almost two-thirds of Irish people were satisfied with the way democracy was developing in their country, compared to less than half in the rest of Europe. The percentage of Irish respondents who gave a high rating to their system of government had risen considerably compared to 10 years

Figure 2.3: *Percentage of Irish adults 'very proud' of Irish national identity in selected age groups, 1982–2003*

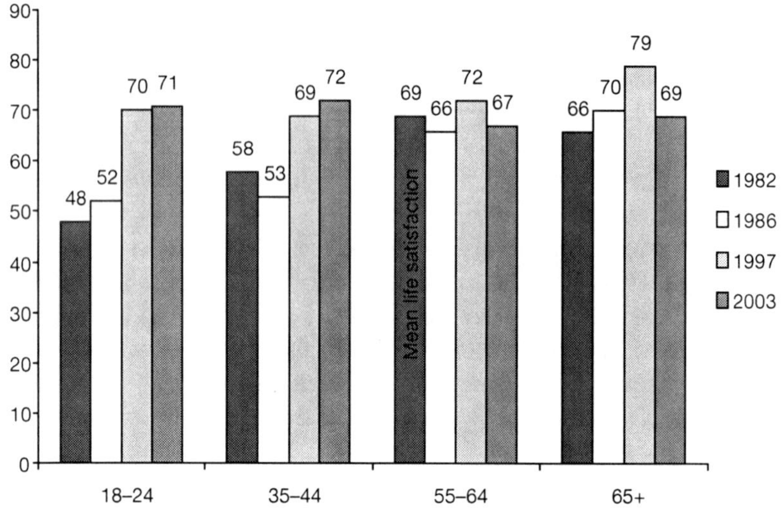

Sources: Mannheim Eurobarometer Trend File 1970–1999, Eurobarometer 60.1, Autumn 2003.

previously, while in most European countries it had fallen (Fahey, Hayes and Sinnott, 2006, pp. 192–202). As the Celtic Tiger advanced, therefore, the attitudes of Irish respondents towards their political system seemed to be more influenced by the positive story of rising living standards and a booming economy than by the bad news of the tribunals of investigation.

Conclusion

As the introduction to this volume has outlined, there are many commentators who assert that the economic boom in Ireland may have made us rich but has also made us miserable – or at least that it has taken away from, rather than added to, our sense of psychological well-being. Such commentary is also found in other countries. It propounds the idea that those who are usually assumed to have benefited from economic advance are more to be pitied than envied. Why? Because for all their material success they are likely to have lost out on happiness and to be living psychologically impoverished lives.

This chapter has taken a sceptical view of such commentary, both as applied to rich countries generally and more particularly to Ireland in the Celtic Tiger era. Certainly, as the critics suggest, economic growth has not produced a long-term improvement in happiness. However, going by the data often used in this area, that is not because we are mired in misery but rather because the majority of people in rich countries are already so high up the scale of subjective well-being that there is little room for further increase. Thus there is no realistic scope for moving on to a higher plane of happiness, since to do so would require that we break out of the constraints imposed by human psychology. The contrast with poor countries is instructive in this regard, since they lie at considerably lower levels on the happiness scales and could reasonably hope for large improvement in the future. These countries reveal what it would mean if rich countries were to find themselves moving down the international scale of relative prosperity. Affluence does therefore seem to give a real boost to how we feel, though we might best appreciate that fact if we suddenly found ourselves lacking the wealth we have come to take for granted.

In this view, the value of sustained economic growth for human happiness is not that it will make us happier in the future but rather that it helps to keep us happy now – it provides the sense of forward movement that seems to be an important underpinning of the quite high levels of morale found in rich countries. This, in essence, is the case made by the American economist Benjamin Friedman in his recent book entitled *The Moral Consequences of Economic Growth*. His central thesis is that steady economic growth is valuable because it supports a generally optimistic and hopeful outlook among the mass of the population and on that basis preserves us from the pessimism, narrowness and proneness to inter-group conflict and hatred that arises when prosperity stalls and people become fearful and insecure about their economic future. He supports this case by examining the links between bouts of economic stagnation or instability and various manifestations of social discontent and conflict over the past 100 years, ranging from upsurges of racism in the US to outbreaks of war in other parts of the world. Speaking of the situation in America, his central conclusion is that 'only with sustained economic growth and the sense of confident progress that follows from the advance in living standards for most of its citizens, can even a great nation find the energy, the wherewithal and most importantly the human attitudes that together sustain an open, tolerant and democratic society' (Friedman, 2005, p. 436).

Beyond that, to charge economic growth with the task of making us ever happier seems unrealistic. If the massive rise in affluence that has occurred in the West in the modern era had constantly translated in ever-rising levels of subjective well-being, the prosperous West of today would have been turned in a Land of Lotus Eaters, with its citizens floating about in a permanent state of wealth-induced bliss, beyond anything that could be counted as a recognisably human experience. That no such euphoric state has or is ever likely to come about could be taken as indication of the limitations of happiness as a yardstick of progress – as if the huge improvements in human welfare that have occurred in the modern world and that may well continue to occur in the future could only be counted as real if they were matched by corresponding increases in emotional uplift. The alternative view is that welfare is a much broader concept than happiness, and that improvements in welfare are worth achieving because they enable us to flourish as human beings, whether or not they make us happier. Thus, it is better to be educated rather than illiterate, to be fit and healthy rather than be cramped by disease and disability, to have a job rather than be unemployed, to have the prosperity that gives us options in life, however badly or well we may use those options, rather than to be hemmed in by material privation. The evidence looked at in this chapter suggests that when these things are in place, we are likely to be somewhat higher up the happiness scale than we would be otherwise – and this rather modest happiness goal is what the Celtic Tiger has helped deliver in Ireland today.

3

Economic Growth and Income Inequality: Setting the Context

Brian Nolan and Bertrand Maître

Introduction

One of the most frequently expressed concerns about Ireland's unprecedented economic boom has been that the benefits have not been shared evenly, that rising living standards have been accompanied by widening gaps, leaving Ireland with a particularly unequal distribution of income. High levels of income inequality can impact on quality of life in a society through a variety of direct and indirect channels, ranging from the social exclusion faced by those near the bottom to the psychological stresses and loss of social cohesion that may be felt throughout the population. It is therefore important to assess to what extent the common understanding of income inequality trends in Ireland is in fact accurate.

This chapter first shows how the spectacular economic growth in the past decade has seen the gap in average income between Ireland and the richer OECD countries narrow dramatically. It then discusses trends in Ireland's income distribution, looking at what happened to income inequality during the boom and how Ireland compares to other rich countries in terms of levels of, and recent trends in, inequality. This reveals that rapid growth has not greatly affected the Irish ranking in terms of income inequality: Ireland continues to have a high degree of economic inequality in comparative terms after the boom, just as it did beforehand. A low redistributive 'effort' is a long-standing characteristic of Ireland's welfare state, and Ireland's new-found prosperity opens up choices that will determine whether this high level of income inequality persists into the future.

Growth and average living standards

We start by describing the dramatic increases in average income that the Celtic Tiger economic boom has produced for Ireland, which form the backdrop, not just for this chapter, but also for the entire book.

T. Fahey et al. (eds.), Quality of Life in Ireland, 27–41.

Starting with GDP per capita,[1] which is very often used in newspaper headlines as a measure of income, over the course of the 1990s Ireland moved from about 60 per cent of the EU average to over 120 per cent of that average (across the 15 countries that were then Member States). Indeed by 2002 Ireland was in the top five countries in the OECD, a broader grouping of 30 rich countries that includes, for example, Australia, Canada, Japan, New Zealand and the USA. Compared with 21 OECD countries for which figures, adjusted both for inflation and purchasing power differences, are available back to 1995, Ireland's GDP per capita swung from about 12 per cent below average in 1995 to 22 per cent above average in 2003.

This remarkable transformation has been attributed to a mix of factors, which it is not our aim to review here. For example, some studies have argued that it should be seen as a belated convergence, one that would have occurred more gradually over the previous 20 years if more appropriate domestic policies had been pursued (on this debate see, for example, Fitz Gerald, 2000; Honohan and Walsh, 2002; Barry, 1999). The growth in productivity and the fall in the rate of age dependency were both important contributors, but all would agree that investment from abroad has been a key factor. This makes GDP per capita problematic as a measure of trends in domestic income, since that inward investment (and foreign labour) generates profits and other revenues, some of which flows back to the countries of origin.

Alternative measures such as Gross National Product (GNP) or Gross National Income (GNI) are therefore more appropriate for our purpose.[2] When these flows in and out of the country are taken into account, outflows of profits and income, largely from multinationals located in Ireland, exceed income flows back into the country.

This means that in a GNI ranking, rather than being in the top five, Ireland in 2002 was only seventeenth in the OECD. While Ireland produces a lot of income per inhabitant, GNI shows that less of it stays in the country than GDP might suggest. Ireland has still been one of the OECD's fastest-growing economies, with a very sharp rise in real income since the mid-1990s. In 1995 this brought GNI per capita from about 20 per cent below

1 In making this comparison it is better to use Purchasing Power Parities (PPPs) rather than current exchange rates. PPPs adjust currency values to take account of differences in purchasing power between countries.

2 GNP adds factor income received from the rest of the world to GDP, and deducts factor payments flowing from Ireland to abroad; however, in addition, GNI adds in subsidies received from the EU and deducts taxes paid to the EU, and thus is a more comprehensive measure of income available to Irish residents (whether institutions or households).

the average for the 21 OECD countries mentioned above to a less pronounced 4 per cent above the average by 2002. This is still quite a leap, but debunks the notion that Ireland is by now one of the very richest countries in the world. We will now examine what has been happening to the distribution of income in Ireland during this period of dramatic growth and convergence.

Trends in income inequality during the economic boom

In order to accurately capture trends in income inequality both reliable data and appropriate methods are required. Different figures from various sources have been used to represent what has been happening to income inequality in Ireland over the period from the mid-1990s, and some care is needed in trying to disentangle the key trends. This illustrates rather dramatically a lesson that has become familiar in research on income inequality internationally, namely that differences not only in data sources but also in the precise way income and its distribution are defined and measured can have major implications for the income inequality levels and trends one finds.[3]

We may start with published results from the Household Budget Surveys (HBS) carried out by the Central Statistics Office in 1994–1995 and 1999–2000, a core source on household expenditure and incomes. These allow us to calculate the share of total disposable household income going to successive groups of households, ranked from the poorest to the richest. These show a clear pattern: the share of the bottom 20 per cent declined by about 0.5 percentage point in total, while the share of the top 10 per cent rose by 1.5 percentage points. So, on the face of it this looks like evidence of substantially 'widening gaps'.

By contrast, an authoritative EU source, the Joint Report by the Commission and the Council on Social Inclusion (2004) presents two widely used summary inequality measures to capture trends in the distribution of income, based on figures from the European Community Household Panel (ECHP) Survey. The first is the ratio of income going to the top versus the bottom one-fifth of the distribution, which for Ireland is shown as declining from 5.1 in the mid-1990s to 4.5 by 2001. The second is the Gini coefficient, an inequality measure widely used in the academic literature that ranges from 0 where there is no inequality to 1 where there is maximum inequality. The EU figures show the Gini for Ireland falling

[3] For a more detailed discussion see Nolan and Smeeding (2005).

substantially from 0.33 to 0.29. So inequality seems to have fallen sharply – gaps have apparently narrowed!

However, both of these sets of figures are actually problematic as far as capturing trends in inequality in Ireland is concerned, for different reasons. The published HBS figures relate to the distribution of income among households, without attempting to take into account that a given income will provide a very different standard of living to a household of say two adults and three children than a single adult living alone. This can make a significant difference not only to the position of different types of household but also to trends in inequality when household size and composition are changing, as in Ireland over this period when average household size fell from about 3.3 to about 3 persons per household.

For this reason, it is now customary when measuring income inequality to focus on persons rather than households as the unit of analysis, to assume that all members of a particular household share a common standard of living, and to measure that by adjusting household income for the number of people depending on it. This is done by the use of what are known as 'equivalence scales'. Rather than just dividing household income by the number of persons in the household – which would treat children the same as adults and ignore 'economies of scale' in household consumption – we calculate the number of 'equivalent adults' and divide household income by that figure. For this purpose we employ an equivalence scale that is widely used in comparative income distribution research, the so-called 'OECD scale'. This assigns a value of 1 to the first adult, 0.7 to each other adult, and 0.5 to each child in the household – so a couple with two children would have its income divided by 2.7.[4]

This makes a big difference to the trends shown by the HBS, as Figure 3.1 illustrates. The share of the top 10 per cent now increases only marginally, by only 0.3 rather than 1.5 percentage points, and the top 20 per cent sees no increase in share, though the bottom does lose out and the middle gain. The ratio of the share of the top to the bottom quintile calculated from these figures increases from 4.7 to 5, while the Gini coefficient is unchanged at 0.31. (Different summary measures can give a rather different impression, even when calculated from the same data source, because they assign different weights to differences observed in various parts of the income distribution.)

---

4 The Central Statistics Office (CSO) kindly produced figures for us from the HBS using person-weighting and equivalising income using this equivalence scale. The HBS micro data lodged in the Social Science Data Archive cannot be used for this purpose because high incomes are 'top-coded' to ensure anonymity.

Figure 3.1: *Income distribution in Ireland 1994/1995–1999/2000 HBS Survey*

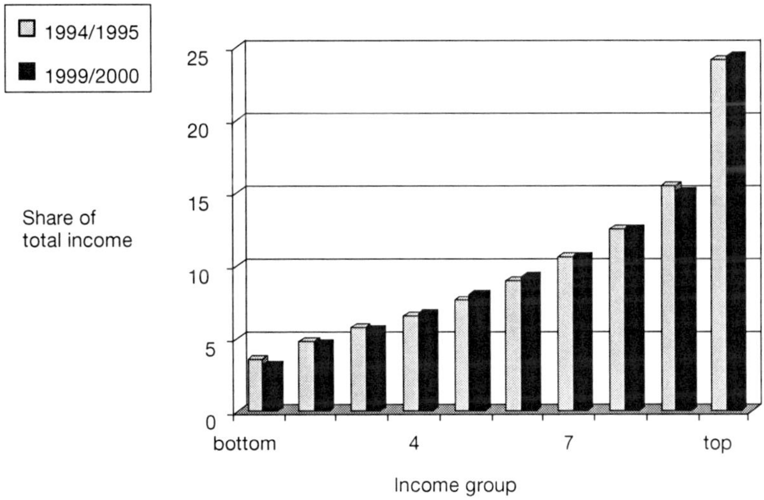

Turning to the figures from the ECHP, unlike the HBS (which draws a new sample each time) this was a longitudinal survey which sought to re-interview the original sample each year. In practice some of the original households inevitably drop out of the sample over time, and this 'attrition' may have a substantial impact on the results, depending on which households they are. It appears that in the case of the ECHP data for Ireland, this served to substantially reduce the share of income measured as going to households towards the top of the distribution.

We know this because the initial sample was in fact substantially supplemented by additional households in 2000 and 2001 in the Irish case, because of the scale of attrition.[5] These additional cases were not included in the ECHP dataset or the figures produced by Eurostat, because no such supplementation was carried out in other countries. The supplemented sample shows a considerably higher share of income going to the top of the distribution than the 'unsupplemented' one, which suggests that the latter is not to be relied on in this context.

This means that the full Living in Ireland Survey (LII), which was the Irish component of the ECHP but includes the supplemented sample from 2000, provides the main alternative to the HBS as a source of data on

---

5 By 2000 a total of 5,500 individuals had been followed since 1994, representing only about 40 per cent of all the adults in the first wave; a new sample of 5,200 persons was then added. See Whelan et al., 2003, Table 2.1, p. 6.

income distribution.[6] Figure 3.2 shows that between 1994 and 2001 the share of the bottom 10 per cent of persons in total (equivalised) income in the LII fell slightly, the middle of the distribution gained substantially, and the share of the top 10 per cent fell by over 1 per cent of total income.

Figure 3.2: *Income distribution in Ireland 1994–2001, LII Survey*

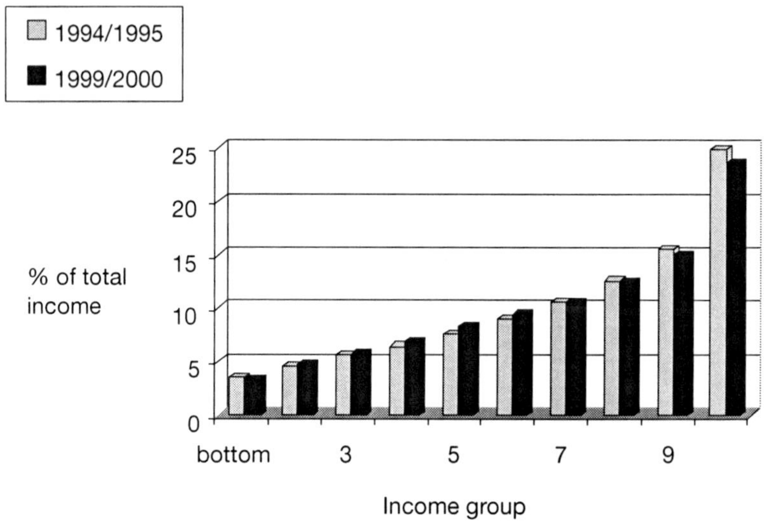

The HBS and the LII both suggest relatively modest declines in shares towards the bottom, but the picture at the top is still something of a contrast, with the HBS showing a marginal increase but the LII suggesting a fall of about 1 percentage point. The LII may still be affected by its panel nature despite sample supplementation and appropriate reweighting, and the HBS has a sample size that is about twice as large, so perhaps most weight should be placed on the latter. The difference in overall trend in inequality between them should not in any case be exaggerated: where the Gini coefficient in the HBS is stable at 0.31, the LII shows a fall from 0.32 to 0.30. What is striking is that neither source suggests the substantial increase in income inequality that many domestic commentators have seen as accompanying Ireland's economic convergence with its higher-income EU partners.

---

6 There are also other differences between the LII and ECHP. The ECHP relies mainly on income in the previous calendar year, whereas in using the Living in Ireland Survey we have mostly focused on income in the previous week or month – like the HBS. Furthermore, Eurostat had its own internal procedures for imputation of missing values, dealing with outliers and weighting the responses.

The figures from the HBS and the LII only bring us up to 2000–2001; published results from the new EU-SILC survey being carried out for Ireland by the CSO give some more up-to-date figures relating to the income distribution. The Gini coefficient shown in the results just published for 2004 is 0.316, and the ratio of the share of the top to the bottom quintile is 5, which does not suggest any dramatic change.[7] However, the pattern of income inequality in this new survey will clearly need to be analysed in depth; and a similar analysis of the forthcoming HBS for 2004–2005 will provide a valuable point of comparison.

While one might expect those towards the top of the income distribution to do particularly well in a boom, general household surveys may not be best placed to capture trends right at the top of the distribution. This is both because it is difficult to be sure that surveys with limited sample sizes will adequately represent any small group in the population, and because those at the top may be particularly elusive from a surveyor's perspective. For this reason it is worth looking at an alternative source of income data for that group, namely incomes reported for income tax.

Top incomes in Ireland during the boom

In the past income tax data was used to study the income distribution in many countries, and there has recently been a resurgence of interest in exploiting such data. This has been focused both on long-term trends going back to the early years of the twentieth century, and – of more direct interest here – on apparently dramatic increases in the share of income going to the very top in some countries in the 1980s and 1990s.[8]

This type of analysis can be carried out for Ireland using figures for the years from 1990 to 2000 published each year by the Revenue Commissioners, showing taxpayers categorised by income range and the mean income for each category.

Using total personal income from the national accounts (crudely adjusted to try to exclude income that does not go to households) and the estimated total number of tax units in the population, we can estimate the shares of tax units and of total income in each range. We then interpolate to produce the estimated income share going to the top 10 per cent and the

---

7 The distribution of pre-tax income among households, without any adjustment for differences in size and composition, can also be derived from the published results, and this does suggest a considerably higher share going to the top decile than the 1999–2000 HBS.

8 See especially Piketty (2001, 2003) on long-term trends in the shares of top income groups in France, Atkinson (2001) for the UK, Piketty and Saez (2003) for the US, and Saez and Veall (2005) for Canada.

top 1 per cent of taxpayers. The results in Figure 3.3 show a substantial increase in the share of the top 10 per cent over the decade, from 33 per cent to 38 per cent. The top 1 per cent saw its share rise sharply in the second half of the decade, and all the growth in share for the top decile was actually concentrated in the top 1 per cent. It means that by the end of the 1990s, the share of the top 1 per cent was more than twice the level prevailing through the 1970s and 1980s. As it happens, most of this growth in turn was concentrated in the top 0.5 per cent.

Figure 3.3: *Shares of top income groups in Ireland, 1989–2000, tax data*

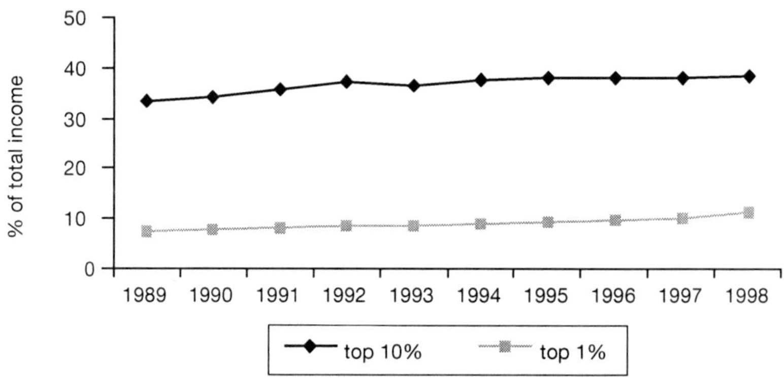

This is very different to the picture suggested by the survey data, and highlights the sensitivity of survey-based estimates of top income shares to what is measured as happening at the very top. On the face of it, the tax data seem to confirm anecdotal assertions that those at the top did particularly well during the economic boom. However, the obvious issue in relation to data from tax records, for Ireland as elsewhere, is how much we should believe them. Some would argue that they are so polluted by attempts by the wealthy to evade and avoid tax that they cannot be relied on.

In the Irish case, one would certainly be concerned that changes in the reporting of top incomes may have played a significant role in the last decade. The rigour with which income tax is administered was certainly tightened significantly, including some high-profile investigations into tax evasion of various sorts, and the marginal rate of income tax has also come down significantly. Both these factors could lead to a greater proportion of income being reported to the taxman, as evasion is seen to become more risky and avoidance less necessary.

It is thus difficult to assess the extent to which the rapid increase in incomes right at the top reflects trends in actual incomes versus reporting behaviour: the likelihood is that both contribute.

Income inequality in Ireland in comparative perspective

In addition to investigating what has been happening to income inequality in Ireland in recent years, it is also very important to have a comparative perspective – is inequality here particularly high or low compared with other countries? Table 3.1 presents the Gini coefficient summary indicator of inequality in the distribution of disposable income among persons in EU Member States in 2003–2004, as reported by Eurostat.[9]

Table 3.1: *Income inequality in the EU, 2003–2004*

Country	*Gini coefficient*
Belgium	0.26
Czech Republic	0.25
Denmark	0.24
Germany	0.28
Estonia	0.34
Greece	0.33
Spain	0.31
France	0.28
Ireland	0.32
Italy	0.33
Cyprus	0.27
Latvia	0.36
Lithuania	0.29
Luxembourg	0.26
Hungary	0.27
Malta	–
Netherlands	0.27
Austria	0.26
Poland	0.31
Portugal	0.38
Slovenia	0.22
Slovakia	0.33
Finland	0.25
Sweden	0.23
UK	0.34
EU–25 average	0.29

We see that inequality is least in the Scandinavian countries, the Czech Republic and Slovenia. It is slightly higher but still below-average in Belgium, the Netherlands, Luxembourg, Germany, France, Hungary and

9 Not all these figures may be as directly comparable as one would like, in terms of sources and definitions, but they are the best available at present.

Cyprus. Ireland is then in a group with above-average inequality, together with Spain, Italy, Greece, Poland, Estonia, Slovakia and the UK,[10] while the Gini is even higher in Latvia and Portugal.[11]

It is also worth noting that when the comparison is extended to include industrialised countries outside the EU, using for example figures from the Luxembourg Income Study database, then Canada and Australia have levels of inequality that are similar to Ireland, but the US invariably displays a considerably higher level of income inequality.

The conclusion to be drawn from this comparative perspective is that Ireland is not really an outlier and is not fairly characterised, as the newspaper headlines sometimes claim, as 'one of the most unequal countries in the EU/OECD'. Instead, it is among a substantial group of industrialised countries, inside and outside the EU, that have relatively high levels of income inequality. This does not represent a new situation: it has been the case since Ireland joined the EU in 1973, which, as it happens, is about as far back as the data allow us to go in measuring overall income inequality in Ireland.

While the factors underpinning the shape of a country's income distribution and producing such differences across countries are highly complex, the scale and nature of the State's interventions via taxation and income support are certainly important factors. 'Redistributive effort' in this sense can be very crudely measured by looking at the reduction in a summary inequality measure such as the Gini coefficient, going from income accruing from the market to income after income tax and including social welfare transfers.

This shows Ireland to have a redistributive effort on roughly the same scale as the UK, slightly less than Canada or Australia but considerably greater than the US; however, other countries in Northern Europe and Scandinavia bring about a larger reduction in inequality via their tax/transfer systems.[12] Similarly, EU figures show that social transfers play a smaller role in reducing the numbers falling below relative income poverty thresholds in Ireland than in many other Member States. This is mostly because the scale of social transfers is more limited than elsewhere:

---

10 These figures show Ireland with a lower Gini coefficient – and so lower income inequality – than the UK, but other sources show the UK with a level of inequality very similar to or even slightly lower than Ireland.

11 From the same source one can also see the top-to-bottom quintile share ratio, an alternative summary inequality measure also mentioned earlier; this gives some different rankings when individual countries are compared, but shows a broadly similar clustering.

12 See Nolan and Smeeding (2005). The Netherlands is interesting in having the same Gini for market income as Ireland but achieving a much larger reduction in inequality by means of its tax transfer system.

Ireland has one of the lowest percentages of national income going on social transfers in the EU. This partly reflects having a low proportion in the population of pension age and a very low unemployment rate, as well as the substantial role played by occupational pensions, but more fundamentally reflects the welfare 'regime' that Ireland has adopted, largely following the British model.

'Welfare regime' refers to the constellation of socio-economic institutions, policies and programmes which countries have adopted to promote their citizens' welfare and in which distinctive combinations of intervention strategies, policy designs and institutional frameworks can be identified. Esping-Andersen (1990) distinguished between 'social democratic', 'corporatist' and 'liberal' welfare regimes; subsequently, a strong case has been advanced for adding a fourth, 'Southern' welfare regime or sub-protective welfare state.

The liberal welfare regime assigns primacy to the market and confines the State to a residual welfare role, social benefits typically being subject to a means test and targeted on those failing in the market. The UK and Ireland are examples of the liberal regime, to which other 'Anglo-Saxon' countries such as the US, Canada, Australia and New Zealand are also assigned.

It can be contrasted with the social democratic regime whereby the welfare state has a more substantial redistributive role, seeking to guarantee adequate economic resources independently of market or familial reliance, and the corporatist regime which views welfare primarily as a mediator of group-based mutual aid and risk pooling, prioritizing those already inserted in the labour market. In Southern Mediterranean countries family support systems play a distinctive role and the benefit system is uneven and minimalist in nature. While there are many important differences between countries within each regime type, the redistributive role of the State is more modest in the liberal and 'Southern' regimes than in the social democratic or corporatist ones. To understand Ireland's level of income inequality in comparative perspective it is the effects of deep-seated institutional differences of this type – rather than the impact of the recent economic boom – that need to be understood.

One of the many factors underpinning such institutional differences across countries is attitudes towards the welfare state and social welfare transfers in particular and, more broadly, what people believe about the relationship between inequality and growth. The notion that there is a trade-off between equality and growth – that at least after a certain point greater equality can only be achieved at the expense of reducing economic growth – has a very long history. In the Irish case there has certainly been a strong emphasis on the need for economic growth in recent years in order to catch up with the higher living standards of neighbouring countries and tackle the high unemployment of the 1980s in particular. However, it is also becoming clear that social protection and, more broadly, the welfare state have key roles to play in a smoothly functioning modern economy, apart altogether from their role in attaining social goals – as evidenced in the National Economic and Social Council's (2005) recent highlighting of the need for a 'developmental welfare state'. Taxation levels have fallen substantially during the economic boom, though whether this is best seen as a cause or a consequence of rapid growth is debated; as people become accustomed to higher living standards their expectations about social provision also rise, but whether they are willing to pay through higher taxes remains to be seen. What is clear is that key decisions about the future direction of Ireland's welfare state will be taken over the next few years, which will have major implications for the level of income inequality.

Widening gaps during the boom?

Much of the public commentary on inequality trends during Ireland's boom has been in terms of 'widening gaps' between the rich and the poor, or between other (often unspecified) groups in the population. So far our focus in this chapter has been on the overall distribution of income, but of course one could think about – and be concerned about – widening gaps in ways that would not necessarily be reflected in the way overall income inequality is conventionally measured. While trends in poverty are discussed in depth in later chapters, it is worth noting here that the numbers falling below relative income thresholds derived as proportions of mean or median incomes have certainly risen over the course of the economic boom.

Taking the commonly used relative income poverty threshold of 60 per cent of median[13] (equivalised) income, for example, about 16 per cent of persons were below that level in 1994 but in 2001 the corresponding figure was 22 per cent (see Whelan et al., 2003 for details). This reflects the fact that social security support rates, though they increased a good deal more rapidly than consumer prices, lagged significantly behind the very rapid rise in incomes from work and property. This meant that the impact of the boom in bringing very substantial numbers from unemployment into work was more than offset by the numbers of long-term pension recipients (notably the elderly) who fell below such relative thresholds.

---

[13] Median income is the income above and below which half the distribution is to be found.

It is important, however, to emphasise that this was taking place in a context where real incomes and living standards were improving throughout the distribution. This is highlighted by the very different picture conveyed by income thresholds held constant in purchasing power terms rather than indexed to average incomes. Suppose, for example, we take the 60 per cent of median threshold in 1997, the middle of the period of very rapid growth, when about 18 per cent fell below that threshold. A threshold with the same purchasing power would have had 36 per cent falling below it as recently as 1994; by 2001, though, only 3 per cent were below the corresponding 'real' threshold. So, over a period of such unprecedented growth, the benchmark used in measuring poverty makes all the difference to the picture one sees; when non-monetary indicators of deprivation are incorporated into the analysis a more complex reality is seen (see also Nolan, 2003; Whelan et al., 2003; Maître, Nolan and Whelan, 2006).

Here though our focus is on income, and it is worth looking at whether gaps between certain groups in the population did indeed widen over the economic boom. We cannot do this in an exhaustive fashion, comparing all possible groups, but a comparison of the position of specific groups in terms of median equivalised income in the 1994 and 2001 Living in Ireland surveys does show certain groups forging ahead as opposed to being left behind.

Figure 3.4 shows that children have been catching up on adults of working age in terms of their household income. Older people, however, aged 65 or over, have fallen a good deal further behind. Men continue to have higher household income than women, but the gap has not widened. Those living in urban areas continue to have higher incomes than those in rural areas, but there was only a marginal increase in the gap between 1994 and 2001. Those in the South and Eastern Regions had higher incomes than those in the Border, Midlands and Western regions, and that gap did widen over the period.

One of the key factors determining how well a household fared over the period was whether its income came predominantly from earnings, self-employment income or social welfare transfers. Social welfare rates rose substantially in terms of purchasing power, but lagged behind average or median household income – partly because the latter were boosted by increasing numbers at work. This meant that although a significant number of households shifted away from reliance on social welfare over the period, those that remained dependent on such transfers did not keep pace with others. Those in households with less than half their income coming from social welfare have median incomes about twice those with half or more of their income coming from social welfare, and this gap widened between 1994 and 2001.

Figure 3.4: *Average income for various groups in Ireland, 1994–2001, LII Survey*

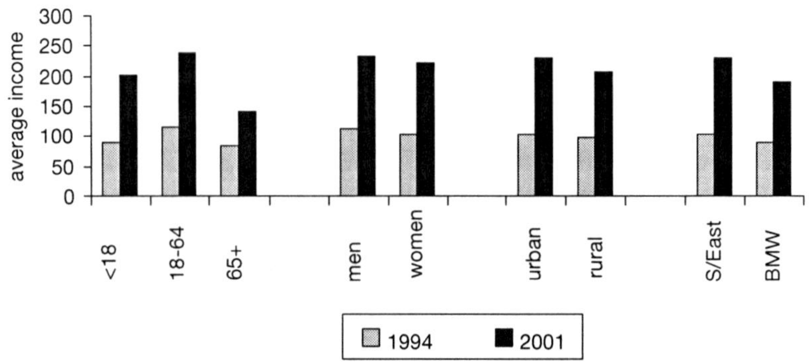

One needs to be careful, however, when thinking about the implications of this widening gap between welfare and other incomes. The gap between households where the main earner (or 'reference person') was unemployed versus working actually narrowed over the period. This reflects the fact that households where the main earner remained unemployed still benefited from the boom, because other adults in those households were much more likely to be employed – the average number of persons in work in these households doubled over the period, so these households became much less dependent on social welfare.[14] Where the main earner was already in work before the boom, on the other hand, there was a less marked increase in numbers at work, and social welfare accounted for only a very small proportion of total income anyway.

Conclusions

Ireland has been one of the OECD's fastest-growing economies since the mid-1990s, with a very sharp rise in real incomes on average. Care has to be exercised in assessing Ireland's ranking by average income per head, because a particularly large proportion of national product flows out again as payments to foreign firms and individuals for their role in producing it. GNI per capita was well below the average for the OECD countries in 1995 and comfortably above that average by 2002 – a remarkable achievement in a very short space of time, even if it did not leave Ireland as one of the very richest countries in the world, as is often asserted.

---

[14] The average number of persons in work in these households rose from 0.5 in 1994 to 1 in 2001, and income from work rose from 20 per cent to 44 per cent of their disposable income.

So, what happened to inequality in the distribution of income in Ireland during this period of dramatic growth and convergence? The available evidence suggests that there was much less change in the shape of the income distribution than is often casually assumed. Household surveys certainly show no dramatic change, though data from the income tax system do show a marked increase in the share of total income going to the very top – the top 1 per cent or even half per cent – of the distribution.

It appears that rapid growth has not greatly affected the Irish ranking in terms of income inequality: the most recent figures suggest that Ireland (like the UK) is in a quite large group of EU or OECD countries with a relatively high degree of economic inequality, compared not just to the Scandinavian countries with their remarkably low levels of inequality but also to countries like France, Germany, Belgium and the Netherlands.

While the overall shape of the income distribution may have been fairly stable, some income gaps did undoubtedly widen over the period – notably between older people and those of working age, but also between those at the top and those at the bottom of the income distribution.

A low redistributive 'effort' is a long-standing characteristic of Ireland's welfare state, and Ireland's new-found prosperity opens up choices that will determine whether Ireland's high level of income inequality and such widening gaps continue into the future.

4

Employment and the Quality of Work

Philip J. O'Connell and Helen Russell

Introduction

How has employment in Ireland been affected by the Celtic Tiger? We are all familiar with the dramatic growth in employment and the equally dramatic fall in unemployment. However some commentators suggest that much of the employment growth during the 1990s was concentrated in households that were already attached to the labour market and that many people were left behind by the boom. This thesis also holds that the Celtic Tiger was accompanied by a deterioration in the quality of work in terms of security, control and skill, and dismisses most employment growth as unskilled. There has been a particular focus on the role of part-time work, with the assumption that part-time work is of poor quality and is casualised.

In this chapter we examine the veracity of this view of the effects of the recent economic boom. In the first half of the chapter we describe some of the major changes in the Irish labour market over the past decade. We also present evidence on the groups who have benefited from the employment growth and consider who has been excluded. Research on work-poverty within households suggests that there has been a steep drop in the number of households without anyone in employment, suggesting that the benefits of growth did extend to these groups. However, there remain groups such as the disabled, lone parents, etc., who still experience difficulties in entering the labour market. This section also draws on existing research to discuss trends in average earnings and earnings dispersion.

In the second half of the chapter we assess the extent to which the quality of work has changed. Trends in the quality of work have been the subject of considerable international debate, so it is of interest to examine the evidence as to whether there has been a deterioration in the quality of work in the Irish economy. To answer this question we examine four aspects of job quality: autonomy, work pressure, security and job satisfaction.

T. Fahey et al. (eds.), Quality of Life in Ireland, 43–66.

Employee autonomy or discretion is chosen as a key dimension of job quality and because there has been some debate as to whether autonomy has increased with the expansion of skilled occupations. Work pressure is included because trends in this job characteristic are particularly important from a quality-of-life perspective as they are strongly related to stress and to work–family tensions.

Employment security is also found to be linked to employee well-being. Figures on short-term/temporary contracts suggest that this form of employment has actually fallen in Ireland since the turn of the century. Moreover, the declining threat of unemployment is likely to make those with permanent and non-permanent contracts feel more secure. However, there may be sectors of the labour market that are experiencing greater external competition and so have experienced greater insecurity. The 'deterioration of work' thesis places a particular focus on the quality of part-time jobs, arguing that many newly created part-time jobs are insecure. It is important therefore to consider the link between part-time work and insecurity.

The final indicator of job quality is more subjective – job satisfaction. This provides a more general insight into employees' assessments of their current job. If there has been a deterioration in job quality we would expect to see this reflected in reduced levels of job satisfaction.

Principal trends in the labour market

Table 4.1 shows summary data on some of the principal changes in the labour market since 1993, a year when unemployment peaked at almost 16 per cent of the labour force, following several years of sluggish growth. Thereafter the labour market impact of the economic boom began to unfold and employment grew very rapidly, by over 650,000 or 55 per cent between 1993 and 2004. The employment rate, expressed in proportion to the population aged 15–64, increased from 51.7 per cent in 1993 to 66.3 per cent in 2004. The Irish employment rate converged with the EU average in 1998, and exceeded it by about two percentage points in 2004.

Unemployment fell below 5 per cent in 2000 and has remained between 4 and 5 per cent ever since. Long-term unemployment has also fallen dramatically, from 8.9 per cent in 1993 to 1.2 per cent in 2004. The past decade or so has seen a fundamental transformation in labour market conditions in Ireland, from a period of labour surplus during the 1980s, which generated mass unemployment and high outward migration, to a situation of booming and virtually full employment, labour shortages and growing inward migration in the late 1990s and early 2000s. The share of

Table 4.1: *Principal changes in the labour market, 1993–2004*

	Source	*1993*	*2004*	*Absolute change*	*% change*
Total employment (000)	1	1183	1836.2	653.2	55.22
Employment rate (% population 15-64)	2	51.7	66.3	14.6	28.2
Unemployment (000)	1	220	84.2	–135.8	–61.7
Unemployment rate (% labour force 15+)	1	15.7	4.4	–11.3	–72.0
Long-term unemployment (000)	1	125.4	26.3	–99.1	–79.0
Long-term unemployment rate (% labour force)	1	8.9	1.2	–7.7	–86.5
Male employment (000)	1	759.0	1084.0	325	42.8
Male employment rate (%)	2	64.8	75.9	11.1	17.1
Female employment (000)	1	435.0	787.0	352	80.9
Female employment rate (%)	2	38.5	56.5	18	46.8
Female share of total employment	1	36.4	42.1	–	–
Part-time employment (% of total employment)	2	10.5	16.8	6.3	60.0
Male part-time employment (%)	2	4.6	6.1	1.5	32.6
Female part-time employment (%)	2	20.8	31.5	10.7	51.4
Fixed-term employment (% of total employment)	2	9.3	4.1	–5.2	–55.9
Male fixed-term employment (%)	2	7.4	3.7	–3.7	–50.0
Female fixed-term employment (%)	2	11.9	4.6	–7.3	–61.3

Sources: 1: CSO, *Labour Force Survey* and *Quarterly National Household Survey (QNHS)*, various years; 2: European Commission, *Employment in Europe, 2004*

non-Irish nationals in total employment in Ireland increased from less than 3 per cent in 1998 to 8 per cent in 2005.

One of the striking features of recent developments in the Irish labour market has been the sharp and sustained increase in women's employment. Total female employment increased by over 80 per cent between 1993 and 2004, almost twice the growth rate among men (43 per cent). These differential growth rates resulted in a shift in the balance of employment between men and women, and women's share of total employment increased from 36 per cent in 1993 to over 42 per cent in 2004. This represents a continuation of a trend from the 1980s: the female share of total employment was only 29 per cent in 1981 and less than 33 per cent in 1988 (O'Connell, 2000). The trend is, moreover, expected to continue, so that women are expected to account for about 45 per cent of total employment by the year 2015 (Sexton, Hughes and Finn, 2002).

Ireland is also in the early stages of the process of population ageing, but already the number of older workers, aged over 45 years, is growing faster than younger workers. Increasing proportions of women and older workers are likely to lead to increased demand for greater flexibility in the organisation of working time in order to facilitate work–life balance in the workplace of the future. It will also pose challenges for both employment policy and policies governing pensions and social welfare provision.

A number of commentators have argued that the impact of the Celtic Tiger has led to increased casualisation or flexibilisation of employment and a deterioration in the quality of work. For example, Allen (2000, p. 5) argues that 'Contract working, job insecurity, constant pressure for flexibility, and systematic efforts to reduce "unit costs" prevail.' He also argues that there has been a dramatic growth in atypical employment, including part-time, temporary and short-term contract employment. In a similar vein, O'Hearn (2001) dismisses most employment growth as unskilled.

Occupational change

Interpretations of occupational trends differ. O'Connell (2000) argues that the relatively rapid process of economic development that occurred over the last four decades of the twentieth century gave rise to a long-term sustained trend of occupational upgrading, although that transformation of the occupational structure was largely complete by the turn of the century. O'Hearn (2001) argues instead that employment growth during the 1990s was concentrated in routine, low-paying services. Part of the difference in interpretation is due to differing time frames, with O'Hearn taking the shorter-term view.

However, even focusing on the 1990s, Sexton, Hughes and Finn (2002) show that between 1991 and 2001 there was growth in both higher-grade occupations (including managers and associate professionals) and in lower-grade occupations (including personal service and sales workers).

Table 4.2 shows employment by occupation for 1998 and 2004, thus allowing us to focus on recent changes in occupational structure. The fastest-growing occupations during this rapid period of employment growth were professionals, associate professionals and technical workers, sales, and personal and protective service occupations. There was also strong growth in the 'other' category, which includes unskilled manual workers as well as 'unstated'. The majority of the growth in sales and in personal and protective services employment involved women.

The more recent trend, entailing an increase in the higher-grade jobs and

Table 4.2: *Employment by occupation, 1998 and 2004*

	1998 Number	%	*2004* Number	%	*Change* Number	% change
Managers and administrators	278,449	19.5	315,708	17.8	37,258	13.4
Professional	144,778	10.2	208,531	11.8	63,753	44.0
Associate professional and technical	116,660	8.2	164,253	9.3	47,593	40.8
Clerical and secretarial	176,218	12.4	213,489	12.1	37,271	21.2
Craft and related	197,916	13.9	242,218	13.7	44,303	22.4
Personal and protective service	125,265	8.8	168,863	9.5	43,597	34.8
Sales	100,126	7.0	131,134	7.4	31,008	31.0
Plant and machine operatives	157,051	11.0	157,166	8.9	115	0.1
Other (includes unskilled and not stated)	129,901	9.1	168,995	9.5	39,094	30.1
Total	1,426,366	100.0	1,770,357	100.0	343,991	24.1

Source: QNHS, 1998 Q2 and 2004 Q2, Special Analysis

some increase also at the lower end of the occupational hierarchy, is consistent with a polarisation process. It should, of course, be acknowledged that the increase in low-skilled employment facilitated the dramatic decline in long-term unemployment and, indeed, the increase in employment in this segment of the labour market may have been influenced by the supply of long-term unemployed with low skills.

One final source of evidence on the changing skill demands of jobs comes from employee characteristics. The educational levels of Irish workers have been increasing consistently over the past several decades. Between 1994 and 2004 there was a marked increase in the educational attainment of the workforce: the share with no qualifications or with just a Junior Certificate level of education dropped from over 40 per cent in 1994 to less than 30 per cent, while the share with a third-level education increased from 25 per cent to 32 per cent.

This does not in itself indicate that there has been any increase in the skills levels of jobs, since there could be a growing mismatch between education levels and job requirements. However, the wage returns to education have been rising alongside the increasing skill levels of the workforce. According to economic theory this means that employers' demands for skills have also been increasing. 'In a standard supply-and-demand model, the joint occurrence of rising returns to education and an increase in skill supply can only be explained by an even faster growth in skill demand' (Tåhlin, 2006).

Figure 4.1: *Educational attainment of those at work, 1994 and 2004*

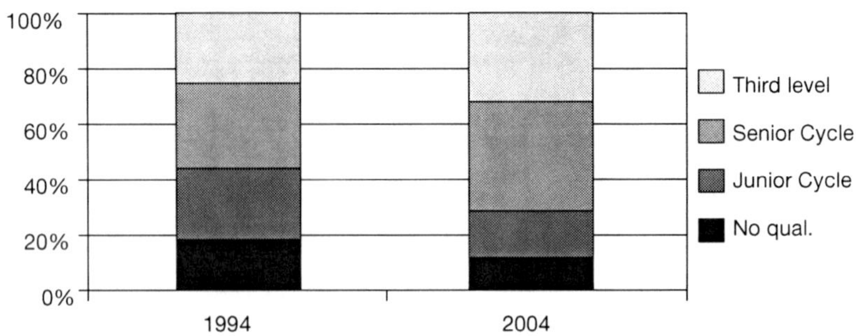

Part-time working

Flexible working arrangements can be advantageous to both employers and workers. For employers, flexibility may offer the capacity to smooth out fluctuations in demand, and, in the context of labour shortages, as experienced in Ireland in recent times, may increase labour supply by tapping new sources of labour, either part-time or temporary, that might not otherwise be available. For workers, flexible working arrangements, particularly part-time work, may offer the opportunity to combine work with other activities, such as education and training or housework and caring commitments. However, the growth of non-standard working arrangements has also been accompanied by increased concern about the quality of part-time jobs, particularly with respect to pay and occupational benefits (Kalleberg, Reskin and Hudson, 2000; Rubery, 1998; O'Connell and Gash, 2003).

In Ireland, part-time work increased sharply from the mid-1980s to the mid-1990s, and indeed accounted for most of the employment growth during that period (O'Connell, 2000). However, since the late 1990s the rate of growth of part-time work has been similar to that of full-time work, so the share of part-time work has remained fairly stable. In 2004 part-time employment accounted for 17 per cent of total employment in Ireland, lower than the EU–15 average of 19 per cent (European Commission, 2005). Part-time working differs sharply by gender: in 2004, about 6 per cent of men worked part-time, compared to 32 per cent of women at work. Accordingly, women account for over three-quarters of all part-time workers, but less than 35 per cent of full-time workers.

The voluntary nature of part-time work is relevant to a consideration of the quality of jobs and to the question of whether part-timers are 'trapped' in these positions. O'Connell, McGinnity and Russell (2003) show that most part-time working is a matter of choice, and that few part-timers are looking and available for another part-time job or a full-time job. They also show that the incidence of such involuntary part-time working fell, from 19 per cent of all part-time employment in 1992 to less than 4 per cent in 2000. Since then the involuntary proportion has fluctuated around 1 per cent of all part-time workers.

Table 4.3: *Total employment (ILO) by occupation, gender and working time, 2004*

	Male Full-time %	*Female Full-time %*	*Male Part-time %*	*Female Part-time %*
Managers and administrators	21.9	14.7	11.9	6.1
Professional	10.4	16.5	6.0	6.7
Associate professional and technical	6.9	13.5	5.7	9.7
Clerical and secretarial	4.9	22.5	5.9	20.1
Craft and related	22.5	1.8	9.4	1.1
Personal and protective service	6.1	12.0	17.4	20.2
Sales	4.9	8.7	16.1	19.4
Plant and machine operatives	12.5	4.5	8.7	2.2
Other (includes unskilled and not stated)	9.9	5.8	18.9	14.5
Total	100.0	100.0	100.0	100.0
Number	1,000,222	524,808	64,932	246,199

Source: QNHS, 1998 Q2 and 2004 Q2, Special Analysis

Table 4.3 shows employment by occupation, gender and working time in 2004. This gives us some insight into the quality of part-time jobs. Among women, part-time jobs are skewed towards the routine and lower-skilled occupations: personal and protective services, sales, clerical and secretarial each account for about 20 per cent of female part-timers and other unskilled occupations for another 15 per cent. This differs markedly from the distribution of full-time jobs among women, where managerial, professional and associate professional occupations are more common. We find a similar contrast between the distributions of full- and part-time male workers.

Fixed-term contracts

The numbers working on fixed-term contracts in Ireland actually fell from a high of 10 per cent in 1995 to 4.1 per cent in 2004, while over the same period, the average incidence of fixed-term contracts across the EU increased from 12 per cent to almost 14 per cent (European Commission, 2005). Thus, with respect to this dimension of labour market flexibility the Irish pattern differs from the European trend. It should, of course, be recognised that Irish employers may have less need of fixed-term contracts than in some other European countries because of the relative weakness of employment protection legislation for those with permanent or open-ended contracts in Ireland. In this context, it is useful to note that fixed-term contracts in the UK, another country with relatively weak employment protection, fluctuated between 6 per cent and 7 per cent over the past decade. These two types of labour market flexibility are related: part-time workers are much more likely to be on temporary contracts than full-time workers.

Working hours

There has been a marked reduction in overall hours worked in recent years. Among men, average hours worked declined from 46.7 in 1989 to 42.3 in 1999 and to 41.1 in 2005. Among women, the decline was from 36.4 in 1989 to 32.7 in 1999 and 31.7 in 2005. This aggregate decline derives from differential trends in both the absolute proportions of men and women working part-time, described in the section above, and in average hours worked by full-time workers.

Figure 4.2 shows the distribution of usual hours worked in all jobs for men and women in 2005. Women are clearly skewed towards the lower end of the distribution, with 13 per cent of women at work working less than 19 hours per week and a further 20 per cent working between 20 and 29 hours.

Figure 4.2: *Usual hours worked, 2005 (ILO employed)*

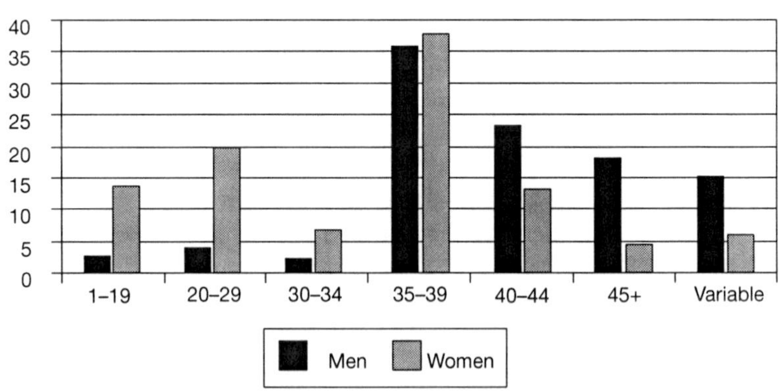

Source: QNHS, 2005 Q2

In contrast, only 6 per cent of men worked less than 30 hours per week. The modal category for women was the 35–39 hour week, with 38 per cent of all women working these hours. Over 18 per cent of all men at work worked more than 45 hours per week, and a further 23 per cent worked between 40 and 44 hours. About 16 per cent of men and 6 per cent of women worked variable hours.

This pattern of working hours appears to share characteristics with both British and continental European patterns of working time. Men have comparatively long average working weeks in Ireland and the UK, as well as in Greece, while average working weeks among women in Ireland are close to the EU average.

However, the share of those working more than 45 hours per week has fallen in Ireland in recent years: from 23 per cent of the total in employment in 1993 to 12 per cent in 2005, and among men the decline was from 31 per cent to 18 per cent. This differs sharply form the trend in Britain, where, notwithstanding a decline in average hours worked, there has been an increase in the proportion of workers, particularly males, working long hours (Edwards, 2005).

Household working patterns

Up to this we have mainly concentrated on individuals. However, the labour market behaviour of individuals, and their standards of living, are crucially affected by the households in which they live and the labour market situation of other household members. Indeed, one of the concerns raised about the impact of the Celtic Tiger is that much of the employment growth during the 1990s was concentrated in households that were already attached to the labour market and that many people were left behind (O'Hearn, 1998; Coulter, 2003).

Table 4.4 shows household employment status for all households with members aged between 18 and 65 for the years 1994, 1997 and 2000, drawn from data collected in the annual Living in Ireland Survey (Russell et al., 2004). The proportion of households in which no member was engaged in paid employment fell from 22 per cent in 1994 to 18 per cent in 1997 and less than 14 per cent in 2000. This represents a very sharp fall in the incidence of workless households after 1994.

The decline in the incidence of workless households was offset by modest increases in the proportions of households in the mixed-work category (where some, but not all adults in the household were at work) and the all-work category (where all adults were at work) between 1994 and 1997. However, between 1997 and 2000 the proportion of households in which all adults were in paid employment increased sharply, from 36 per cent in 1997 to 49 per cent in 2000.

Table 4.4: *Household employment status, 1994 and 2000 (Population aged 18–65 only)*

Household Employment Status	*1994* %	*1997* %	*2000* %
No work	22.1	17.6	13.6
Mixed work	42.9	46.1	37.1
All work	34.9	36.4	49.3
Total	100.0	100.0	100.0

The proportion of households in which some, but not all adults were at work declined from 46 per cent in 1997 to 37 per cent in 2000. So, the expansion in employment opportunities in the later years of the 1990s led to a very substantial increase in work-rich households, a continuation of the decline in workless households, which had begun in 1994, as well as some reduction in the proportion of households with a mixed work pattern. These trends over time are consistent with trends in individual employment and unemployment over the period and suggest that the recent period has been characterised both by increasing household prosperity as well perhaps as increased pressure faced by individual workers in balancing work and life roles, an issue we explore in greater depth below.

Earnings

During the 1990s earnings in Ireland lagged well behind those of our north-western European neighbours (O'Connell, 2000). However, given the rapid growth in employment as well as the emergence of skill and labour shortages, particularly in the years around the turn of the century, it is perhaps not surprising that compensation per employee and earnings before deductions (including employer-provided benefits) increased in Ireland by almost 36 per cent between 1999 and 2004, a substantially faster rate of growth than in most other countries (National Competitiveness Council, 2005). Compensation grew by less than 20 per cent in Germany, France, Italy, Finland and Denmark over the same period. As a consequence, Irish rates of compensation per employee are now broadly similar to those in other north-western EU countries.

Rising inequality in the distribution of earnings has been a prominent feature in many industrialised societies in recent years and often occurs during a period of rapid economic growth. Table 4.5 shows trends in the dispersion of gross hourly earnings – employee pay before tax or social insurance contributions are deducted – for all employees in Ireland in 1994 and 2000. The table shows the earnings of those at different points in the distribution expressed as a proportion of median income – the earnings of the individual right in the middle of the distribution.

Table 4.5: *Distribution of hourly earnings, all employees, 1994–2000*

	1994	*2000*
	Hourly earnings as proportion of median	
Tenth percentile	0.48	0.58
Ninetieth percentile	2.23	2.11
Ratio: Top decile / bottom decile	4.70	3.65

(Nolan, 2003)

The earnings of individuals at the lower edge of the top decile were 2.23 times the median in 1994 but had reduced to 2.11 times the median in 2000. Similarly, the earnings of individuals at the upper edge of the bottom decile were closer to the median in 2000 than in 1994. Thus, during this period, there was some decline in earnings dispersion, even though it remained wide in 2000, with the individual at the ninetieth percentile earning 3.65 times the hourly wage of the person at the tenth percentile. The narrowing of earnings dispersion during the latter part of the 1990s is in contrast to the widening which, as previous research has shown, occurred in the previous decade, that is, at the beginning of economic expansion between the mid-1980s and mid-1990s (Barrett, Fitz Gerald and Nolan, 2000). Thus, the rapid growth of the 1990s in Ireland seems to have reduced wage inequalities, perhaps due to the strong supply of highly skilled workers, both from domestic sources and immigration in this period (Barrett, Fitz Gerald and Nolan, 2002). More recent data on earnings have become available from the National Employment Survey 2003 (CSO, 2006). This provides a particularly robust measure of employee earnings collected from a very large sample, and is likely to become the benchmark for future earnings series. At the time of writing, however, the NES results for 2006 are not yet available, so this source cannot inform us about recent trends in earnings over time.

Table 4.6 shows additional evidence on relative earnings by educational attainment. The ratios provide no support for suspected polarisation in earnings by qualification levels during the boom years 1997–2002. Among those with income from employment, the earnings gap between those below upper secondary education, compared to those with upper secondary remained virtually constant at about 25 per cent. Similarly, the earnings premium for those with tertiary education, compared with those with upper secondary education was close to 45 per cent in both years.

Table 4.6: *Relative earnings of the population with income from employment by level of educational attainment for 25–64-year-olds (upper secondary and post-secondary non-tertiary = 100)*

	1997	*2002*
Below upper secondary	75	76
Tertiary	146	144

Source: OECD, 2006, p. 138

Remaining disadvantage

Notwithstanding the dramatic expansion in employment and the fall in unemployment, labour market disadvantage has not entirely disappeared. A recent National Economic and Social Form (NESF) report argues that 'labour market vulnerability is not an aberration or a left-over from the early 1990s – rather it continues to be generated today, even in a tight labour market' (NESF, 2006, p. x).

The most disadvantaged are those who combine skill and educational deficits with health and disability problems, and in some instances, additional problems such as homelessness, substance addiction, etc. For example, in 2003, over 55 per cent of the unemployed had either no formal qualification or had only completed lower secondary education to a Junior Certificate standard, compared to about 30 per cent of those in employment (O'Connell, 2005).

The proportion of school leavers who leave before completing upper secondary education has remained at about 20 per cent since the mid-1990s, so the ranks of those who are likely to experience labour market problems are being continually augmented. A recent report by the Disability Authority shows conclusively that people with disabilities are far less likely to have a job, or to participate in the labour force than other people of working age (National Disability Authority, 2006). Many lone parents also experience difficulties in the labour market, though the employment rates of lone parents increased substantially over the course of the 1990s (Russell et al., 2004). Nonetheless, major barriers to employment remain for lone parents seeking to enter employment, including the high cost of childcare, as well as the potential loss of rent supplement and other secondary social welfare benefits.

The quality of employment in Ireland – the best of times?

In the previous section we explored how the structure of employment has changed with the economic boom. We have described the nature of change in hours of work, contract types, as well as changes in occupational distributions and sectors. However, these indicators provide only a partial insight into the nature of work experienced by Irish workers in the 2000s. There is a substantial and long-standing body of international literature about the changing quality of work. Debates about whether work has become more or less skilled go back to the 1960s when authors considered whether automated production processes reduced the autonomy and skills of workers or freed them from more of the repetitive and dull elements of their jobs (Blauner, 1964; Braverman, 1974).

In more recent times the debate has continued around the introduction of new technology and whether this has led to greater monitoring, increased work demands (e.g. by speeding up throughput of work) or, on the positive side, whether it has increased the skill levels and opportunities for skill use among workers (Gallie et al., 1998).

The implications for the quality of work of the growth in part-time work and flexible working have also received attention in the international literature, however, the extent to which atypical work is linked to poorer work conditions is found to vary across countries (Esping-Andersen, 1999; Gornick and Meyers, 2003; O'Reilly and Fagan, 1998). Changing work conditions are also addressed in the literature on industrial relations and human resource practices. This literature considers whether new practices, such as performance-related pay, team-working, etc., improve or disimprove the conditions of workers. In the Irish case, Geary (1999) argues that the extent of these new practices has been exaggerated. He further argues that where these practices are used they have resulted in more responsibility for workers, but that overall control of work organisation and team composition remains with management. Concern about changing conditions of work, particularly levels of work intensity, have also arisen in the literature on work–life balance.

Empirical studies reveal a multifaceted picture of working conditions and suggest that the direction of change varies across different dimensions of work quality and across countries and time. For example, levels of autonomy/task discretion increased in Britain between the 1980s and 1990s and subsequently declined. International comparisons show divergent trends in task discretion (Gallie et al., 2004). The evidence on work intensity is somewhat more consistent. Green and McIntosh (2000) use data from the European Survey on Working Conditions to show that work effort increased across Europe between 1991 and 1996, especially in Britain, Ireland and France. However, using European data, Gallie et al. (2004) found increases in work intensity were greatest between the 1980s and the mid- to late 1990s and have levelled off since then. The evidence of change in job quality is therefore rather inconclusive and suggests that change in Ireland is unlikely to follow a neat progressive or regressive path as suggested in more global theories of the changing nature of work.

Here we focus on four key dimensions of job quality: autonomy, work pressure/stress, security and job satisfaction. There is a lack of reliable long-term data on quality of work in Ireland, although the macro-level changes in the occupational structure outlined in the preceding section suggest that there may well have been some change in these dimensions of work.

Drawing on results from the 2003 Changing Workplace Survey (CWS) (O'Connell et al., 2004), we examine conditions across different occupational groups, focusing in particular on the three most rapidly expanding groups outlined above, namely: professional, associate professional, and personal service/sales. We also look at the growing part-time workforce and compare their conditions of work to those of full-time employees. As the CWS was the first national dedicated employee survey in Ireland we do not have many reliable measures of change over time. Where available, we cite information from EU surveys such as the International Social Survey Project (ISSP), Eurobarometer, and the European Working Conditions Surveys; however, it should be noted that the Irish sample sizes for these surveys are relatively small and therefore there may be significant errors around these estimates.

Worker autonomy

Autonomy refers to the level of control that workers have over work tasks, effort and timing. A more expansive measure of autonomy would also include the extent to which a person can influence higher level decisions about the organisation and the nature of work (this is explored in the high-performance work practices literature). Worker autonomy or discretion is viewed by many as a central element of skill and of the nature of the employee–employer relationship (Gallie, forthcoming).

The Changing Workplace Survey contained a six-item measure of employee autonomy which addresses both task discretion and control over working time.[1] Autonomy levels vary widely across occupational groups

---

1 Respondents were asked how often the following applied (almost always, often, sometimes, rarely/almost never): (1) You decide how much work you do or how fast you work during the day. (2) Your manager decides the specific tasks you will do from day to day. (3) You decide when you can take a break during the working day. (4) Your manager monitors your work performance. (5) You have to get your manager's OK before you try to change anything with the way you do your work. (6) You can decide to take on new work or new contracts or initiate new projects. Respondents' average scores on these six items were calculated to form a scale of autonomy that ranges from zero for those who have no autonomy to three indicating full autonomy.

(see Figure 4.3). Two of the three occupations where most jobs have been created since 1998 (professional, and technical/associate professional) record high levels of autonomy. Employees in personal service/sales occupations have below-average levels of autonomy. Both task discretion and discretion over work time are low for these workers; for example, just over half of this group always/often decide on their own pace/volume of work, and only 44 per cent decide their own breaks, and 56 per cent always/often need their managers' approval to change the way they work.

Figure 4.3: *Level of autonomy by occupational group and part-time status*

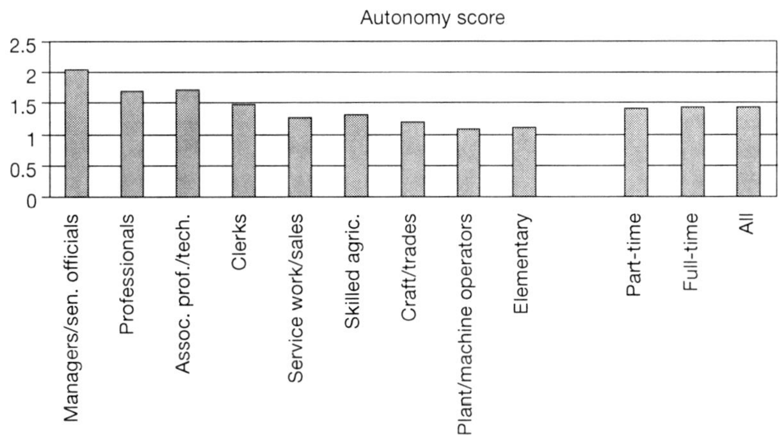

Source: Changing Workplace Survey, 2003 (part-time defined as less than 30 hours per week)

Those working less than 30 hours per week report the same level of autonomy as full-timers. However, if we switch from an hours-based measure to a self-defined measure of part-time status we find that part-timers score lower on the autonomy scale than full-timers (1.4 versus 1.5). Multivariate analysis of this group (O'Connell and Russell, 2005) found a small negative effect of part-time work on autonomy levels when education, tenure, sex and age were controlled, but this disappeared with the addition of occupational and organisational controls. This suggests that part-time work is linked to lower autonomy because of the concentration of part-timers in certain sectors and jobs.

There is relatively little direct information on change in employee discretion over time. According to Eurobarometer surveys, the proportion of Irish workers who said it was very true that they had a lot of say over what happened in their job declined from 32 per cent to 27 per cent between 1996 and 2001 (Gallie et al., 2004). The European Working Conditions Surveys suggest that the levels of task discretion in 2000 were the same as in 1991, with the intervening level in 1995 being somewhat higher.[2] Levels of control over working time (breaks and holidays) were also relatively stable between 1995 and 2000 in these surveys.

When employees are asked on an individual basis whether their level of discretion has changed in the previous two years, just over one-third of workers say that their level of decision-making 'in their own day-to-day work' has increased (Figure 4.4), while only 1 per cent say that their autonomy has declined. Very similar proportions of workers report that the skill level of their job has increased in the last two years.

Figure 4.4: *Change in work conditions in the last two years*

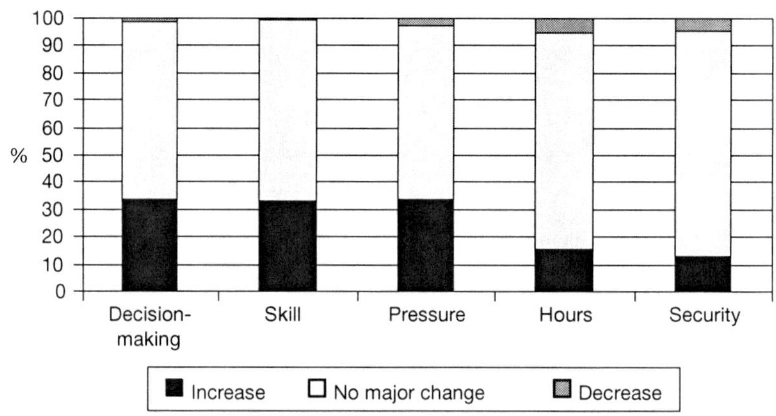

Data source: Changing Workplace Survey, 2003.

Work pressure/stress

While there has been disagreement about the nature of skill change in recent decades there is more general agreement at the theoretical (if not empirical) level that work pressure is rising. Some have argued that increased skill demands, growing task complexity and the greater responsibility that comes with increased autonomy all accentuate the pressure of work (Gallie et al., 1998; Capelli et al., 1997). Others argue that factors such as globalisation, increased competition and greater exploitation of workers have intensified work pressures (Kirby, 2002). The work–life balance literature further suggests that factors outside of work,

2 For example, the proportion reporting control over the speed of work went from 70 per cent in 1991 to 72 per cent in 1995 to 68 per cent in 2000. Given the small sample sizes it is unlikely that these changes are statistically significant.

such as the rise in female employment, have also led to increasing strain within the workplace. This issue is addressed in Chapter 10 and therefore is not considered in detail here.

The proposition that work pressure is increasing is consistent with employees' perceptions of change in their own jobs. Figure 4.4 above shows that one-third of employees feel that the level of pressure they work under has increased over the last two years. However, the pattern is less clear if we compare trends over time between 1996 and 2003 (Figure 4.5).

Figure 4.5: *Changes in work intensity 1996–2003: percentage that agree/strongly agree*

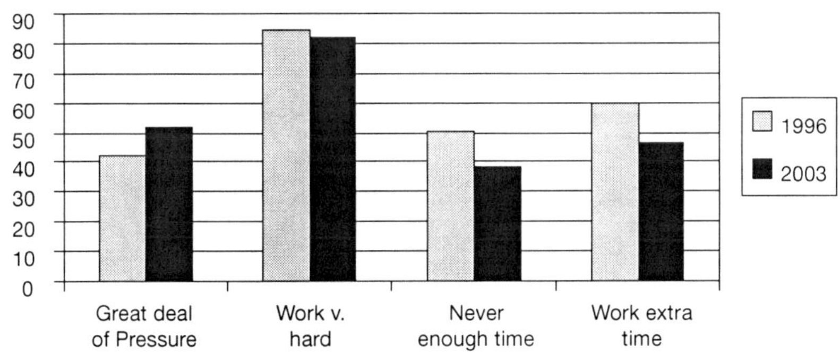

Source: 1996 Eurobarometer 44.3; 2003 ESRI/NCPP Changing Workplace Survey

While there has been an apparent increase in the proportion of workers who say they are under a great deal of pressure, there was virtually no change in the proportion agreeing that they 'work very hard'. On the two time-pressure measures ('never enough time to get things done' and 'I often have to work extra time over and above formal hours to get through the job or help out'), the trend appears to be downwards. However, it should be noted that the response categories differ somewhat at the two time points and this may account for some of the variation observed. The European Working Conditions Surveys carried out in 1991, 1995 and 2001 show a more consistent upward trend in the work effort indicators included there. The figures for Ireland show that the proportion of workers working at high speed increased from 24 per cent in 1991 to 33 per cent in 1996 to 37 per cent in 2000. Similarly, the percentage reporting working to tight deadlines increased from 36 per cent to 48 per cent to 53 per cent across the three surveys.[3]

---

3 For both indicators the figures refer to the percentage experiencing these conditions at least 50 per cent of the time.

A somewhat longer time series, from 1989 to 2003, is available for two further items relating to work intensity – stress and exhaustion (Figure 4.6). These show a downward trend in stress between 1989 and 2001 and a subsequent increase in 2003. The proportion of respondents who come home exhausted increased between 1989 and 1996 and has since decreased. While these figures do not accord with popular accounts of increasing work strain, they are consistent with the decline in both average hours and the proportion of workers working very long hours described above.

Figure 4.6: *Proportion always/often finding work stressful or coming home exhausted*

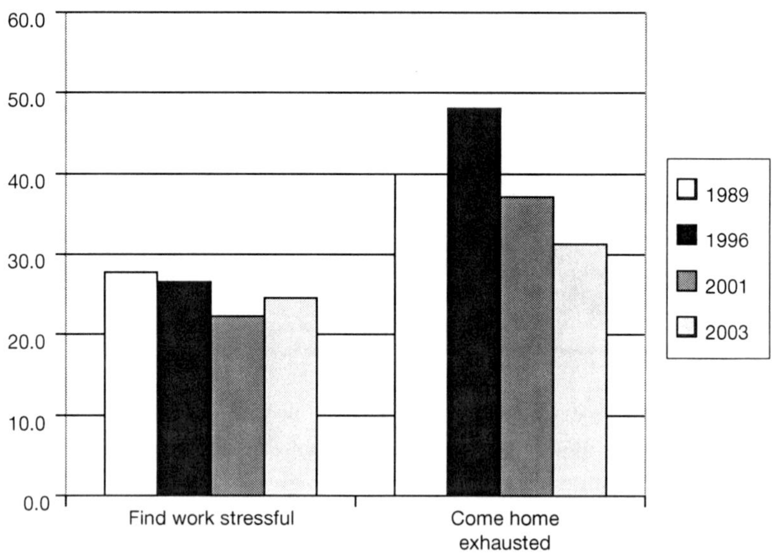

Data sources: 1989 ISSP, 1996 Eurobarometer, 2001 ISSP, 2003 Changing Workplace Survey.

Work pressure is strongly associated with occupational status; however, unlike autonomy and insecurity this aspect of job quality is worse in the higher occupational groups, including the fast-growing professional and associate professional/technician occupations (Figure 4.7). The increase in sales/personal service occupations and growth in part-time work may, however, provide a countervailing influence, as these groups experience significantly lower levels of work intensity.

Job security

The third aspect of job quality that we consider is job security. The statistics outlined under 'Principal trends in the labour market' provide

Figure 4.7: *Work pressure scores by occupational group and part-time status*

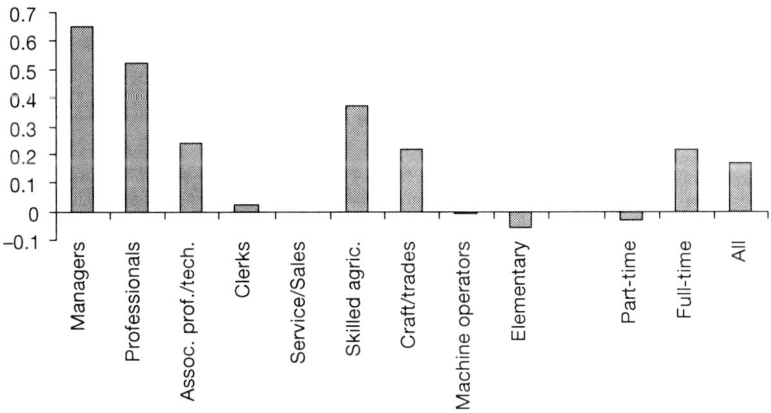

Source: The Changing Workplace Survey, 2003 (This is a composite score of the four items outlined in Figure 4.5. The scale ranges from −2 to +2 with higher scores indicating greater pressure.)

evidence that there has been a decline in the proportion of workers on fixed-term contracts. Moreover, the positive economic conditions and low unemployment should enhance feelings of job security more generally. In most sectors of the economy, those on permanent contracts face little fear of the redundancies and closures that characterised the 1980s.

Figures for 1996 and 2004 show that the proportion of respondents who felt the statement 'my job is secure' was very true increased from 38 per cent to 43 per cent over that period.[4] This upward trend in perceived job security is confirmed by the ISSP surveys carried out in 1989 and 2001, which show the proportion strongly agreeing with the statement 'my job is secure' increased from 20 to 24 per cent while the proportion disagreeing fell from 23 to 17 per cent. At the individual level, 13 per cent of employees believe their own job security had increased in the preceding two years (see Figure 4.4 above) which also suggests a modest upward trend in security.

Perceived job security is linked to occupational status but the relationship is not as linear as for some of the other aspects of job quality. Those in the expanding managerial and professional classes are indeed the most secure; however, the associate professional group feel less secure

---

4 Source for 1996 is the Eurobarometer 44.3. The source for 2005 is the European Social Survey 2004.

Figure 4.8: *Job security by occupation and part-time status*

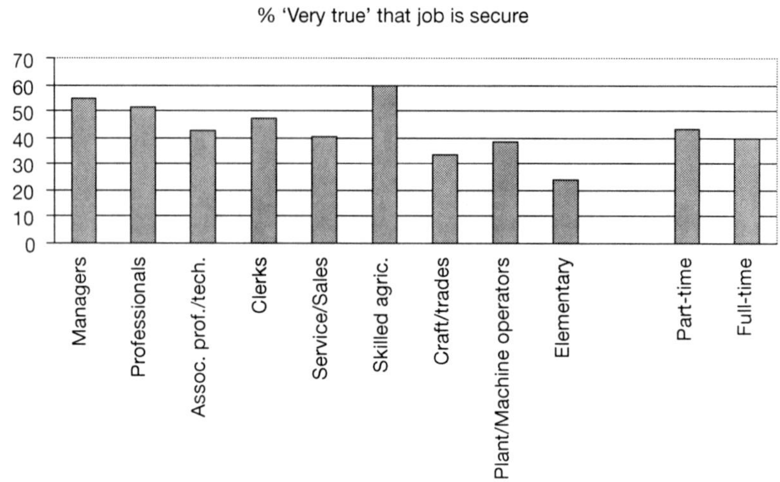

Source: European Social Survey 2004, Irish data.

than clerical workers and are closer to the sales and services group. Part-time workers feel marginally less secure than full-timers, but this gap is less than might be expected given the higher proportion of part-time workers who are on non-permanent contracts.

Job satisfaction

In the 2003 Changing Workplace survey we included a number of measures of job satisfaction. One item asked respondents about their overall job satisfaction, and additional items investigated satisfaction with different job dimensions such as the physical working conditions, hours of work, commuting time, and earnings.

In general we see that Irish employees express a high level of satisfaction, with over 90 per cent of respondents agreeing or strongly agreeing that 'in general' they are satisfied with their job. High levels of satisfaction were also recorded on the other work dimensions, with over 85 per cent expressing satisfaction on each measure with the exception of earnings where the proportion fell to 70 per cent (see O'Connell et al., 2004). These responses were combined to form a satisfaction scale, and the distribution by occupation and part-time status is outlined in Figure 4.9. Again, in three of the four occupational groups which have shown the greatest expansion in recent years, there are relatively high levels of job satisfaction, while those in the expanding service/sales occupations are not so content with their employment.

Those working part-time are found to express higher levels of job satisfaction than those working full-time. Further analysis shows that part-time employees remain marginally more satisfied than full-timers when sector, occupation, firm size, age and sex are controlled (O'Connell et al., 2004).

Figure 4.9: *Mean job satisfaction by occupation and part-time status*

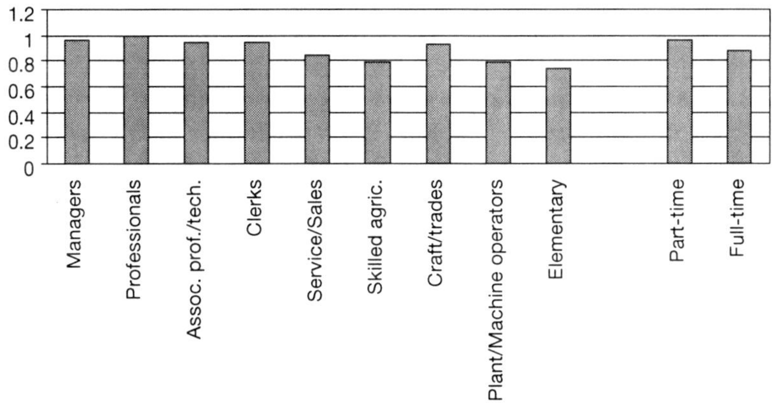

Trend data on job satisfaction in Ireland is inconclusive. The Eurobarometer surveys carried out in 1996 and 2001 suggest that the proportion of employees who were completely satisfied increased from 17 to 20 per cent. However, the ISSP work orientation modules fielded in 1989 and 2001 suggest that the proportion of workers who are completely satisfied remained stable at 16 per cent (as did the average satisfaction score).

In summary, following a period of rapid economic expansion the Irish workforce displays high levels of job satisfaction and increasing job security. However, the majority of employees feel under pressure of some sort and autonomy is restricted in a number of respects – the majority of employees can control their pace of work and timing of breaks but almost one-third do not have any control over their tasks and cannot change their way of working on their own initiative.

The available trend data do not suggest that the economic boom has caused any overall deterioration in the quality of employment as suggested in more pessimistic accounts of change. Feelings of security have increased while levels of autonomy and satisfaction have fluctuated but do not show any conclusive evidence of improvement or deterioration. Nor is there evidence of the much-heralded increase in work stress and work pressure over time. Many workers do feel under pressure but this has not intensified with the recent boom. Moreover, those under most pressure tend to be in the most rewarding jobs both intrinsically and financially.

There remain strong occupational differences in the quality of employment. The expansion at both the upper and lower ends of the occupational hierarchy in the professional and associate professional occupational groupings and service/sales groupings between 1998 and 2004 is likely to have had a countervailing impact on worker autonomy, work pressure, satisfaction and security. A growing proportion of part-time workers fare worse than full-timers in terms of discretion and security but display low levels of stress/pressure and high satisfaction. High satisfaction among part-time workers suggests a trade-off between job quality and flexibility (this issue is discussed further in O'Connell and Russell, 2005) and is consistent with the figures presented under 'Principal trends in the labour market' that part-time working is now almost entirely voluntary.

Conclusions

The labour force and employment grew very strongly in Ireland over the past decade or so. Perhaps the most impressive achievement over that period was the virtual elimination of unemployment. An important element of the expansion in employment has been the surge in women's employment over the past decade. Women are expected to account for about 45 per cent of total employment by the year 2015.

Rapid economic development over the final four decades of the twentieth century gave rise to a sustained long-term trend of occupational upgrading, which entailed the expansion of professional, technical and managerial occupations and increased the importance of education and skills. While this long-term transformation was largely complete by the turn of the century, professional and associate professional and technical occupations continued to expand into the 2000s. We also observe an increase in personal service, sales and unskilled manual occupations since 1998. So, parallel with the expansion of higher-grade jobs there has also been some expansion in lower-skilled occupations, providing some support for a polarisation process. Arguably, however, it was the expansion of low-skilled jobs that made possible the dramatic decline in long-term unemployment achieved since the mid-1990s.

As in other European countries there has been an increase in part-time working in Ireland in recent decades. In Ireland, as elsewhere, the large majority of part-time workers are women. We have shown that the distribution of part-time jobs is skewed towards lower-skilled occupations.

In contrast, the numbers working on fixed-term contracts in Ireland actually fell after the mid-1990s. Thus, with respect to this dimension of labour market flexibility, the Irish pattern of fixed-term working differs from the European trend, although, given the weakness of employment protection legislation in Ireland, employers may feel less need to rely on fixed-term contracts to achieve flexibility.

The proportion of households in which no one was in paid work fell sharply over the course of the 1990s, while the proportion in which all adults were at work increased sharply. This reflects the employment boom and suggests that employment opportunities became much more widely dispersed over the course of the 1990s. An increase in work-rich households entails greater pressure on support services, for example, childcare, and may increase the demand for working arrangements that provide a more favourable balance between work and other life-roles.

Average earnings increased relatively rapidly since the late 1990s, with the result that average employee compensation converged with north-western European averages in the early 2000s. While earnings dispersion increased between the mid-1980s and the mid-1990s, the rapid growth in Ireland during the 1990s was associated with some decline in earnings dispersion. This may have been due to the strong supply of skilled workers to match demand during the employment boom. Despite these gains in average compensation, real unit labour costs have fallen in Ireland compared to the EU, suggesting that, on average, Irish labour costs remain competitive.

In order to explore further the issue of the quality of the jobs created in the booming economy we examined the available evidence on four key dimensions of job quality: worker autonomy, work pressure/stress, job security and job satisfaction. In particular we examined how the expanding occupational categories fared on these dimensions of job quality. We also looked at how the growing part-time workforce compares to full-time workers along these dimensions.

Of the three occupational groups that grew most rapidly between 1998 and 2004, two were towards the top of the occupational structure: professionals, and associate professionals and technical occupations. The other, personal and protective services and sales, was lower-skilled. We found that at the upper end of the occupational structure professionals and technical occupations were characterised by high levels of autonomy and job satisfaction but also by increased work pressure.

On the other hand, we found that the other expanding groups, personal and protective services and sales, were characterised by low levels of job autonomy and lower levels of job satisfaction, but also low levels of work pressure. These differences between the expanding occupations suggest some polarisation of job quality. We also found that part-time work is characterised by lower levels of job pressure and higher levels of job satisfaction. More generally, we found that there has been some increase in perceived job security over the last decade We concluded that there was little evidence of a deterioration in job quality in recent years or indeed of a significant improvement over time.

The most important changes in the Irish labour market have been the dramatic rise in employment, the fall in unemployment, the expansion of high-skilled occupations, and the steep increase in the numbers of women at work. Other positive but less dramatic developments have been the decline in involuntary part-time working, and the fall in the number of non-permanent jobs. These positives are somewhat tempered by the groups who remain disadvantaged in the labour market and the concurrent rise in lower-skilled service jobs, but even this latter 'negative' may have been important in providing opportunities for the reintegration of the unemployed. On balance, our assessment of the impact of the boom on employment is that it has been largely positive.

5

Opportunities for All in the New Ireland?

Christopher T. Whelan and Richard Layte

Introduction

The past decade of economic growth has vastly changed the employment opportunities available to Irish workers. As the next chapter of this volume will show, Ireland has more and better jobs available than ever before, yet it is still not difficult to find both media and academic discussion which argues that this growth masks a persistent and deepening problem of marginalisation and blocked mobility. Writers such as Kirby (2002, 2006) and O'Hearn (1998, 2000) argue that not only has employment growth been largely in unskilled and dead-end jobs, but they also suggest that some groups are finding it increasingly difficult to get into good occupational positions. This argument moves well beyond the notion that inequalities in income or conditions are increasing. Instead it argues that less advantaged groups are increasingly marginalised and they and their children are unable to break into the more advantaged occupations. If true, such a situation would run counter to most people's concept of equity. Few would argue that equality of conditions irrespective of individual effort is appealing – let alone attainable – and most would agree that Irish society should strive to foster equality of opportunity and would be unhappy if opportunities to rise on one's own merits were becoming increasingly rare. Such inequality would also be a serious problem for Irish society since it would entail a mammoth waste of human talent and possibility.

In fact, as we show in this chapter, the real picture is very far from being as pessimistic as that painted by some commentators. The available evidence shows that the proportion of Irish people in professional and managerial occupations has grown substantially since the 1970s and, if anything, this trend has intensified over the past decade. At the same time the proportion of the population in low-skilled occupations has fallen steadily. As a consequence, the majority of Irish people are in jobs involving better conditions and prospects than those of their parents.

T. Fahey et al. (eds.), Quality of Life in Ireland, 67–85.

Debates about equality of opportunity are complex, however, and, even as the absolute chance of rising up the hierarchy increases, it is possible that those from more privileged backgrounds may sustain and even enhance their relative advantage. This chapter shows that, while those at the top of the class structure have enjoyed considerable success in maintaining an unfair advantage, in some important respects there has been a move towards a more open society. So, although Irish society continues to exhibit substantial inequality of opportunity, with the affluent and comfortable still enjoying a substantial advantage, this advantage does seem to have decreased over the years of the boom.

The boom, inequality and meritocracy

As Chapter 2 of this volume argues, Ireland has always had a more unequal distribution of income than other European nations, but there is no evidence that such inequality has increased during the economic boom. Ireland has developed a particular social model which Rhodes (1998) has labelled 'competitive corporatism'. Irish competitive corporatism has used centralised bargaining between government, employers and trade unions to set national wage agreements, taxation and social policies. Unlike traditional forms of the model, Irish corporatism has not prioritised 'equity' as an objective. Successive agreements have increased the real value of social welfare payments and spending on social services, but there has been no concerted attempt to equalise incomes through taxation and redistribution. If anything, policies may have copper-fastened existing differences between better and worse off groups in areas such as health care by introducing subsidies to middle- and higher-income groups to buy private medical care.[1]

Irish 'competitive corporatism' also includes widespread intervention in the labour market by the government. The strategy of maximising employment participation through low direct taxation and employment creation substantially increased the level of employment in Ireland with a consequent decline in unemployment from 16 per cent in 1994 to less than 4 per cent currently.

In the course of a decade the Irish labour market moved from a significant labour surplus to a labour shortage. Over the same period, as shown in Chapter 2, the trend in neither earnings nor household income

---

1 Ó Riain and O'Connell (2000) distinguish between the role of the State in shaping both developmental and distributional outcomes and argue that each may have a relatively autonomous logic but that developments in one institutional sphere may be critical to the ability to pursue strategies in the other.

had been towards greater inequality, although it should be kept clearly in mind that Ireland was a comparatively unequal society before the economic boom.

Given these trends in employment and income inequality, it is not at all obvious what the consequences might be for equality of opportunity between social groups. It does not appear that overall inequality has increased, but existing large inequalities in Irish society have remained largely undiminished. As already argued, the growth in employment of the past decade means that there are now far more jobs available involving higher pay and better conditions than ever before. The important question is whether this absolute increase in the scale of opportunities has been distributed across Irish society in a relatively equal manner, or whether some groups have had less benefit from the overall opening-up of opportunities than others. In sociological research the term 'meritocracy' has been used to describe a notional society in which success is entirely dependent on the combination of personal endowments (usually signified by IQ) and effort rather than the social and economic endowments that people inherit from their parents or favours from social networks. Though a thorough going meritocracy may be impossible, even undesirable,[2] it is important to establish whether the economic growth of recent years has been accompanied by a growth in opportunities for those from all sections of Irish society on the basis of merit.

Ireland managed to avoid acute labour shortages through the boom because of the initial influx of migrant Irish workers and the subsequent inflow of other nationalities, but it remains true that employers have not been able to draw on a ready pool of unemployed people with the requisite skill. This could mean that employers have had to employ individuals from all backgrounds and with lower skills/qualifications, whereas in the past they may have been choosier. In such circumstances those from less advantaged backgrounds, who tend to have lower levels of formal education and less of the 'social capital' on which better connected groups can draw, may be more successful in entering previously unattainable jobs.

In the following sections we bring empirical evidence to bear on these issues using research that has been carried out by the ESRI.[3] Before doing so, however, we first need to define what exactly we mean by increasing 'meritocracy'.

---

2 The sociologist Michael Young (1958) satirised a fictional meritocracy in his book *The Rise of Meritocracy* and showed that it may not necessarily be the equitable democracy that many envisage.

3 See Whelan and Layte, (2002, 2004, 2006) and Layte and Whelan, (2004)

Marginalised groups, social classes and equality of opportunity

Up to this point we have been less than precise about what we are referring to when we speak of equality of opportunity and to whom such equality should apply. Individuals differ across a multitude of different dimensions that are potentially relevant for their well-being and long-term life chances. It is clear, for instance, that some groups experience substantial marginalisation as a result of belonging to specific groups such as refugees or Travellers, while others may have personal characteristics (such as a disability) which reduce their life chances. However, the focus of our analysis in this chapter is on inequalities of opportunity between groups defined by a wider set of criteria.

Our attention will therefore centre on groups in the general population who are defined in more general socio-economic terms. The best indicator of general socio-economic position is an individual's present or past occupational position. This categorisation has the benefit of providing us with a stable measure that can be compared across time and has demonstrable associations with other forms of disadvantage. To measure the extent of success in reaching more advantaged positions we need to have a starting point, so here we examine the relationship between the social class of individuals at the time at which a survey was carried out and that of the main 'breadwinner' in the household when they were growing up.

Using occupational class takes us to the heart of the debate about equality of opportunity. This revolves around the likelihood of individuals moving into better (or worse) positions over time. Such movement is of crucial importance because social class groups defined by occupational position differ in a systematic fashion in terms of other dimensions of advantage and disadvantage and this makes them appropriate as groupings that summarise general life chances.

Occupations can be grouped into social classes in a number of different ways. The Irish Central Statistics Office (CSO) clusters occupations according to whether someone is in a manual or non-manual occupation, the level of skill required in the job and whether the person is a manager or an employer. Other classifications use similar groupings but defined in terms of whether the person is self-employed or, if employed, the extent to which they enjoy promotion opportunities, pension provisions and discretion in relation to working arrangements. An example of the latter is the Erikson/Goldthorpe (EG) classification. In this chapter we use both the CSO and EG classifications, both of which use seven different classes, although our discussion of comparisons between individuals and parents relies on the EG classification. Parents' class is defined using an individual's recall of the occupation of the 'main breadwinner' when they 'were growing up'.

What do we mean by equality of opportunity? At its most basic, equality of opportunity implies equality in access to the paths leading to higher occupational and social class positions. True equality of opportunity would thus occur where children face identical obstacles (and costs) and come equipped with identical resources.

Unfortunately, it is very difficult to measure the opportunity structure presented to children and their parents since it is a complex mix of many dimensions. So we examine equality of opportunity by focusing on 'outputs' rather than the 'inputs', that is, in terms of the achieved social class positions of offspring and how these relate to those of their parents. In this sense we are more interested in equality of outcomes rather than equality of opportunity, strictly speaking. This assumes that individuals from different class origins place an equal value on access to higher social class positions. There is some evidence that preferences for certain occupational niches vary depending on one's origins, with farming providing the most obvious example.

However, such effects tend to be modest in comparison with those derived from differences in resources associated with such origins and barriers to entry to class destinations, such as the need for minimal levels of educational qualifications or the appropriate forms of capital. Thus, in general, we assume that all differences in outcome stem from differences between groups in resources. The available evidence does suggest that educational differences are a good deal more important than IQ differences in determining one's class destination and, as we will see, even where those from different social classes attain the same educational level, working-class children are still less likely to attain the better occupational position than their middle-class peers. Ability and effort count, but working-class children require more of both to prosper.[4]

The position we adopt gives relatively little weight to the negative role that cultural factors can play and takes as its starting point the assumption that individuals from all social class origins act rationally within the context given by the resources they can draw on, their perceptions of the risks and advantages associated with different choices and the barriers they confront.[5]

---

4 Breen and Goldthorpe (1999, 2001)

5 For a discussion of the failure of the 'cultural' approach to explain long-term trends in educational participation and, in particular, social class and gender differences in such levels and a detailed discussion of the 'rational action approach', see Goldthorpe, 1987, and Breen and Goldthorpe (1997, 1999).

Consistent with this view, there is very little evidence that social mobility per se impacts negatively on individuals' well-being or social networks.[6] Our measure of equality of opportunity focuses on the relative success of those from the lowest and least rewarded social classes in entering the highest and most rewarded social classes compared to those originating in those classes. In this sense perfect equality of opportunity would involve a situation where there is no systematic relationship between the class of parents and that of their offspring. In reality of course, this has never come close to being the case in any of the societies that sociologists have studied. However, examination of trends in the strength of the association across generations can tell us a great deal about whether equality of opportunity is increasing or decreasing in Ireland.

The changing pattern of social classes in Ireland

A country's social class structure tends to change in a rather predictable fashion as it moves from an agricultural to an industrial and on to a 'post-industrial' form of economic organisation. Although Ireland may be thought to have skipped important parts of the 'industrial' phase, the order of changes in class structure is an extremely familiar one. In the early 1970s Ireland was still very much in transition from an agricultural to an industrial society, whereas by the end of the century it had clearly made the transition to being a post-industrial society. The transformation involved two distinct phases. The first, running from the early 1960s to the early 1980s, involved a rapid reduction in the numbers in agriculture and unskilled manual work and significant increases in the level of employment in white collar and skilled manual work. The second phase, running from the early 1980s to the early years of the new century, was characterised by a continuing decline in relation to agricultural and unskilled manual work, although at a slower pace. Skilled manual work also declined and increased opportunities were concentrated in the professional and managerial sector.

As shown in Figures 5.1 and 5.2, using the CSO classification, we observe a substantial amount of change in the class structure even between 1991 and 2002, with a dramatic increase in the proportion in professional and managerial jobs for both men and women. For men the proportion in these jobs increased by approximately 50 per cent and for women by some 40 per cent. Since the numbers in work increased substantially during this period the absolute increases were even more dramatic. The increase at the

---

6 See Goldthorpe (1987)

top of the class structure was compensated for by a decline in agriculture and in unskilled manual work. For women a reduction in the proportion in skilled manual work was observed together with a corresponding increase in the number in clerical work. Thus, contrary to claims by authors such as O'Hearn (2000, pp. 78–81) that employment growth has been concentrated in routine low-paying services, the available evidence strongly supports O'Connell's (2000, pp. 75–76) conclusion that there has been a general upgrading in the quality of positions in the labour market.

Figure 5.1: *CSO social class groups for men, 1991 and 2002*

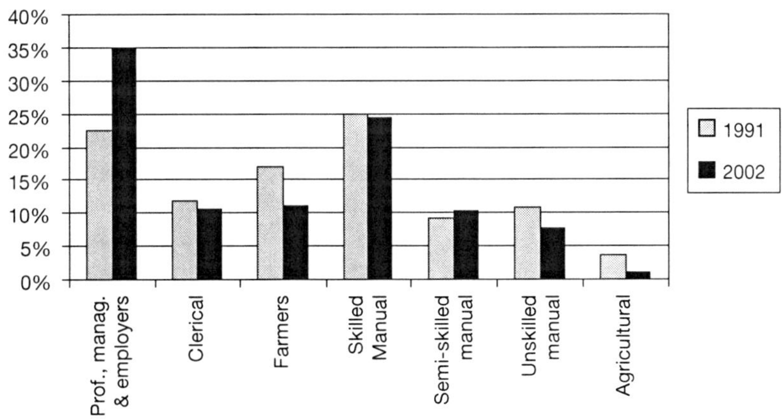

Figure 5.2: *CSO social class groups for women, 1991 and 2002*

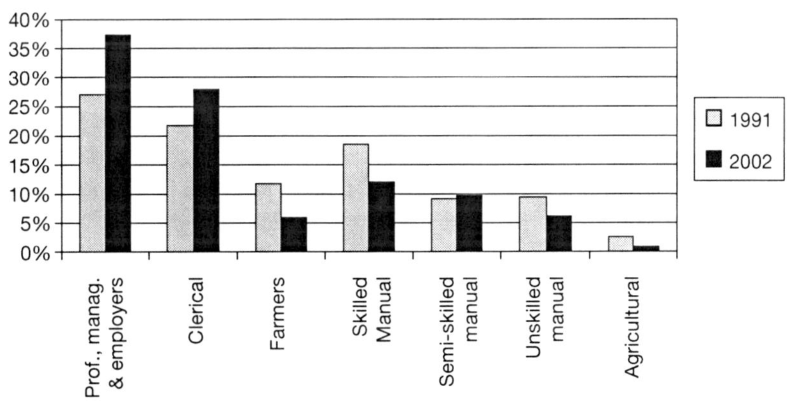

The increase in jobs in the professional and managerial classes and the decrease in the unskilled manual social class created 'structural' pressure on those from manual and farming backgrounds to move into the higher social class locations. Such changes promote what sociologists term 'absolute social mobility' arising from 'push' and 'pull' factors associated with the changing contours of the class structure. Of course the number and type of class positions is not independent of, for example, the educational qualifications of the individuals available to fill them, but the trend would suggest that opportunities were becoming available to those from lower social class backgrounds.

Did we see an increase in upward movement over recent decades in Ireland? The contexts in which such trends emerged are rather different for men and women. For women our analysis relates to those active in the labour market since otherwise we would be classifying many individuals on the basis of positions that they occupied many years previously. The most recent period was one in which participation in the female labour market rose dramatically. In addition, there was a significant shift in the balance between full and part-time work over the period. In the earlier phase women active in the labour market among the older age groups were a rather select group in that the better educated were much more likely to remain in the labour market, while at the later stage this was much less true.

The changing composition of women participating in the labour force makes it particularly difficult to reach unambiguous conclusions regarding trends in social fluidity among women. In addition, it is necessary to take into account that in most cases, the class origins of women are measured by the occupation of their fathers and this has a significant impact on the pattern of mobility observed for women. The fact that very few women inherit farms or small businesses, or enter traditional skilled manual occupations, inevitably leads to large-scale mobility for those originating in those class origins. Thus, 'push' factors play an even greater role for women than for men.

The version of the EG class schema that we employ places both non-skilled manual workers and routine service-type non-manual occupations in the same class. For convenience, in our subsequent discussion we will refer to this class as the non-skilled class. This decision has a particularly significant effect on the class distribution of women. It also has a substantial effect on estimated levels of mobility for women. A failure to distinguish between different types of 'white collar' work would have the consequence of producing spuriously high estimates of upward mobility and corresponding underestimation of downward mobility. Figures 5.3 and 5.4 show, respectively, the proportions of men and women who are mobile, upwardly mobile, mobile into the professional and managerial class and, lastly, mobile into that class from the working classes.[7]

---

[7] For a detailed discussion of our definitions of 'upward' and 'downward' mobility see Layte and Whelan (2004).

Figure 5.3: *Absolute class mobility in 1973–2000 for men*

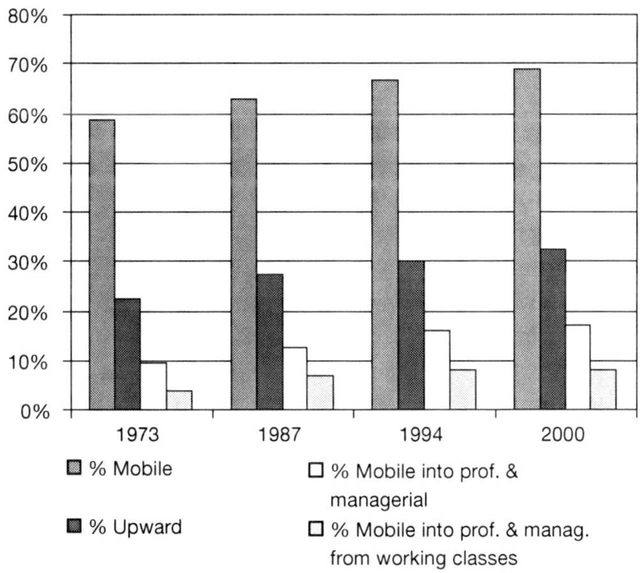

For men the figures cover the period between 1973 and 2000, while for women they span the period 1987 to 2000. If we focus first on men in Figure 5.3, it is clear that mobility – the number of offspring who are not in the class of their parents – has been increasing from 1973 through to 2000 and has been sustained through the recent years of growth. It is also clear that the sharper increase was in upward rather than downward mobility, with the former rising from 22 per cent in 1973 to 32 per cent in 2000 (i.e. 45% increase). Although it is not shown in Figure 3, downward mobility actually decreased over the same period for men. As a consequence, whereas in 1973 the overall probability of moving into a class lower than your parents for men was about the same as moving into a class above them, by 2000 the average Irish male was almost twice as likely to move up as to move down.

Mobility into the professional and managerial class also rose gradually from 10 per cent in 1973 to 17 per cent in 2000. Similarly, mobility from the working class to the professional and managerial class almost doubled, rising from 4 per cent in 1973 to 8 per cent in 2000. The pattern is not shown in Figure 3 but the increase in mobility into the professional and managerial class was matched by a corresponding decrease in downward mobility into the non-skilled class from 15 per cent in 1973 to 13 per cent in 1987 and 12 per cent by 2000. The consequence of these changes was that while men located in the professional and managerial classes were increasingly drawn from a diverse set of class origins, the non-skilled class came increasingly to form a self-recruiting bloc with very few of its members being drawn from outside the working class.

The profound changes in the class structure created a situation whereby working-class men were much more likely to rise up through the social class structure and an increasing proportion were making it to the most rewarded professional and managerial positions. At the same time, those groups outside of the working classes were also able to substantially reduce their risks of falling into the non-skilled manual class.

As is clear from Figure 5.4, the picture is rather different for women. They are more mobile then men in each year, but there is relatively little change in such levels over time. The situation for women is also very different in that they experience almost equal levels of upward and downward mobility. This arises both from their exclusion from farming, self-employment and traditional skilled manual employment, and their substantial over-representation in lower-level personal service occupations. Over time, women have upward mobility levels that are similar or even greater than men's, but they display substantially higher downward mobility rates. The situation for women also differs from that of men in that the balance between upward and downward mobility changes little over time. These findings are likely to be closely associated with the dramatic changes in the scale and pattern of labour force participation for women.

Figure 5.4: *Absolute class mobility in 1987–2000 for women*

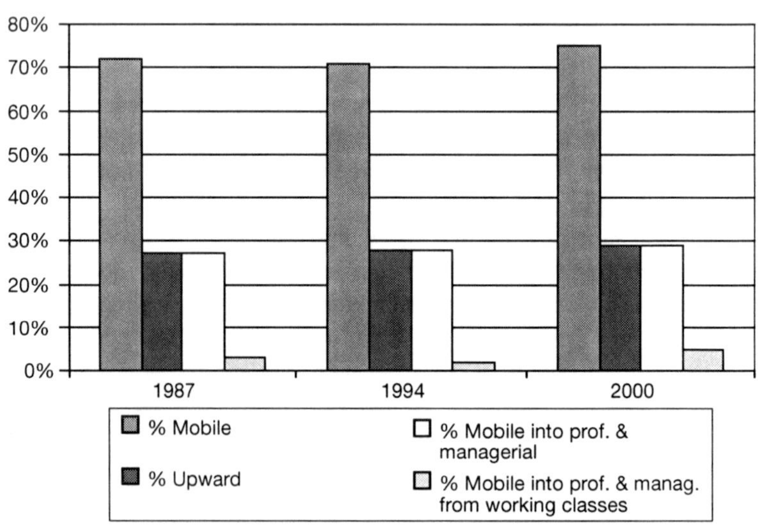

Is increasing mobility accompanied by increasing equality of opportunity?

The previous section showed that not only were Irish people more likely to move into a job with better conditions and prospects than their parents in 2000 than they were in 1973, but that this was also true of those in working-class groups. The rate at which those from working-class groups were moving into the professional and managerial class doubled between 1973 and 2000. However, it was also apparent that those outside of the working-class were also able to consolidate their positions during this period and this highlights a key issue in the study of equality of opportunity: All classes may experience an increase in the chances of promotion, but some may have an advantage in reaching higher social class occupations. All classes may see an improvement in 'absolute' terms in their chances of progression, but the offspring of working-class groups may still be relatively disadvantaged in comparison to the offspring of middle-class groups and the professional and managerial classes in particular. This is demonstrated for both men and women in Figures 5.5 and 5.6 where we show the proportions that were immobile (i.e. not moving from the class of their parents) and the proportions entering the professional and managerial class broken down by the class of their parents.

Figure 5.5: *Proportion of men immobile and entering the professional and managerial class by class of parents in 2000*

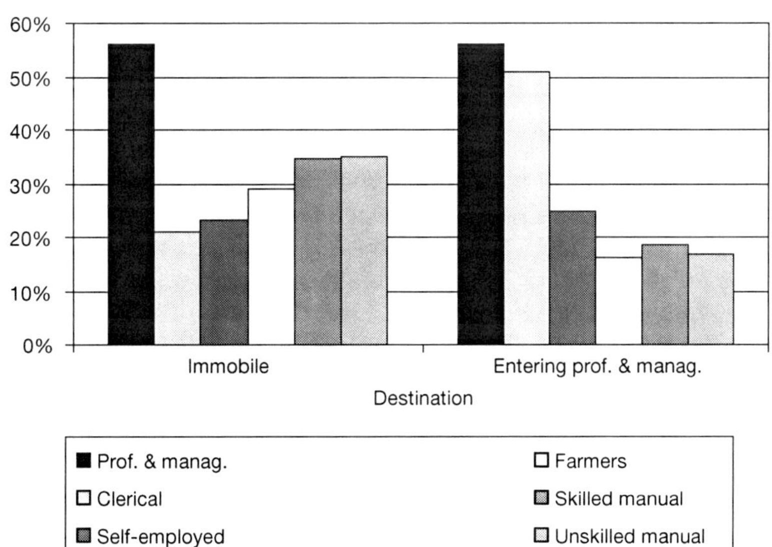

Figure 5.5 shows that the highest proportion of men who were immobile is observed for those from professional or managerial backgrounds. This proportion is almost one and a half times as large as that for the next highest group, those men who come from the manual classes.

Figure 5.6: *Proportion of women immobile and entering the professional and managerial class by class of parents in 2000*

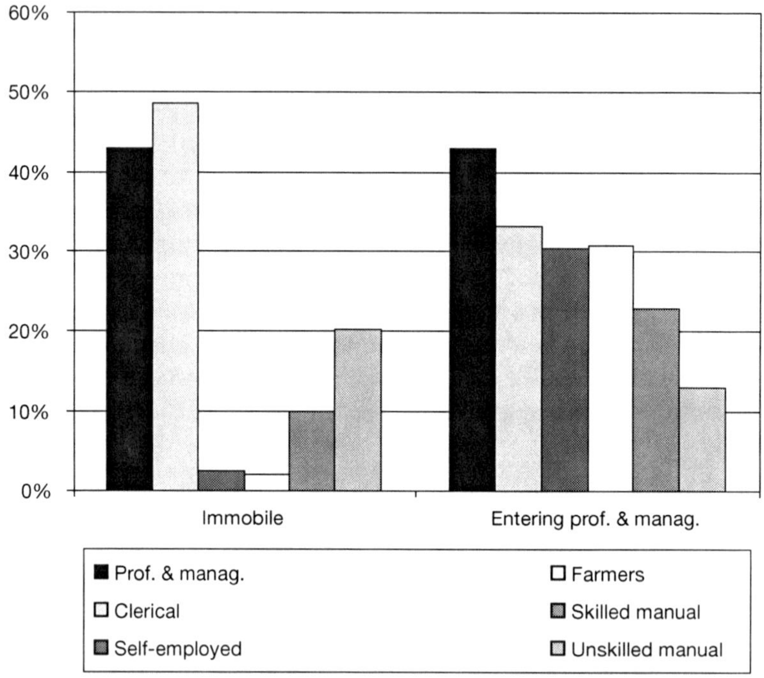

If we look at Figure 5.6 we see a somewhat different pattern for women. Immobility in the professional managerial class is somewhat lower than for men although almost one in two remain in their class of origin. For the clerical group (office workers) immobility levels are rather higher for women, with one in two being found in their class of origin compared to one in five men. On the other hand, immobility in the farming and small business classes is almost non-existent and in the skilled manual class is modest in comparison with men. In contrast, immobility in the clerical class is almost as high for women as it is for men in the professional and managerial classes, with almost one in two remaining in the same class as their parents. This undoubtedly reflects the limited opportunities for women for mobility into classes associated with the ownership of property and the skilled manual classes.

Together, these patterns show that those from the most advantaged class are far more likely than those from the least advantaged to be in the same classes as adults. Sons and daughters of doctors, lawyers and company managers are far more likely to make their way back into these positions than are the sons and daughters of plumbers, bus drivers, shop workers and cleaners; in itself this not undesirable. What is crucial is whether the ability of those from the higher social classes to maintain their privileged position is at the expense of those from less favoured origins.

We can look at the evidence presented in Figures 5.5 and 5.6 regarding the proportions entering the professional and managerial classes by class of origin. This shows that the proportion located in the most advantaged classes is highest for those coming from such origins. For example, the proportion of those from a professional and managerial class background who entered that class is over three times higher than the comparable figure for those from the non-skilled manual class for both men and women. While the general hierarchy of class advantages is broadly similar for men and women, there are a number of important differences. Men from clerical origins, for instance, are a good deal more likely to be found in the professional and managerial class than their female counterparts. Conversely, women from farming origins are twice as likely as men from such backgrounds to be upwardly mobile into the professional and managerial class. This finding is entirely consistent with the well-known fact that farmers have always adopted quite different strategies for sons and daughters.[8]

The available evidence consistently shows that differences in outcomes for men and women are not due to different patterns of class inequalities. Instead they are a consequence of occupational segregation by gender and the consequent distribution of class destinations. Within those structural constraints class processes appear to be gender-blind.[9]

It is clear that the overall level of upward mobility in Irish society has increased substantially since the early 1970s and that this trend has been maintained in the recent period of accelerated growth. The available evidence shows that skilled and unskilled working-class families have been increasingly successful in scaling the class structure and gaining access to well-rewarded and coveted jobs in the professional and managerial classes. However, this does not mean that equality of opportunity has been achieved, since the offspring of professionals and managers still enjoy very substantial advantages over those from working-class backgrounds in gaining access to more favoured positions and in

8 See Hannan and Commins, 1992

9 See Breen and Whelan (1993) and Layte and Whelan (2004)

being buffered against the risk of being found in the less favoured positions. The final questions we wish to address relate to whether this advantage has increased or decreased over time and to what we can attribute the differential in outcomes for working-class children.

Explaining inequality of opportunity

We saw in the previous section that there is a strong association between an individual's current social class and that of their parents. The ability of those from more favoured class origins to maintain their positions across generations clearly suggests that these groups possess advantages that they use to good effect in getting their children the most coveted jobs. Initially this sounds rather conspiratorial, suggesting that well-off and connected parents are colluding to give their children an advantage, but in reality the diverse processes are both more mundane and subtler.

At a basic level, parents who are professionals or managers occupy jobs that are well-rewarded in terms of salary and fringe benefits and so these households are much more likely to be able to provide an environment where a child can thrive and develop to their potential. This advantage influences all areas of the child's life, with increased resources providing a better diet leading to better physical and mental development. Data from the Living in Ireland Survey show, for instance, that men from professional and managerial backgrounds are on average 3 cm taller than men from unskilled manual backgrounds and this reflects their living standards during childhood. Even children growing up now exhibit this difference. The ESRI survey of sports participation among children carried out in 2005 found that 16-year-olds from professional and managerial backgrounds were on average 2 cm taller than their classmates from unskilled manual homes. Inequality of opportunity parallels inequality of material conditions.

Education is often the main pathway to occupational success, and better physical and mental development may be one reason why the children of higher social class families tend to get better educational results on average than those in other social classes and particularly the manual working classes. But better physical and mental development probably plays a substantially smaller role in educational success than the fact that middle-class parents have more books and resources from which children learn plus higher levels of education themselves.[10] The proportion of

[10] Middle-class households are also more likely to send their children to schools whose intake is predominantly middle-class and this tends to lead to a more favourable academic environment.

professional and managerial parents with third-level qualifications will be far higher than in any other group and this means that these parents are more knowledgeable about the education system and more vocal in their relationship with schools. Middle-class parents may also put a higher value on education and so are more likely to push their children to stay longer in education and work harder.

Sociological research is rather divided about the underlying processes that produce class differences in educational attainment. Some place particular emphasis on the relationship between the functioning of the educational system and class-specific cultures. This includes explanations that see the educational system as a conservative force or as arbitrarily rewarding one class over another but also extends to explanations that simply identify class differences in aspirations and parental differences in the value placed on education. An alternative perspective places predominant emphasis on material disadvantage.

Of course such explanations are not mutually exclusive and, in particular, material disadvantages at one stage of the life cycle may have an impact on values, beliefs and aspirations at later points.[11] Thus, as indicated earlier, while not denying class differences in culture in the aforementioned sense, the position we adopt sees working-class children as attempting to behave rationally given the resources available to them and the manner in which such resources impact on their understanding of the education system and their perceptions of the costs and benefits of particular choices. This approach seems more consistent with long-term trends towards increased participation rates and the changing gender differentials in such rates.[12]

Research suggests however that even where working-class children have an identical IQ and educational qualifications to middle-class children, they are still less likely to make it into the most advantaged occupations and social classes. Education may be the most important factor in social class differences in occupational attainment but the impact of their family of origin persists even when we have taken educational differences into account. The direct inheritance of property or other forms of capital continues to play a significant role.[13]

Over and above such visible class differences there exist 'softer' and often unmeasured differences between individuals from different

---

[11] See Breen (2004) for further discussion of these issues.

[12] See Breen and Goldthorpe (1997)

[13] The model that has been most frequently applied to the analysis of social mobility in Ireland is labelled the 'Agriculture, Hierarchy and Property (AHP)' model. (Breen and Whelan, 1992 and 1994)

backgrounds relating to social skills and social capital, but it is clear that working-class children need to show significantly more 'effort' to achieve the same occupational level as a middle-class child.[14]

Increasing equality of opportunity?

The discussion above suggests some reasons why working-class children are less likely to make their way into the most advantaged jobs, but is this differential in opportunity stable or have there been changes over time? Strong demand for labour in the economic boom of recent years has made it far more difficult for employers to be choosy about the individuals that they recruit and this may have decreased the disadvantage of candidates from working-class origins.

In analysing such issues we focus on men. Unfortunately we do not have data for women for 1973 so it is impossible to look at long-term trends for women. Furthermore, the rapidly changing situation in relation to both the extent and nature of women's participation in the labour force makes it difficult to offer unqualified conclusions regarding changes in class inequalities with regard to equality of opportunity. However, what we do know is that at any point in time the manner in which class inequalities operate is very similar for men and women.

Research from the ESRI has examined trends in the differential between men from different class origins. In broad terms, this research is in line with a large body of international findings in showing the general stability of class differentials over time. In fact what is striking about comparisons across societies is not the manner in which they differ, but the remarkable similarity in the core pattern of inequalities of opportunity.[15] However, differences do exist and in the Irish case some interesting changes have been observed over time.

The most striking finding is that the relative disadvantage which those from non-skilled manual backgrounds faced in entering the professional and managerial class, compared to those originating in that class, had decreased significantly between 1973 and 2000. In Figure 5.7 we take the 1973 level of disadvantage as the reference point and allocate it a value of 100 per cent. We then show the values for later years as a percentage of the 1973 value. From Figure 5.7 we can see the disadvantage experienced by the non-skilled class had by 1987 fallen to 78 per cent of its 1973 value.

---

[14] Breen and Goldthorpe (1999, 2001)

[15] See Erikson and Goldthorpe (1992) and Breen (2004)

Figure 5.7: *The disadvantage faced by men with unskilled manual origins in moving into the professional and managerial class, 1973–2000*

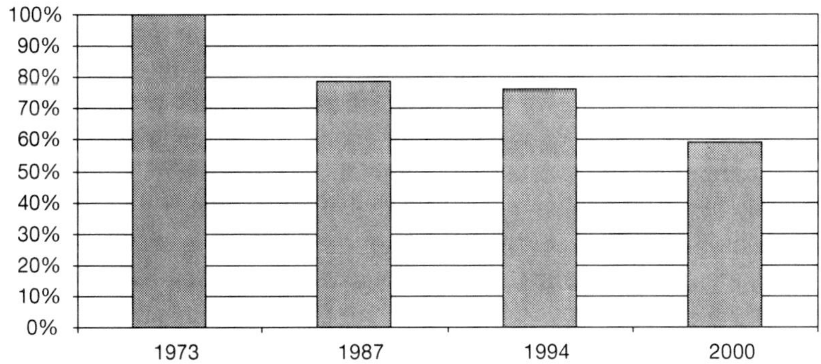

By 1994 there was a further reduction to 76 per cent. Finally, there was a very substantial decline to 59 per cent by 2000. It should be said that sociological research provides very few instances where the barriers faced by disadvantaged classes have actually decreased over time and so this Irish finding is striking. It is also interesting that the largest fall in differentials faced by those from non-skilled origins came between 1994 and 2000, exactly the period in which the Irish labour market was growing most quickly and demand for labour strongest.

How did the observed reductions in inequality of opportunity come about? One common explanation put forward is that educational achievement has come to play a greater role. This theory holds that employers are increasingly choosing candidates for jobs because of their educational achievements rather than other criteria such as having the 'right' social class background. Clearly educational expansion has been one of the key factors promoting economic growth in Ireland.

Without such expansion the Irish class or occupational structure would not have its current shape. In that sense expansion of educational opportunity is intimately linked to increased opportunities for mobility. Furthermore, the cost of educational failure has increased and investment in education remains a perfectly rational choice for the individual. However, Irish research has demonstrated conclusively that the role of education in the transmission of relative class advantage has actually declined rather than increased.[16]

If education was not the key to the trend towards the increased equality of opportunity observed, how are we to account for this phenomenon?

[16] See Whelan and Layte (2002, 2004, 2006, for further details)

While there is no necessary relationship between economic growth and increased equality of opportunity, the pattern of change over time in Ireland suggests that both long-term factors, associated with the upgrading of the class structure, and short-term factors reflected in the tightness of the labour market have played a role.[17] In the absence of empirical studies of employer behaviour with regard to recruitment and promotion, the manner in which change has come about constitutes something of a black box. If employers pay increased attention to characteristics other than education that either directly or indirectly tap social background or family and community affiliations this could go together with constant or indeed reduced levels of inequality of opportunity. However, the background in the Irish case was one of increasing labour shortages and an institutional context whereby employers, not withstanding social partnership at the national level, enjoyed increased discretion at the workplace level.[18]

Against this background, the fact that a weakening impact of education has gone together with increased social fluidity suggests that employers, both in recruitment and promotion, may have paid increased attention to performance-related attributes and in a manner that has been to the advantage of those from less favoured backgrounds. Breen and Whelan (1991) showed that levels of intra-generational mobility were particularly low in Ireland and suggested that this may have been related to the absence of large-scale industrial enterprises. Unfortunately the 1994 and 2000 datasets do not contain information on first occupation. However, it is entirely consistent with the evidence that we have presented that a significant increase in work–life mobility may have contributed to the higher levels of absolute mobility and social fluidity that we have observed.

Conclusions

The unprecedented growth of the last decade or so has utterly changed the Irish economy and Irish society. A country which once had the highest rates of unemployment in Europe now has labour shortages and income growth rates which far outstrip most other European nations. Yet increasing relative income poverty rates and stubbornly high levels of income

---

17 See Breen and Luijkx (2004)

18 Some of the newer sectors, especially in high-tech manufacturing and in private sector service industries proved difficult to unionise. Private sector unionisation is estimated to be 30 per cent (Hardiman, 2000). Roche and Geary (1998) concluded that where change in work-place practices have taken place it tends to be in line with Anglo-American industrial systems that are not very favourable towards consultative or inclusive forms of decision-making.

inequality in Ireland are just two indications that such changes do not mean that poverty and marginalisation are curiosities from the past. It is this contrast of intense growth and undiminished inequality that has led many to suggest that, contrary to expectations, economic growth in Ireland has actually been accompanied by widening gaps between social groups and decreasing equality of opportunity.

In this chapter we have sought to examine this analysis using evidence from a range of studies. Our overall finding is a good deal less pessimistic than that just discussed. Employment growth has actually been strongest in better-paid and -rewarded occupations in the professions and there has been a substantial growth in managerial and technical occupations. This increase in available positions at the 'top' of the occupational hierarchy has been accompanied by a decrease in the total number of unskilled and semi-skilled occupations.

All this means is that the majority of intergenerational mobility in Ireland over the last three decades has been upward and Irish people are now likely to work in a better job than their parents in terms of rates of pay and benefits.

Such absolute changes in opportunity need not, however, be accompanied by equality of opportunity between social groups. It is perfectly possible for more working-class children to progress into the most coveted jobs whilst at the same time middle-class children remain relatively more successful if the overall number of 'higher' positions has increased. This is exactly the scenario that has occurred in Ireland over the last three decades. The occupational playing field remains substantially tilted in favour of children from more advantaged households even as the flow of children from working-class origins into middle-class positions has dramatically increased. However, there is evidence of a reduction in such inequality over time.

6

Consistent Poverty and Economic Vulnerability

Christopher T. Whelan, Brian Nolan and Bertrand Maître

Introduction

One of the common criticisms of the 'Celtic Tiger' is that it left the poor further behind: even if they did not become poorer in absolute terms, what they got were mere crumbs compared to the bounty gained by the well-off. Increased marginalisation and social exclusion amid growing affluence has been a recurring theme. One of the problems with this argument is that it has relied, to a substantial extent, on trends in relative income poverty where households are counted as poor if their incomes fall below a certain fixed proportion of mean or median household income, adjusted for family size and composition. However, accurate income data are hard to collect and even when accurate do not always give a good indication of households' command over resources.[1] Therefore, a picture of poverty based on relative income alone is inadequate. Furthermore, as Chapter 3 has shown, particular difficulties arise in circumstances of exceptional growth, such as have characterised the recent Irish situation, where it is possible for the poor to gain quite substantial increases in income but at the same time continue to be classed as poor in relative income terms.

In order to arrive at a clearer picture, we have to recall what 'poverty' means. The language used by the EU throws some light on this question. It speaks of poverty not simply as lack of money but as 'social exclusion', that is, as an inability to participate in the normal life of the society to which one belongs. The question therefore is whether we can identify a

1 See Nolan and Whelan, (2005), Whelan, Layte and Maître (2004)

T. Fahey et al. (eds.), Quality of Life in Ireland, 87–103.

sub-set of the population who can be considered as cut off from the living standards and lifestyles of the social mainstream.[2]

Our contention in this chapter is that it is possible to categorise the population in this way, though not necessarily in simple dualistic terms – the 'haves' and the 'have nots'. Rather, based on detailed analysis of data for a number of dimensions of living conditions, we propose an 80:10:10 classification. Four out of five of the population can be described as reasonably secure, well-off and insulated from a range of economic stresses and strain to which the remaining one-fifth of the population is vulnerable. This economically vulnerable group can be further divided into two almost equally sized groups. Just less than one in ten of the population simultaneously experience the combination of low income and extreme material deprivation that we refer to as 'consistent poverty'. A further one in ten, while avoiding such poverty, continue to experience a heightened risk of income poverty, material deprivation and economic stress that marks them off from the more secure four-fifths of the population. Furthermore, we would suggest that among the economically vulnerable there is a smaller sub-set that is multiply deprived in that they are exposed to high risks of deprivation across a wide range of dimensions, including health, housing and quality of neighbourhood.

Irish society can be characterised as having a tiered set of deprivation levels. The size of the consistently poor, economically vulnerable and the multiply deprived groups is significant and reflects the considerable level of inequality found in Irish society. However, the available evidence leads us to the conclusion that both the levels and depth of deprivation in Ireland are a good deal more modest than suggested by radical critics of the Celtic Tiger experience.[3]

Our argument will proceed as follows. Under 'Incorporating measures of lifestyle deprivation' we will focus on combining indicators of deprivation with income measures of poverty and demonstrate how trends in consistent poverty that incorporate such indicators differ from those relating to purely income poverty estimates.

Under 'Reconfiguring the measurement of consistent poverty' we show how the measurement of consistent poverty has been reconfigured in the light of changed economic circumstances and important changes in the

---

2 In answering this question the data available to us forces us to focus on residential households. We therefore miss out on groups such as the homeless and the Travelling community who are undoubtedly characterised by high levels of poverty and economic vulnerability. However, given the proportion of the total population constituted by such groups, our estimates of overall risk and incidence figures are unlikely to be seriously affected.

3 The detailed analysis on which these conclusions are based can be found in Whelan and Maître (2007a, 2007b).

data from which our estimates are derived. Under 'Economic vulnerability' we extend our concern beyond consistent poverty in order to focus on a broader conception of economic vulnerability that incorporates both multidimensional and dynamic concerns. Having identified three groups that we refer to as the 'non-vulnerable', 'the economically vulnerable but not consistently poor' and the 'consistently poor'. Under 'Income poverty, material deprivation and economic pressures profile by economic vulnerability and consistent poverty' we explore the consequences, in terms of income poverty, material deprivation and the experience of economic pressure of membership of such groups.

Incorporating measures of lifestyle deprivation

In everyday use, poverty in developed countries is often seen as an inability to attain a decent or adequate standard of living. Since what is seen as adequate is likely to change over time and differ across societies, this means that the definition is essentially relative. This relative approach to thinking about poverty has been officially adopted in Ireland in the definition set out by the National Anti-Poverty Strategy (NAPS) in 1997:

> People are living in poverty if their income and resources (material, cultural and social) are so inadequate as to preclude them from having a standard of living which is regarded as acceptable by Irish society generally. As a result of inadequate income and resources people may be excluded and marginalised from participating in activities which are considered the norm for other people in society.[4]

This definition implies that those measured as poor should be experiencing various forms of what their society would regard as serious deprivation. Income on its own does not provide a satisfactory basis for capturing such exclusion. When low income and deprivation approaches are employed to identify the most disadvantaged they are seen to identify distinctively different groups in terms of their socio-demographic profiles.

This has been shown to be true across a wide range of EU countries.[5] However, the Irish case is particularly complex because the very rapid growth in average incomes since 1994 poses particular problems in capturing what is generally regarded as exclusion. Measures that incorporate actual living standards or levels of lifestyle deprivation

---

4 National Anti-Poverty Strategy, 1997, p. 3

5 See Whelan et al. (2001, 2004) and Whelan and Maître (2005)

produce outcomes closer to the real income measure results, referred to in the previous chapter, than to those relating to relative income thresholds.[6]

The widespread adoption of the terminology of social exclusion/inclusion in Europe reflects *inter alia* the concern that focusing simply on income misses an important part of the picture. Our intention is to look beyond notions of relative income poverty in order to develop rather broader concepts of economic vulnerability and consistent poverty that seek to incorporate concern with the dynamic and multidimensional character of deprivation and social exclusion. A measure of poverty combining both low income and manifest deprivation was developed at the ESRI initially using results from a household survey carried out in 1987.[7] Those below relative income poverty lines and reporting what was termed 'basic deprivation' were identified as experiencing generalised deprivation due to lack of resources. This 'consistent' poverty measure was subsequently the basis for the global poverty reduction target adopted in the NAPS. Figure 6.1 shows the percentage of households in the sample that is deprived of one or more items on the basic deprivation index and falls below 70 per cent of median income. It reveals a very different trend to that found earlier (in Chapter 3), which focused on relative income poverty lines: 'consistent' poverty at the 70 per cent line fell from almost 15 per cent to under 5 per cent between 1994 and 2001.

Figure 6.1: *Percentage of persons below 70 per cent of median income and experiencing basic deprivation in 1994 and 2001, Living in Ireland Surveys*

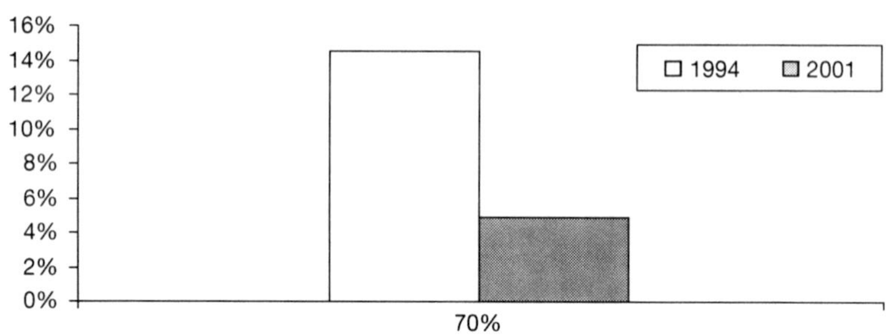

Reconfiguring the measurement of consistent poverty

Unfortunately it is not possible to extend this comparison to the later period because the manner in which the information relating to deprivation was collected in the European Union Statistics on Income and Living

6 Layte, Nolan and Whelan (2004), Whelan, Nolan and Maître (2006)

7 See Callan, Nolan and Whelan (1993) and Nolan and Whelan (1996)

Conditions (EU-SILC), which is the source of such information since 2003, differs sufficiently from the procedures employed in the earlier Living in Ireland Surveys to make the results non-comparable. However, we will proceed to make use of data from the first full wave of EU-SILC conducted in 2004 to provide as up-to-date as possible a picture of economic vulnerability and consistent poverty. The availability of this new data also allows us to reassess the measurement procedures relating to consistent poverty. The Irish approach has attracted a good deal of international attention.

A number of in-depth national poverty studies have applied the combined income poverty and deprivation approach and Austria has followed Ireland in the use of a 'consistent poverty' measure for official national reporting.[8]

In the Irish case the precise manner in which basic deprivation and consistent poverty are measured, in terms of the specific non-monetary indicators used for that purpose, was initially established using data for 1987 and then 1994, and has been re-examined in several studies since then using more up-to-date information. However, over the past decade Ireland has experienced unprecedented economic growth, accompanied by profound change in standards of living, points of reference and the broader societal context. Important issues arise as to how this has affected the extent and nature of poverty and whether the original 'consistent poverty' is still adequate for the purposes of answering such questions.[9]

Criticisms of the original basic deprivation index focused particularly on the narrow range of deprivation indicators incorporated. Some saw it as being appropriate to a more frugal era and implicitly accepting an absolutist view of poverty. After a period of unprecedented growth and with the recent availability of the EU-SILC it would appear ripe for re-evaluation. It was clear from the outset that, as living standards rose, the specific items employed in the consistent poverty measure would need to be revised at some point, in light of changing notions of what is minimally adequate. The intention was never to measure poverty in an 'absolute' manner but rather in a 'less relative way'. In focusing on a set of basic deprivation items it was not considered to be a problem that respondents reporting an enforced lack of such items were in possession of apparently non-essential items.[10]

---

8 Specific studies include Lollivier and Verger (1997) for France, Perez-Mayo (2004) for Spain, Gordon et al. (2000) for Britain and Förster (2005) for a range of European countries.

9 See Honohan and Walsh (2002) and Blanchard (2002)

10 See Mc Kay, 2004, for a discussion of the interpretation of respondents' reports of lacking items because they cannot afford them.

If we were to impose such a condition then households possessing DVDs, videos or stereos, or indeed spending money on cigarettes or alcohol, could never be deemed to be poor. In what follows we will refer to our key set of deprivation indicators, comprising the deprivation component of the new consistent poverty measure, as 'economic strain'. This label is chosen in preference to the earlier one of 'basic deprivation'. This is done for two distinct reasons. The first is that Eurostat has taken to referring to such measures by this label and it seems desirable, in developing measures based on EU–SILC, that we should endeavour to achieve as much consistency in terminological usage as is possible. The second is that given our earlier argument that we do not wish to use the possession of 'non-essential' items as a basis for excluding individuals from consistent poverty, we accept that the labels 'basic' and 'secondary' deprivation have the potential to be misleading.

Using the EU-SILC data, researchers at the ESRI have developed new indices of consistent poverty that incorporate income poverty thresholds and enforced absence due to inability to afford two or more items from an 11-item index of economic strain.[11] The 11 items included in the economic strain dimension in the EU-SILC index are set out in Table 6.1. These include six items from the set on which the NAPS consistent poverty targets were based – shown in the first part of the table – referring to deprivation in relation to food, clothing and heat. Two items included in the original basic deprivation set are now dropped. The item relating to 'being unable to afford a substantial meal because of a lack of money' is omitted because the statistical analysis shows that its relationship to the underlying dimension we are trying to tap is a good deal weaker than for the other items. We have also chosen to omit the item relating to 'going into debt to meet ordinary living expenses' because it is rather general and unspecific and open to different interpretations. As Mc Kay and Collard (2003) note, debt is a rather emotive term that can be used to describe two quite different situations. The first relates to consumer credit while the second refers to financial difficulties involving arrears in payments.

As can be seen from Table 6.1, the new measures involve a broader conception of deprivation than the earlier index. In particular, a number of the items focus specifically on adequate participation in family and social life. They include being able to afford to entertain family and friends, buy presents for family or friends once a year, and have an afternoon or evening out. Further, additions relate to keeping the house warm and buying new furniture.

[11] For more detailed discussion of these issues see Maître, Nolan and Whelan (2006) and Whelan, Nolan and Maître (2006).

Table 6.1: *EU-SILC basic deprivation items*

Items retained from original basic set
Two pairs of strong shoes
A warm waterproof coat
Buy new rather than second-hand clothes
Eat meals with meat, chicken, fish (or vegetarian equivalent) every second day
Have a roast joint (or its equivalent) once a week
Go without heating during the last 12 months through lack of money
Items now added to basic set
Keep the home adequately warm
Buy presents for family or friends at least once a year
Replace any worn-out furniture
Have family or friends for a drink or meal once a month
Have a morning, afternoon or evening out in the last fortnight, for entertainment
Items now dropped from original basic set
Going without a substantial meal due to lack of money
Going into debt to meet ordinary living expenses

In constructing a consistent poverty measure incorporating the items comprising the original basic deprivation index, the ESRI researchers argued that, given the extremes of deprivation captured by such items, the enforced absence of even one item together with income poverty was sufficient to fulfil the conditions for consistent poverty. In developing the economic strain index one of our objectives was to develop a measure of consistent poverty where the poverty rate was not dependent on any one item. Detailed analysis shows that a threshold of 2+ is appropriate for the new index.[12]

In the 2004 EU-SILC survey 9 per cent of the population were found to be consistently poor in that they were living in a household where net disposable income adjusted for family size was below 70 per cent of median income (the point below which half the population is found) and they reported an enforced absence of two or more items from our 11-item index.[13]

[12] See Maître, Nolan and Whelan (2006) and Whelan, Nolan and Maître (2006)

[13] At the 60 per cent line the figure is just less than 7 per cent.

Evidence for the importance of taking both income and lifestyle deprivation into account is provided in Figure 6.2 in the manner in which being above the economic strain threshold of 2+ items discriminates among those below the 70 per cent relative income poverty line in terms of the subjective economic pressures they experience. Six out of ten of those above the deprivation threshold report inability to meet unanticipated expenses compared to two out of ten of those below the threshold. For housing expenses the respective figures are eight out of ten and two out of ten. Just less than half of those above the threshold report difficulties in relation to arrears compared to one in twelve of their counterparts below the line. Finally, three-quarters of the former report difficulty in making ends meet compared to just over one in four of the latter. The consistently poor are very sharply differentiated from those who are below the 70 per cent income line but are not exposed to such deprivation, being between two to six times more likely to report economic pressure depending on the specific indicator on which one focuses.

Figure 6.2: *Economic pressure by income poverty (70 per cent median) and the EU-SILC 11-item measure*

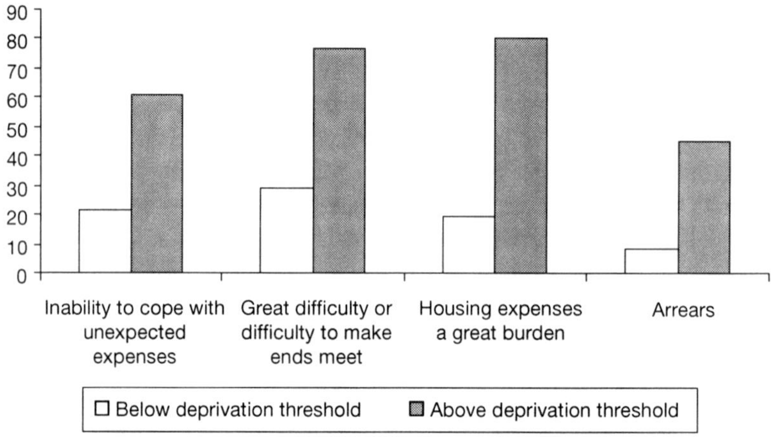

Economic vulnerability

The consistent poverty approach allows us to take an important step in the direction of the multidimensionality of poverty. However, in addition to directing our attention to such multidimensionality, the social exclusion perspective also places particular emphasis on the processes or mechanisms by which exclusion comes about. Notions of vulnerability are closely associated with the social exclusion perspective.[14] We can define vulnerability as not necessarily involving current deprivation either in income or other terms but rather insecurity and exposure to risk and shock.[15]

One goal in developing a measure of vulnerability is that it should serve as a point-in-time proxy for risk of exposure to persistent disadvantage. This dynamic objective is combined with a concern to go beyond measures based on single indicators. The IMF, the UN and the World Bank have developed a range of approaches to measuring vulnerability at the macro-level.

Consistent with the approach developed here, the World Bank sees vulnerability as reflecting both the risk that a household or individual will experience an episode of poverty over time and a heightened probability of being exposed to a range of risks.[16] However, most attempts to measure vulnerability have operated at the macro-level.[17] Such approaches must confront the usual issues relating to the aggregation of indicators. How do we combine measures relating to such factors as life expectancy, income poverty rates, unemployment levels and educational standards? As a consequence of such difficulties and in contrast to the UNDP's Human Development Index (HDI), the EU Laeken indicators were very deliberately presented individually with no attempt to produce an overall 'score' across dimensions – indeed Atkinson, Marlier and Nolan (2002) argue that this should be avoided precisely because the whole thrust of the European social agenda is to emphasise the multidimensionality of social disadvantage.

Our notion of economic vulnerability is applied by identifying a group of individuals who are sharply differentiated from the rest of the population, not only in terms of income poverty but also in terms of exposure to economic strain and the subjective experience of economic stress. In what follows we apply the concept of vulnerability to the EU-SILC 2004 data survey. Applying appropriate statistical techniques we succeed in identifying a group constituting 20 per cent of the population that we designate as economically vulnerable.[18] The crucial elements by which these groups are distinguished are: risk of being in income poverty, probability of experiencing an enforced lack of two or more of the 11 items making up our economic strain index and being more likely to report that

---

14 See De Haan (1998)

15 See Chambers (1989)

16 See World Bank (2000)

17 World Bank (2000), UN (2003)

18 For statistical details see Whelan et al., 2007a, 2007b

their household is experiencing difficulty or great difficulty in making ends meet. In Figure 6.3 we set the distinctive profiles of both the vulnerable and non-vulnerable groups. While 19 per cent of the latter are income poor at 70 per cent of median income this is true of 70 per cent of the former.

Figure 6.3: *Economic vulnerability profiles*

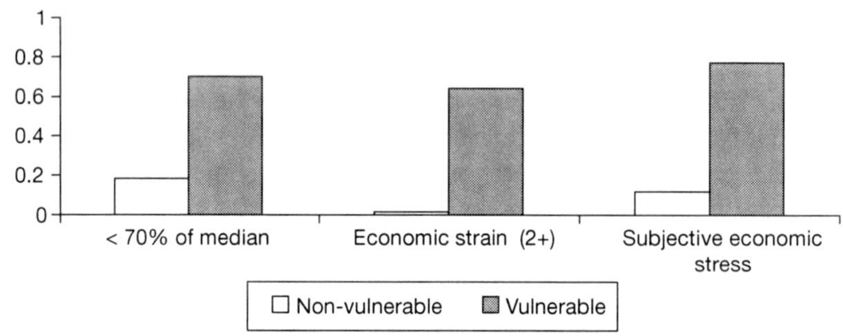

While this involves significant differentiation, it is relatively modest in comparison to that relating to the other dimensions incorporated in the measure of vulnerability. Seventy-eight per cent of the economically vulnerable report that their households have difficulty in making ends meet compared to 12 per cent of the non-vulnerable. However, even such polarisation is modest in comparison with that relating to the deprivation items that make up our measure of economic strain. While 65 per cent of the vulnerable group experience an enforced lack of two or more of such items, this is true of only 1 per cent of the remainder of the population. In summary, a clear pattern of multidimensional differentiation emerges as between the vulnerable and non-vulnerable. The most striking contrast relates to the basic deprivation items that make up our index of economic strain, followed by that involving the subjective experience of economic strain and, finally, the differential risk of income poverty.

While our statistical procedure for establishing economic vulnerability identifies a group very close in size to that of the income poor at 60 per cent of median income, the overlap between these groups is small. Only one in two of those below 60 per cent of median income are identified as economically vulnerable. This provides a striking contrast with the situation in relation to consistent poverty where all of those located in this group are also found in the economically vulnerable cluster. The consistently poor thus form a subset of the vulnerable group.

As we illustrate in Figure 6.4, we can thus identify three distinct groups. The first, which constitutes 80 per cent of the population, is largely buffered against income poverty, economic strain and subjective economic stress. Such groups may experience specific difficulties in relation to factors such as health or housing or neighbourhood environment but they are not subject to any form of generalised economic disadvantage. The second, who make up 10 per cent of the population, are distinctive in terms of economic vulnerability. Finally, 9 per cent of the population is identified as both vulnerable and consistently poor.

Figure 6.4: *Typology of economic vulnerability and consistent poverty*

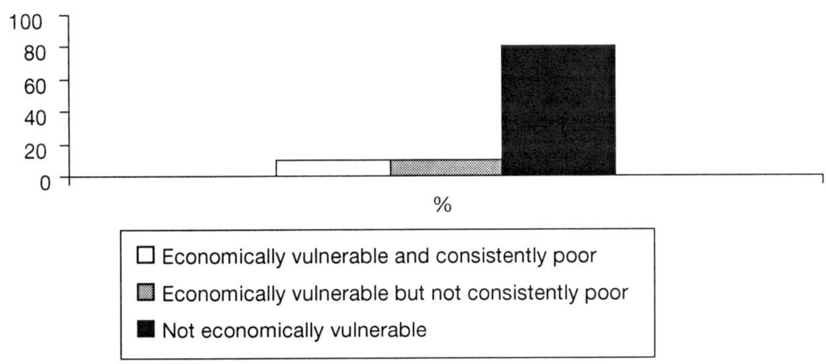

Income poverty, material deprivation and economic pressures profile by economic vulnerability and consistent poverty

In this section we wish to explore the consequences of being located in the three categories identified in the previous section. We start by illustrating in Figure 6.5 the extent to which such groups report deprivation in relation to key elements of the economic strain index. In particular we focus on the items relating to a warm waterproof overcoat, new rather than second-hand clothes, presents for friends and family once a year, and inviting family and friends for a meal or a drink once a month.

Not surprisingly the non-vulnerable are effectively insulated from risk of exposure to such deprivations, with the highest level observed being 1 per cent for the final item relating to entertaining family and friends. In contrast, between one out of five and two out of five of the consistently poor report deprivation in relation to the first three items and almost seven out of ten with regard to the final item. The economically vulnerable but not consistently poor group occupies a position almost halfway between the first two groups. The level of deprivation rises from 8 per cent for a warm coat, to 11 per cent for presents for the family, to 16 per cent for new clothes and, finally, to 37 per cent for having family for a meal or a drink.

Figure 6.5: *Deprivation by typology of economic vulnerability and consistent poverty (% lacking item)*

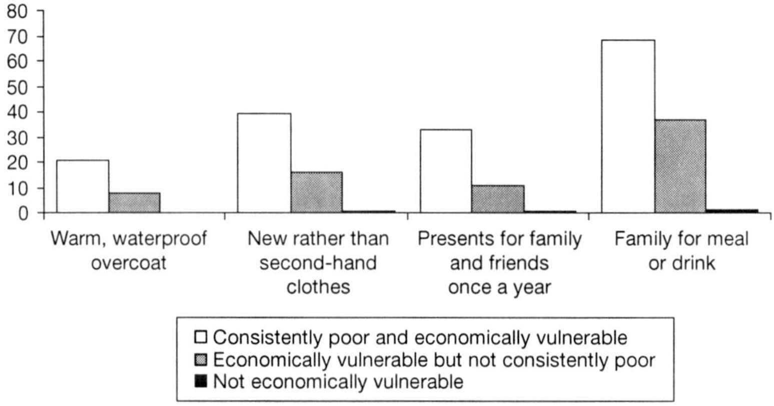

In Figure 6.6 we set out the comparable pattern in relation to the experience of a range of economic pressures. Specifically, we focus on inability to cope with unexpected expenses, debts in relation to routine expenses, arrears in relation to housing and utilities and experiencing housing costs as a great burden. The broad pattern of differentiation is rather similar to that observed in the case of economic strain. However, it is somewhat less sharp, particularly with regard to the contrast between the consistently poor and the economically vulnerable. Only in the case of experiencing housing costs as a heavy burden do the non-vulnerable report any significant level of economic pressure, with the relevant figure reaching 15 per cent. The figure for inability to cope with unexpected expenses falls to 10 per cent and that for the remaining two items to 4 per cent.

For the consistently poor, in contrast, eight out of ten report difficulty in coping with unexpected expenses. Three out of five indicate that housing costs are a burden. Just above two out of five report problems with arrears and one-third have incurred debts in relation to routine expenses. Experience of day-to-day economic pressures is pervasive among the consistently poor. Such experiences are also not unusual among those who are economically vulnerable but not consistently poor. In fact, felt pressure arising from housing costs is almost as high for the economically vulnerable as for the consistently poor. In addition, almost half report inability to cope with unexpected expenses, and one in four experience pressure in relation to debts and arrears.

In relation to the question with which we started regarding the extent of marginalisation in Irish society, the crucial question that remains to be

Figure 6.6: *Subjective economic pressures by economic vulnerability and consistent poverty typology*

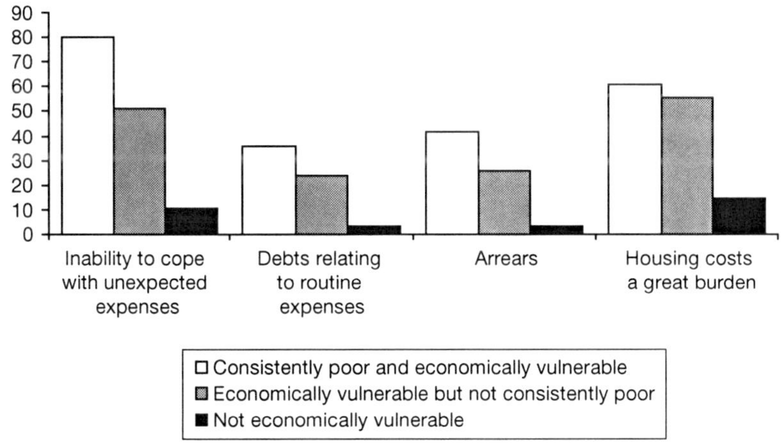

answered is how clear is the distinction between the consistently poor and those who are economically vulnerable but not consistently poor? Is there a case that the label 'consistent poverty' should be extended to cover both groups? As we have seen, the evidence in relation to the distribution of economic pressures is less decisive than in the case of the deprivation items making up the economic strain index.

In order to shed further light on this issue, in Figure 6.7 we focus on a set of consumer durables that are possessed by virtually all non-vulnerable households. These include a telephone, a video recorder, a CD player and a microwave. In developing an index of consistent poverty, we have never considered that possession of such items should automatically exclude households from being defined as poor. In fact, a substantial majority of the consistently poor possesses each of the items. However, the number deprived in relation to such items is significantly higher than for the remaining groups. Thirty per cent report such deprivation in relation to a phone, 25 per cent do so with regard to a CD player and 20 per cent to a video recorder. Finally, 15 per cent report enforced deprivation of a microwave.

In contrast, the non-vulnerable group reports close to zero deprivation on all four of these items. As in the case of economic strain, while the economically vulnerable but non-poor are very sharply differentiated from the non-vulnerable, their deprivation levels are less than half those observed for the consistently poor.

One final factor differentiating the consistently poor from the vulnerable is the risk of being below a range of income poverty lines. By definition, all of the consistently poor are found below 70 per cent of median income.

Figure 6.7: *Consumer durables by economic vulnerability and consistent poverty typology*

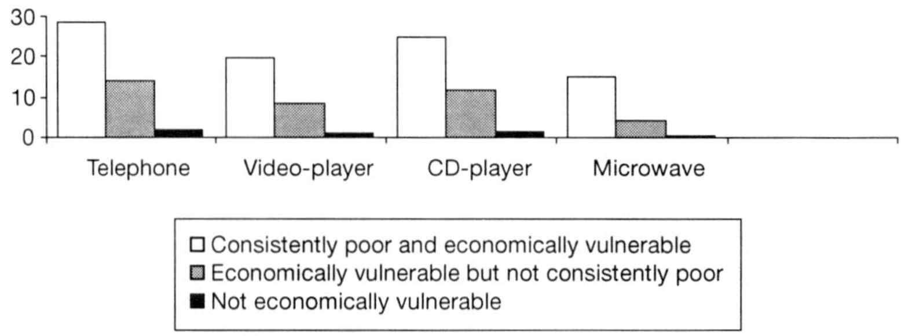

As set out in Figure 6.8, for the vulnerable but not poor this falls to just over one in two and for the non-vulnerable to less than one in five. Even at the 60 per cent line seven out of ten of the consistently poor are below the threshold compared to almost two out of five of the vulnerable and one in ten of the non-vulnerable. At the 50 per cent line over two out of five of the consistently poor remain below the income poverty line. This figure falls to one out of five for the vulnerable but not poor and to just above one in twenty for the non-vulnerable.

Figure 6.8: *Income poverty by economic vulnerability and consistent poverty typology*

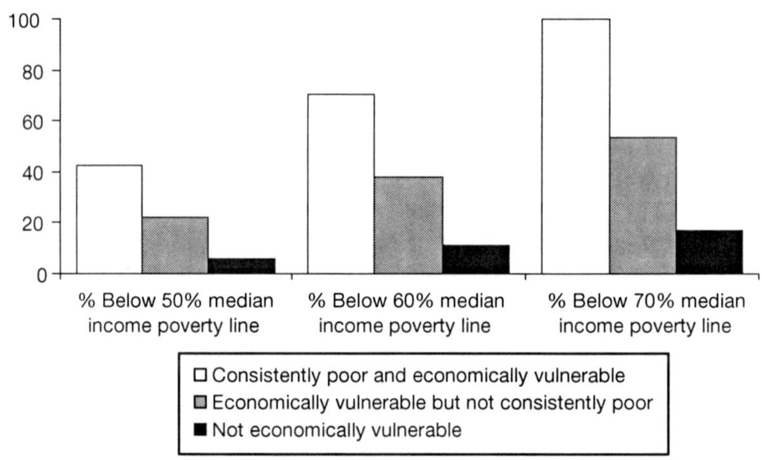

The pattern of differentiation in terms of income poverty, economic strain, widely available consumption items and subjective economic pressures suggests that the threefold distinction we have made is worth maintaining. Those economically vulnerable but not consistently poor suffer substantial disadvantages in comparison with that broad stratum of the population that make up the non-vulnerable group. However, the contrast between this group and those we currently designate 'consistently poor' is such as to make us reluctant to extend this label to the economically vulnerable category as a whole.

Before offering our final judgement on this issue, however, we proceed to look at the composition of the three segments of the population that we have identified in terms of some key socio-economic distinctions.

Socio-economic status by economic vulnerability and consistent poverty

From Figure 6.9 we can see that almost only one in four of the consistently poor are in households where the reference person is at work and just over one in three is either at work or retired. Thus, almost two-thirds are in households where the reference person is excluded from the labour market – being unemployed, ill or disabled, or involved in full-time home duties. By far the largest category is comprised of those involved in home duties who make up almost one-third of the consistently poor. The unemployed and the ill/disabled each account for one-sixth. The profile of the consistently poor contrasts sharply with those who are not economically vulnerable, where almost seven out of ten are in households where the household reference person is at work and eight out of ten are either at work or retired. The economically vulnerable, as we would expect, occupy an intermediate position. Almost one in two of the relevant reference persons are at work and almost six out of ten are at work or retired. They are almost as likely to be retired as the consistently poor but are only half

Figure 6.9: *Composition of economically vulnerable groups by labour force status*

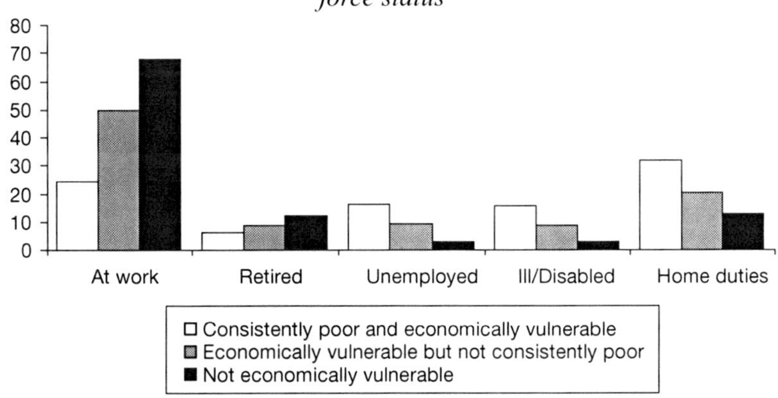

as likely to be ill/disabled and one-third less likely to be involved in home duties.

Turning to housing tenure, as set out in Figure 6.10, we find that over one in three of the consistently poor are local authority tenants and one in two are found either in such housing or in private tenancy. In contrast, little more than one in ten of the non-vulnerable are found in these categories. The economically vulnerable but not consistently poor are a slightly more heterogeneous group, with two-thirds being owners and one-third tenants. Overall, both the deprivation and stress profiles and the socio-demographic composition of the respective groups provide considerable justification for maintaining a clear distinction between the consistently poor and those vulnerable but not consistently poor.

Figure 6.10: *Composition of economically vulnerable groups by tenure*

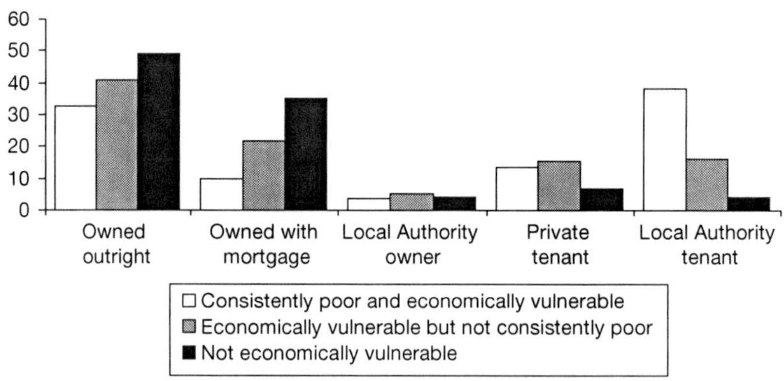

Conclusions

In this chapter we have sought to assess the consequence for poverty and economic vulnerability of the unprecedented growth experienced by the Irish economy over the past ten years. The answer to this question, as we have made clear, depends on the indicator on which one focuses. If relative income poverty is the benchmark then, as shown in Chapter 3, matters have worsened over time. However, such measures are least suited to precisely the sort of rapidly changing economic circumstances found in Ireland in recent times.

This should make us extremely reluctant to place undue emphasis on poverty measured in purely relative income terms. Where the focus is on income measures that capture improvement in real living standards, or indices that capture inadequate living standards directly, the observed trend is unambiguously towards an improvement over time.

The economic vulnerability measure distinguishes groups that display different profiles in terms of material deprivation rather than simply being above or below a particular income threshold. The population can be split on an approximately 80:20 basis as between non-vulnerable and vulnerable. The latter are sharply differentiated from the former in terms of income poverty but even more so in terms of subjective economic stress and, most particularly, with regard to the experience of enforced absence of the basic deprivation items making up the economic strain index.

The consistently poor, who are currently both below 70 per cent of median income and lacking two or more of the basic deprivation items that make up our economic strain index, constitute just less than one in ten of the population. Those individuals who are currently vulnerable but not consistently poor also make up one-tenth of the population. Both of these groups are sharply differentiated from the more than four-fifths of the population who are buffered against any form of generalised deprivation.

The weight of the evidence points conclusively towards maintaining the distinction between the consistently poor and the remainder of the vulnerable segment. The latter clearly operate under substantial economic pressures relating to housing expenses, experience of debt and inability to cope with unexpected expenses. They also experience standards of living significantly below the broad stratum of the society that make up the non-vulnerable group. We also anticipate that they are likely to be characterised by significantly higher risk of falling into consistent poverty. However, they experience substantially lower levels of deprivation than the consistently poor in relation to both items such as participation in family and community life and widely available consumer durables. Equally strikingly, only half of them are found below 70 per cent of median income.

Irish society after the Celtic Tiger is characterised by a set of tiered levels of deprivation. Both the scale and pattern of deprivation vary depending on whether one focuses on economic vulnerability, consistent poverty or the combination of low income and multiple deprivation.

We have no desire to minimise the degree of social stratification involved in such differentiation or to minimise the stresses and strain experienced by those exposed to these forms of deprivation and vulnerability. However, we are forced to conclude that both the levels and depth of such deprivation are a good deal more modest than suggested by radical critics of the Irish experience of globalisation.

7

Health and Health Care

Richard Layte, Anne Nolan and Brian Nolan

Introduction

Health plays a central role in people's perceptions of their quality of life, and access to good health care is a key ingredient in an overall sense of security and well-being. This chapter examines how health and health care have evolved over the course of Ireland's economic boom. Media coverage highlights the negatives: increasing suicide, road deaths, binge drinking and obesity, together with over-crowded accident and emergency departments and the perception that the health-care system is a 'black hole', absorbing ever-increasing resources for no return. Our aim is to assess the more complex reality, where some aspects of health and health care have been improving and others standing still or deteriorating, and to examine the role that public perceptions of those trends play in attitudes towards quality of life in Ireland. We look first at trends in health, and then how the health services and their use have evolved.

Are the Irish becoming healthier as well as wealthier?

The relationship between economic growth and health is complex. Research shows that average life expectancy increases with the average wealth of a country, but more income buys progressively less extra life expectancy, and average income in itself is probably not the crucial factor. As little as 10 per cent of the improvement in life expectancy across countries since 1970 may be directly attributable to increasing incomes, with other more structural changes accounting for the remaining 90 per cent (Wilkinson, 1996). The impressive economic growth of the last decade might be expected to have some impact on death rates and life expectancy in Ireland, but longer-term structural and economic changes may have as much or more of an influence. Furthermore, even if life expectancy increases people may not feel healthier: improvements in medical technology mean that once life-threatening illnesses such as heart

T. Fahey et al. (eds.), Quality of Life in Ireland, 105–122.

disease and diabetes can now be managed effectively, but the person living with a chronic condition may not regard themselves as healthy.

Some developments in Irish lifestyles accompanying economic growth over the last decade could also have a negative impact on health. For example, worries about alcohol consumption have been very prominent in the Irish media and the subject has attracted some public health research interest too. Research links the high levels of Irish alcohol consumption to a range of outcomes as varied as suicide, mental illness, visits to accident and emergency departments, unprotected sex and road traffic accidents. Moreover, reports also directly link increasing alcohol consumption to increasing income in a culture that encourages binge drinking. Alcohol consumption increased by over 40 per cent between 1989 and 1999, whereas in most other countries in the EU–15 consumption fell. Interestingly, the majority of this growth in consumption occurred after 1995, which strongly suggests that rapidly increasing real incomes in the economic boom played a role, although per capita consumption had been increasing for far longer.

Increased alcohol consumption and particularly binge drinking have also been implicated in the rapid increase in sexually transmitted infections (STIs) which has occurred since 1989. Between 1989 and 2003 reported STIs increased from 2,228 to 11,153 (NDSC, 2004), and research (Rundle et al., 2004; Layte et al., 2006) has shown that alcohol plays a significant role in unprotected sex, particularly among younger people for whom growth rates in STIs have been highest. Growth in STIs may also be related to the higher number of sexual partners experienced by younger Irish people compared to previous generations. There may be a link between this change and higher levels of alcohol use but the change may also be related to a general reorientation of sexual mores among Irish people.

There is also some evidence that the Irish population, like those in the UK and US, is increasingly likely to be overweight and obese. Results from the National Health and Lifestyle Surveys show that the proportion of the population classified as overweight increased by 2 per cent between 1998 and 2002, with the proportion obese increasing by 3 per cent over the same period. Excess weight and obesity in particular increase the risk of outcomes such as heart disease and type II diabetes.

Given such trends, it is not at all clear that the health of the Irish population would necessarily have improved over the boom period. What, then, does the evidence about health suggest? There are two basic types of health measures. First, there are 'objective' indicators of health such as death rates or the reported prevalence of particular diseases/conditions. Ireland has accurate statistics on frequency only for a limited number of diseases, so death rates/life expectancy are the primary 'objective' source of data on trends in health. The second type of health measure is self-reported, generally collected via social surveys asking individuals various questions about their health. Such 'subjective' assessments give a picture of how people perceive their own health, but have to be treated carefully, as they are likely to be influenced by factors other than underlying physical and mental condition. We now look at trends in death rates and life expectancy, and then at subjective evaluations of health.

Changing Irish death rates

Life expectancy from birth is significantly affected by infant mortality, so life expectancy at 65 is often a better indicator of the health of the adult population. Figures from the first census of the newly founded Irish State in 1926 show that average life expectancy at 65 for both men and women was among the highest in Europe. Yet, whereas life expectancy in other European countries rose through the remainder of the century, for Irish men it remained flat for most of the century, and for women it lagged behind the European average. In 1960 life expectancy for Irish men at 65 was 12.6 years compared to the European average of 12.7, whereas by 1990 the European average had increased to 14.6 while the Irish figure was 13.4. Irish women in 1960 had a life expectancy at 65 of 14.4 years compared to a European average of 15.1, while by 1990 the corresponding figures were 17.1 versus 18.4.

Though it is difficult to pin down exactly why life expectancy in Ireland failed to match that of other European countries during most of the twentieth century, the disparity in living standards is likely to have played a significant role. Lower living standards impact on life expectancy through many different paths, including poorer housing conditions and nutrition. High smoking rates also meant that Ireland had one of the highest death rates from diseases of the circulatory system in Europe. In 1980 Ireland's death rate from this cause was 40 per cent higher than the average of the old 15-country EU.

However, it is clear from Figure 7.1 that even in 1980 the trends for all causes and for circulatory diseases were on a downward path, and this continued up to the present with the death rate for circulatory diseases in 2002 50 per cent lower than in 1980. Moreover, the gap between Irish death rates from circulatory illness and the average for the 15-country EU closed significantly over the same period, with the Irish rate falling to 120 per cent of the EU average by 2002.

The downward trend in deaths from circulatory causes was clearly already in place before the economic boom, and the rate of decrease did not quicken in the 1990s compared to the 1980s, so longer-term changes in Irish society seem the primary cause. Just as the economic reforms of

Figure 7.1: *Death rates from diseases of the circulatory system 1980–2002*

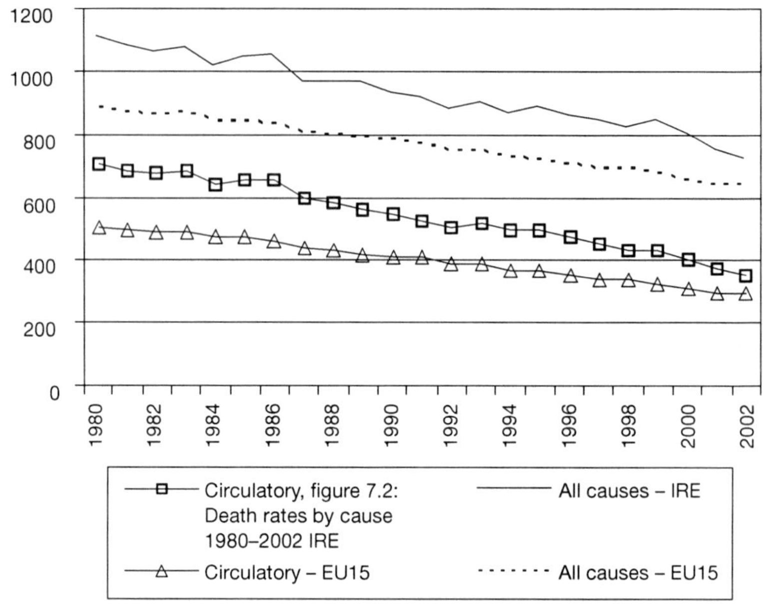

the 1960s and 1970s opened the economy up to foreign competition and investment, the same process may also have occurred for social and cultural influences as Ireland looked outward and absorbed influences from Britain, the US and the European Community.

Although economic living standards did not begin to converge with the European average until the 1990s, the convergence of lifestyles had begun much earlier, and this is likely to have included changes in a host of areas of Irish life that impacted on levels of premature mortality. For example, heart disease is strongly influenced by diet, smoking and level of exercise and these lifestyle factors changed significantly after the 1960s. Whereas the staple Irish diet had previously consisted of meat and potatoes in different guises with an emphasis on fried food, this changed substantially in the decades after 1970 as consumer choice and prosperity increased and the mass media highlighted the lifestyles of other cultures. The impact of growing health awareness should also not be underestimated. The dangers of smoking became public knowledge in the 1970s and smoking rates in Ireland dropped off precipitously between 1975 and 1980, particularly among higher-income groups, and continued to fall until the end of the century.

In the 1980s health awareness and health improvement became a major business and this message was delivered across an ever-expanding number of media outlets. Bennett et al. (2006) have estimated that almost 30 per cent of the fall in deaths from heart disease between 1985 and 2000 can be explained by healthier eating habits, and that better diet and exercise allied with decreases in smoking account for 62 per cent of the decrease, with improvements in medical and surgical therapies the other key contributor.

The high level of deaths from heart disease led to a concerted policy response in the 1990s, and by 2002 the Irish rate was only 12 per cent higher than the EU–15 average, compared to 26 per cent higher in 1986. Diseases of the circulatory system and cancers, the two biggest causes of premature death, also fell but much more slowly. Cancer deaths, for example, decreased from 215 to 194 per 100,000 between 1980 and 2002.

As Figure 7.2 shows, death rates were also falling across most other causes over the same period. The decrease in accidents shows that the improvements in living conditions were not confined to diet and lifestyle alone. Irish society was becoming a less harmful place generally as best practice from other nations was adopted and health given a greater prominence generally. The only exception to this downward trend is suicide, which Figure 7.2 shows rose from 7.7 per 100,000 in 1980 to a peak of 13.5 in 1998 before decreasing to 11.2 by 2002.

Figure 7.2: *Death rates by cause 1980–2002*

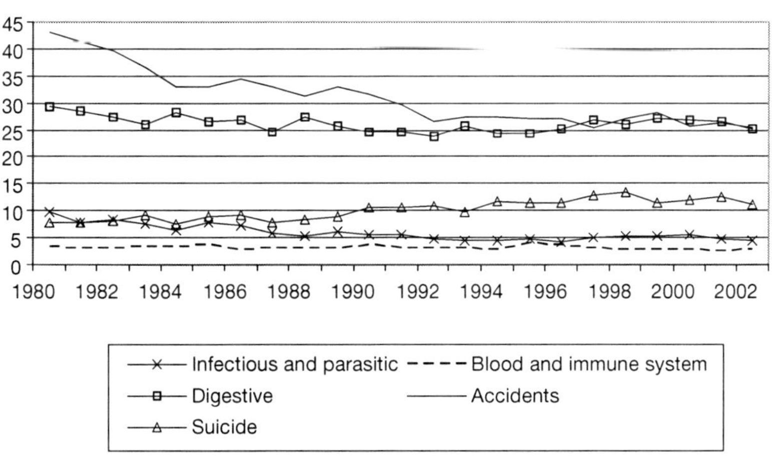

This masks different patterns for men and women, with women's suicides on a shallow downward path and men's on a much steeper upward path. The male suicide rate in Ireland has been increasing since at least 1970 and surpassed the EU average in 1995. However, since 1998 it has been falling back toward the EU average and may be another instance of Irish patterns converging with our EU neighbours, albeit in a less positive fashion.

Social class differentials in death rates

The overall pattern of death rates also masks differentials between groups in Irish society, social class groups in particular. In 1981, men from the unskilled manual social class between the ages of 30 and 65 had a death rate 2.7 times greater than men from the higher professional social class after we adjust for age. Measuring class for women is more problematic as a large proportion of women would not have been employed at death and so could not be assigned a social class grouping. Nonetheless, if we carry out the same exercise as among men we find that women in the unskilled manual social class had a death rate 2.6 times higher than women in the higher professional class in 1980.

This large differential in death rates across social class groups has been observed in many countries and Ireland's level of inequality does not appear unusual in an international context (Kunst et al., 1996), although direct comparisons are difficult. Between 1981 and 1991 the social class differential between unskilled manual and higher professional men fell to 1.9 and the corresponding differential among women fell to 2.0, suggesting that social class differences may be weakening.

Unfortunately changes in the occupational classification system in the 2002 census mean that we cannot see if this continued through the growth years of the 1990s.

Improving health?

Death rates and life expectancy are useful barometers of population health, but falling death rates do not mean that the prevalence of certain diseases is falling too. Indeed, the 44 per cent reduction in death rates from heart disease discussed in the previous section means that a higher proportion of those with heart disease will be alive but living with a serious chronic heart condition. Bennett et al. (2005) show a significant increase in the prescription of drugs for heart disease between 1990 and 2002, though this is more likely to reflect better detection and more uniform treatment than an increase in the prevalence of the condition.

Measuring the 'health' of a population is problematic. The World Health Organisation defines health as: 'a state of complete physical, mental and social well-being, not merely the absence of disease or infirmity'. 'Health' is not then just the absence of disease, although the absence of disease or injury should clearly be taken into account.[1] The definition also makes it clear that people's self-assessment of their health or broader well-being is also important.

Actually measuring such a complex concept is difficult. In social survey research there are three main types of population health measures: 'medical', 'functional' and 'subjective' measures. The first defines health in terms of deviation from some physiological 'norm' and asks about specific diseases or whether the person has a 'chronic illness'. 'Functional' measures define ill health in terms of inability to perform 'normal' tasks and roles. Lastly, subjective measures ask individuals to rate their overall health in a generalised fashion.

Results for all of these measures can be found in Irish social surveys, and here we focus on responses to the Living in Ireland Panel Survey which ran from 1994 to 2001. Looking first at 'chronic' illness (i.e. a long-standing illness or condition), these data show that the proportion of men and women reporting a chronic illness was stable between 1995 and 2001. However, patterns varied across age and sex groups. For example, men up to age 35 were around twice as likely to report a chronic illness in 2001 as they were in 1995, whereas men aged 65 or more are less likely to do so.

Among women, those aged under 25 or 65 or more were less likely to report a chronic illness by 2001, whereas those between 25 and 44 were more likely to do so. It is hard to give specific reasons why patterns vary across age groups, but as we will see shortly, other data have also suggested improvements in the health of older Irish people and this may be reflected in the proportions reporting a chronic illness. On the other hand, 'functional' measures of the extent to which those reporting a chronic illness are 'limited' (derived from questions asking 'are you hampered in your daily activities by this physical or mental health problem, illness or disability?') show small but significant decreases in limiting physical and mental illness between 1994 and 2001 for all population groups.

Lastly, we have broad self-assessed health measures such as the one in the Living in Ireland survey which asks 'in general, how good would you say your health is?' Although very simple, this question has been shown to perform well in research on health differences between social groups and to be a very good overall predictor of health status.

Responses to this question between 1994 and 2001 show a small worsening of self-assessed health overall, although patterns differ substantially between age and sex groups. Both older men and women report a better level of health by 2001, whereas young men are

---

[1] The opposite also applies, i.e. the absence of disease does not necessarily imply 'health'.

significantly more likely to have poorer self-assessed health in 2001 than they did in 1994.

How can we explain the differing trends in interview data from surveys compared to death rates? As already argued, a decrease in death rates does not necessarily translate into better health status for the population.

Better lifestyle or fewer accidents may result in less illness, but improved surgical and medical treatments could mean that more people are living with chronic health conditions. The age profile of the population also matters, of course, since older people are more likely to have a chronic condition than younger people, but the probability of ill-health at any given age may also be falling over time.

There is some evidence from studies of older people in Ireland, the UK and the US that levels of disability are falling, reflecting real increases in health status. The recent survey of Health and Social Services for Older People (McGee et al., 2005) showed that disability had fallen significantly between 2000 and 2004 among the Irish population aged 65 or more and this finding has been replicated in the UK and US. This is based on very specific questions about the person's physical abilities rather than a broader self-assessment.

How then do we explain the stability or worsening of broad self-assessed measures of health? The mental, social and emotional costs of increased economic growth could conceivably play a role.

Although average working hours have decreased over the last decade, there has been an increase in employment rates particularly among women and this may have placed increased time constraints on households. In the last decade increases in house prices and a lack of transport infrastructure also mean that many Irish people now commute long distances on a daily basis. Such factors could lead to a fall in perceptions of quality of life and of health.

If that was the case, however, one would also expect to see a sharp increase in perceived stress for individuals. Figure 7.3 divides the population into three groups for whom differences emerge and shows that mental stress, as measured in social surveys, fell sharply between 1987 and 1994 and also – though much less sharply – between 1994 and 2001.

Economic uncertainty and deprivation are among the main influences on this indicator of stress (Whelan, Hannan and Creighton, 1991) and these fell significantly across the period as levels of employment rose, unemployment fell and real incomes increased. If work intensification and longer hours away from home are generating higher levels of stress, this is not evident or is at least outweighed by the decrease in stress arising from high unemployment and poverty.

Figure 7.3: *Average psychological stress by age group and year*

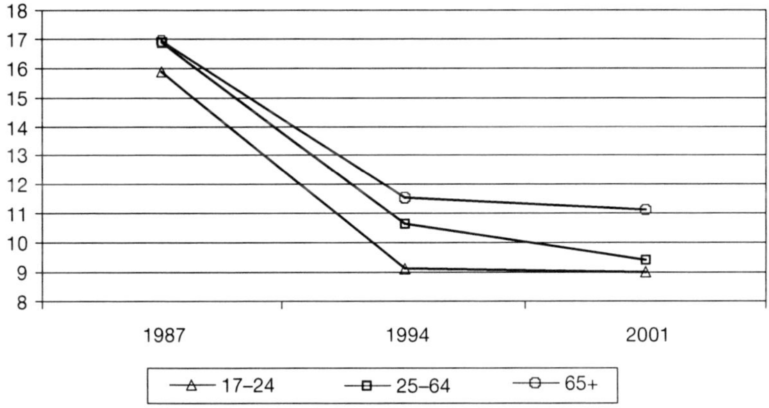

An alternative answer may lie in the attitudes Irish people now have towards their own health. Increased interest in health improves self-care and health-seeking behaviours, but it also makes the individual less likely to ignore conditions or problems that would have been dismissed or assumed to be part of 'growing older' in previous decades. This increased health consciousness may have been exacerbated in the last decade by the increasing 'consumerisation' of Irish society where increased wealth and choice mean that people are less tolerant of problems in their life that they believe they can rectify. Even as objective health status improves, people may become more sensitive to smaller health issues and adjust their overall sense of 'health' accordingly.

Changing health care in Ireland

Having looked at the health of the Irish population, we now turn to an examination of changes in health care in the last decade and a half. The economic growth witnessed in Ireland has meant that far more resources have been available for investment in health care and the sector has seen increased spending on a grand scale. But how has this expenditure been distributed across the health-care system and has it had any real impact on the quality and quantity of services provided?

Health expenditure since 1990

Public expenditure (capital and non-capital) on the health services has increased greatly since 1990, increasing by 200 per cent in real terms, with most of this increase occurring since 1997. This is in contrast to the experience during some years of the 1980s when public health expenditures fell in real terms. When the substantial involvement by the private sector in finance and delivery of health services in Ireland is included, total health expenditure (both public and private) amounted to over €10.3 billion in 2002, an increase of 180 per cent in real terms over 1990. The proportion of total health expenditure accounted for by the private sector declined from 25 per cent in 1990 to 18 per cent in 2002, reflecting the proportionately larger increase in public sector expenditure (see Figure 7.4).

Figure 7.4: *Public, private and total health expenditure 1990–2002 (Constant 2002 prices)*

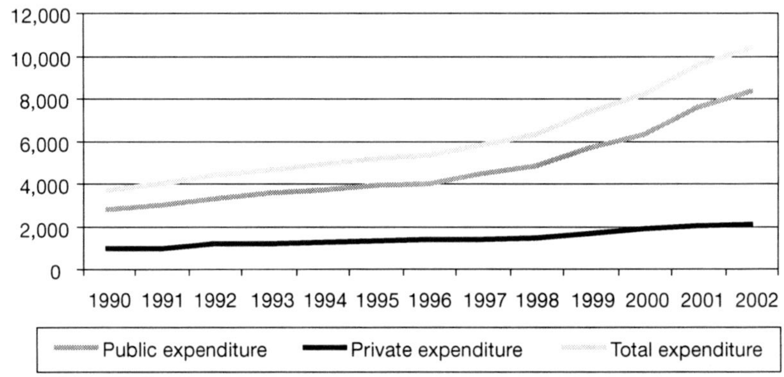

Comparative perspective

How does Ireland's spending compare with other developed countries? Comparing Ireland with the old EU–15 and some other industrialised countries, Irish health spending as a proportion of GNP was 6.9 per cent in 1990,[2] with only Spain, Portugal, the UK and Japan spending less on health as a proportion of GNP. By 2002 (see Figure 7.5), Ireland had moved up to fourteenth place, with 9.0 per cent of GNP devoted to health spending, just below the OECD–22 average of 9.3 per cent. In terms of health spending per head of population, health spending in Ireland grew by the largest percentage between 1990 and 2002 among the 22 countries examined (by 9.6 per cent on average each year). In 2002, Ireland was ranked twelfth out of 22 countries in terms of per capita health spending, compared with second lowest in 1990.

[2] While expressing health spending as a proportion of GDP is the conventional way of comparing expenditure across countries, the use of GDP as the reference point may be misleading in the Irish case, since repatriation of profits abroad by multinationals based in Ireland is both very high and variable from one year to the next. (See also Nolan and Nolan, 2004)

Figure 7.5: *Total health expenditure as a percentage of GNP, 2002*

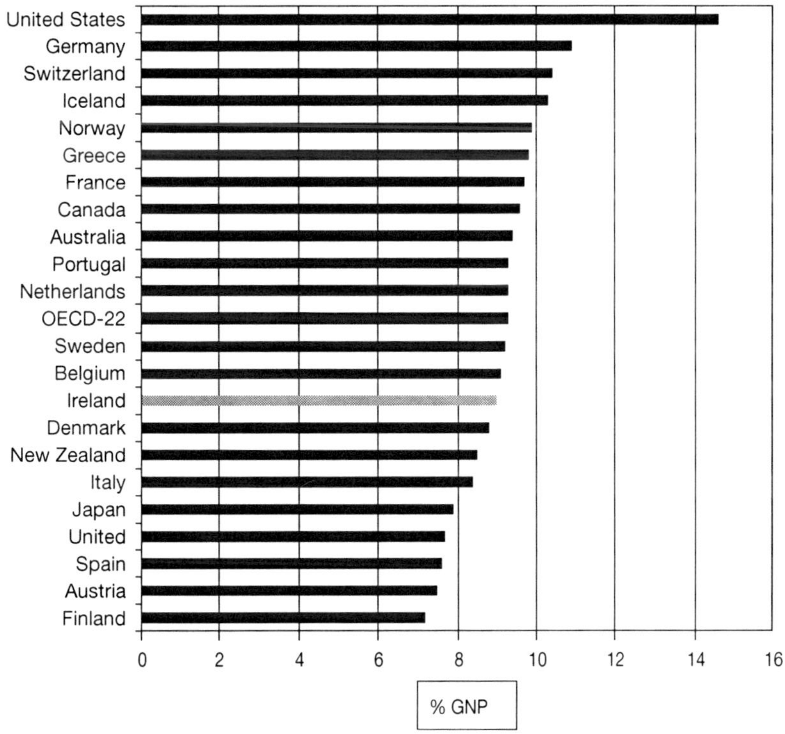

Components of non-capital public health expenditure

Towards what type of services has this increased health spending been devoted? The Department of Health and Children distinguishes a number of different programmes in its spending,[3] and the hospital and community health programmes accounted for nearly two-thirds of its non-capital expenditure in 2002 (see Department of Health and Children, 2002). Some spending by that Department is more properly regarded as social spending, in particular most of the 'community welfare' and 'handicapped programmes' which comprise about one-fifth of its current spending (see Wren, 2004; these are not included in the OECD figures on health spending in Figure 7.5). When these are excluded the hospitals programme accounts for more than 60 per cent of total current public health spending, while community health services make up about 20 per cent.

[3] The Department of Health classifies non-capital public health expenditure into seven different programmes: the community protection programme, the community health services programme, the community welfare programme, the psychiatric programme, the programme for the handicapped, the general hospital programme and the general support programme (see Department of Health and Children, various years).

Between 1990 and 2002 current expenditure on public hospitals rose by 168 per cent, with little change in the distribution of expenditure across different hospital types. In the community health programme the highest rates of expenditure growth were for the provision of pharmaceuticals under the Drugs Payment Long Term Illness Schemes. The community protection programme also recorded very high rates of growth over the period, whereas the psychiatric programme saw its share of total public non-capital expenditure fall substantially as patients were transferred from institutional to community care.

To what extent have increases in expenditure been accounted for by increases in pay and pensions costs rather than additional services? While the health component of the public sector pay and pensions bill increased from 31 per cent in 1990 to 40 per cent in 2002, the proportion of total non-capital public health expenditure accounted for by pay and pensions declined from 64 per cent in 1990 to 59 per cent in 2002.[4] However, recent controversy over the suspension of the PPARS (Personnel, Payroll and Related Systems) computer payment system and the cost of extension of medical card eligibility to all over-70s in 2001 fuel concerns over the extent to which expenditure increases are delivering value for money.

In terms of staff numbers and composition, the number of full-time equivalents employed in the public health service has increased by 60 per cent since 1990. The number of health and social care professionals grew most rapidly, by 193 per cent, followed by management and administrative staff, which increased by 113 per cent. Medical and dental staff numbers rose by 68 per cent. While accounting for the majority of public health employment, nursing staff grew by only 35 per cent over the period, so that their share of total employment fell from 42 per cent in 1990 to 35 per cent in 2002.[5]

However, the proportion of total public health employment accounted for by medical/dental, nursing and other health and social care staff remained stable over the period, accounting for 55 per cent of the total in both 1990 and 2002.[6]

---

4 Overtime costs are a significant component of health sector pay. An examination of the ratio of gross to basic pay for non-consultant hospital doctors in 2002 suggested that the ratios ranged from 185 per cent for senior registrars to 215 per cent for interns (Department of Health and Children, 2003).

5 This was largely due to cutbacks in nurse training places in the 1990s and the consequent difficulty in recruiting nursing staff (see Wren and Tussing, 2006)

6 The Brennan Report in 2003 could find no evidence to support the contention that the majority of new positions in the health sector had been taken up by administrators, rather than those involved in providing direct patient services (Department of Health and Children, 2003).

Service provision

While documenting changes in expenditure over time is relatively straightforward, tracking changes in service provision and assessing the extent to which changes in expenditure are associated with changes in service levels is much more difficult. Because they account for the majority of expenditure and also because of the availability of data, we focus here on acute hospital and GP services.

Acute hospital services

Over the period 1990–2002 the number of in-patient beds in public acute hospitals fell by 13.5 per cent, from 13,730 to under 12,000. As a consequence of declining average length of stay per patient treated, from 6.9 days in 1990 to 6.5 days in 2002, the number of in-patient discharges (including deaths) increased by almost 6 per cent over the period. The number of procedures carried out on a day-care basis – where the patient did not have to stay in overnight – more than doubled. While these accounted for 22 per cent of total in-patient discharges in 1990, they accounted for 37 per cent in 2002 (Department of Health and Children, 2002). The number of out-patient and A&E attendances at public hospitals also increased, by 20 per cent and 8 per cent, respectively.

How did patients feel about the care they received? Findings from the National Patient Perception of the Quality of Healthcare Surveys in 2000 and 2002 suggest that over 90 per cent of respondents were either satisfied or very satisfied with the overall quality of care that they received in public hospitals.[7] One area of concern was the tendency for surgery to be cancelled due to staff or bed shortages, and concerns regarding the provision of information and the level of discussion with staff were also frequently articulated, attributed primarily to lack of time on the part of staff. Patient satisfaction with the cleanliness of the hospital was high in both years.

This contrasts sharply with the findings of a 2005 audit of hygiene standards in 54 acute public hospitals in Ireland, which found that 48 per cent of hospitals scored poorly, 43 per cent fair and only 9 per cent were classified as good (Health Services Executive, 2005). Publicity about such findings, and about the risks associated with hospital stays due to the MRSA (methicillin-resistant Staphylococcus aureus) 'super-bug', might well have negatively affected patient attitudes of late.

The perceptions of the public at large, and whether and how these differ from those with recent experience of the health services, are also of

---

7 See Irish Society for Quality and Safety in Healthcare, 2001 and 2003

interest. A 1999 survey found that 43 per cent of a random sample of the population regarded the quality of care in the public health system as good or very good, 34 per cent regarded it as adequate and 23 per cent as bad or very bad. While certain aspects of the public hospital system, such as quality of the facilities, are viewed negatively by a majority of respondents, the quality of medical care was rated more highly, with 52 per cent of respondents regarding the quality of medical care in the public hospital system to be very good (Watson and Williams, 2001).

GP services

The 2001 Primary Care Strategy highlighted the need to further develop a team-based approach to the provision of primary care services. From 1997 to 2001, the number of GPs per practice remained constant at 1.7, suggesting that prior to the Strategy, little progress has been made in moving towards a team-based practice approach to the provision of GP and other primary care services. In addition, a 1996 survey of GPs found that 75 per cent of GP practices employed no other health professionals such as counsellors, public health specialists or physiotherapists (Indecon Economic Consultants, 2003). The Strategy also highlighted the need for a comprehensive out-of-hours service, in particular to reduce dependence on A&E services. However, over the period 1995 to 2000 the proportion of emergency admissions to hospital increased from 67 per cent to 71 per cent (Department of Health and Children, 2003).

Despite this, levels of satisfaction with GP services are high (see Department of Health and Children, 2001). The Primary Care Strategy has not been implemented to any significant degree as yet, with lack of funding cited as the main reason.

Issues of concern

While levels of health expenditure are now broadly comparable with other developed countries, and levels of activity in the acute hospital sector have increased greatly, issues of equity of access and of quality of service – particularly in A&E departments – continue to dominate public discussion.

GP services and medical card eligibility

There is ample empirical evidence in Ireland that the pattern of utilisation of GP services across the population does not simply reflect differences in 'need' (see Nolan, 1991; van Doorslaer et al., 2000; Nolan and Nolan, 2004; Layte and Nolan, 2004; Madden, Nolan and Nolan, 2005; and Nolan, 2005). In particular, the difference between those with and without medical card cover is significant; those with medical cards have free GP care and report on average 1.6 more GP visits per annum than those who have to pay, even when differences in other socio-economic characteristics and measured health status are taken into account (Nolan and Nolan, 2004). Unmeasured differences in need may contribute to this differential but seem unlikely to explain it fully. It is difficult to say whether medical cardholders 'overconsume' GP services or non-medical cardholders 'underconsume' them, or indeed both. Research elsewhere on the impact of charges on the utilisation of health services suggests, however, that charges reduce the use of both 'appropriate' as well as 'inappropriate' services (Keeler, 1992).

Eligibility for a medical card is primarily dependent upon income and is decided on the basis of a means test vis-à-vis income thresholds set nationally. Rapid economic and employment growth and lagging behind of the thresholds meant that the proportion entitled to a medical card fell sharply from the mid-1990s. In 2001, entitlement to a medical card was extended to all individuals aged 70 years and over regardless of income.

In December 2004, the Minister for Health and Children announced the introduction of a 'GP Visit' card, to cover the cost of GP visits but not the associated prescription costs. The income thresholds are 25 per cent higher than for the standard medical card, and it is expected than an additional 200,000 individuals will become eligible for the new cards.[8] Together with the substantial increase in the income thresholds for a medical card announced in October 2005, this reflected concerns about the significant financial burden that the cost of GP visits (and the accompanying prescriptions) places on individuals just above the income threshold. However, it is not clear that proximity to the income threshold is the critical factor. Comparing all those without medical card cover and controlling for other influences on GP visiting, such as age and health status, little difference in visits was found across the income distribution except towards the top (Nolan and Nolan, 2005).[9] This suggests that the costs of GP visits and prescriptions are a significant factor for those on middle incomes, not just those marginally above the income threshold.

Acute hospital services and private health insurance

The rapid rise in the proportion of the population with private health insurance has exacerbated the 'two-tier' nature of the Irish hospital system.

---

8 By December 2005, between 2,716 (Primary Care Reimbursement Service estimate) and 4,685 (HSE estimate) GP Visit cards had been issued (*The Irish Times*, 10 January 2006).

9 The extent to which those on high incomes are able to bypass the GP and go directly to a private medical specialist may partly explain this pattern.

Almost half the Irish population now pay for private health insurance, primarily to cover the costs of private hospital care, much of which is actually provided in public hospitals.[10]

Attitudinal surveys provide some insight into why individuals perceive the need to take out private health insurance, in the context of universal entitlement to free or heavily subsidised public hospital care. In a 2000 survey the most commonly cited reasons were to avoid large medical bills, to ensure quick treatment and to ensure good hospital treatment (Watson and Williams, 2001). Issues such as being able to have a private bed or a private room were perceived as much less important. These responses highlight the perception that patients with private insurance have shorter waiting times and are guaranteed consultant care, in comparison with those who must rely on the public system. A 2001 CSO survey found that public patients did face substantially longer waiting times than those with private health insurance. The National Treatment Purchase Fund (NTPF), which was established in 2002, has attempted to deal with waiting lists for public patients. Public patients who are waiting a year or longer for treatment (or children waiting for six months or longer) are encouraged to register with the NTPF, which then purchases private care on their behalf. While waiting lists for many elective procedures have now been reduced, significant equity and efficiency concerns in relation to public patients remain.

Statistics on patient discharges from public hospitals reinforce this picture. In public hospitals, 20 per cent of in-patient beds are 'designated' as being for private patients, but those patients account for a larger proportion of elective and emergency in-patient discharges (see Nolan and Wiley, 2001, Wiley, 2005). Access to hospital for elective procedures in particular may not be distributed according to need, but rather influenced by private insurance cover and ability to pay. Extending the activities of the NTPF and ensuring that public beds are not used by private patients would not deal with the underlying structural problems aggravated by the complex interrelationship between the public and private sectors in the provision of acute hospital services.

Even if private hospital care were provided solely in private hospitals, the existence of tax relief for private health insurance and tax breaks for the construction of private facilities gives rise to concerns over the fairness of the State subsidising private health care for the better-off. When much of private care is actually provided in public hospitals, the two-tier nature of access is all the more striking.

---

[10] In 1990, 34 per cent of the Irish population had private health insurance, increasing to 40 per cent in 1998 and 50 per cent in 2003 (Health Insurance Authority, 2003, and Department of Health and Children, 1999).

Accident and emergency services

In 2001, 71 per cent of all in-patients in acute public hospitals were admitted through A&E departments (Department of Health and Children, 2003). It is therefore one of the most visible components of the health service and, consequently, the media attention devoted to the quality of care received in A&E is extensive. The relationship between GP and A&E services is particularly important in this regard. Individuals without a medical card who present at A&E without a recommendation from their GP currently pay €60; this charge has been gradually increased in recent years, in part due to concerns that those without medical cards were using A&E rather than the more costly GP services. While the charge is currently slightly above the average fee for a GP consultation, the poor provision of out-of-hours services may still encourage individuals to go to A&E rather than their GP. In addition, all patients who are referred to hospital by their GP must enter hospital via A&E. A number of bodies[11] have highlighted the strain this places on A&E departments, in that such patients are effectively examined twice, and have recommended that Acute Medical Units (AMUs) be established in all departments to cater for such admissions.

Findings from the National Patient Perception of the Quality of Healthcare Surveys in 2000 and 2002 for patients admitted to hospital through A&E suggest some deterioration over that period. In 2000, 79 per cent of respondents who were admitted to hospital through A&E reported being seen by a doctor within one hour of arrival, but by 2002 this had fallen to 64 per cent. In 2000, 66 per cent were told they would be admitted within one hour of arriving, and after this 79 per cent of respondents were waiting 6 hours or less for a bed. The respective figures for 2002 were 47 per cent and 87 per cent. Overall, 91 per cent of those admitted to hospital through A&E in 2000 were either fairly satisfied or very satisfied with the care and service received in the A&E department, and this was 86 per cent in 2002. Of the ten per cent who were dissatisfied with their experience in A&E in 2000, the most commonly cited reasons were delays in admission, followed by poor facilities and hygiene, low staffing levels and the lack of attention to the pain experienced at the time. While media reports and the attention received by A&E services more recently would suggest further deterioration after 2002, the evidence does not allow that to be evaluated.

---

[11] Irish Medical Organisation (2004) and Comhairle na nOspidéal (2004)

Summary

In this chapter we have seen that there has been considerable improvement in the health of the Irish population, measured in terms of indicators such as death rates and life expectancy, but that this trend began well before the onset of the economic boom. There have been particularly pronounced reductions in the number of deaths attributable to circulatory diseases such as heart disease. However, people's subjective assessments of their health showed only small improvements or even worsened. Rather than arising from increased work intensity and work life stress, this seems most likely to reflect changes in attitudes to, and expectations about, one's health.

The economic boom has enabled Ireland to devote substantially more resources to the health sector, and Ireland now spends about the OECD average on health. Activity in the acute hospital sector has risen substantially but that system is clearly under severe strain, while primary care services have not been expanded as rapidly as intended, despite clear recognition of its potential to reduce pressure on acute hospitals and on A&E services in particular. Equity of access remains a key concern, both in terms of the affordability of GP services and the two-tier access to hospitals associated with the unique Irish mix of public and private health care.

8

The Housing Boom

Tony Fahey and David Duffy

Introduction

The boom in the Irish housing market began in 1994 and has yet to run its course. Having been born with the Celtic Tiger, it is often taken as emblematic of the social and economic transformation that has happened since the mid-1990s. Surging house prices and expanding residential construction are not unique to Ireland over the past decade but have spread through much of the developed world, including many economies that have a weaker demographic and economic performance than Ireland. Thus the housing boom in this country is but a local variant of a wider international phenomenon. The Irish variant has indeed been bigger than elsewhere but the fundamentals that are driving it, such as the growing population, the rapidly expanding economy and the competitive mortgage market, have also been stronger, so that the Irish experience is in many respects no more difficult to account for than that of other countries.

In any event, the statistics of house prices and housing construction in Ireland since 1994 have been remarkable. In some senses they are positive, not least in the sheer scale of housing output that has been achieved and the substantial rate of new household formation that has been facilitated. But housing trends also cause unease, as they sometimes seem to be careening out of control and to threaten the long-term balance and health of the economy. They are also interpreted by some as epitomising problems of inequality in Irish society. On the one hand, house price rises have made existing home owners rich, at least on paper, but on the other hand, the criticism is made that many poorer people and younger households have difficulty accessing any housing at all – a problem that some have called a crisis of the housing system (see, for example, Drudy and Punch, 2005).

The long-term *economic* impact of these developments cannot yet be judged, since it is only from a vantage point of the future that we will know whether the boom phased out in a gradual and manageable way or ended in an abrupt crash. Our concern here is with the more immediate *social*

T. Fahey et al. (eds.), Quality of Life in Ireland, 123–138.

impact, in regard to such things as the affordability and quality of housing, its implications for household and family formation, and its significance for social inequality. While these too are in constant transition, some social features associated with the housing boom can be outlined and assessed, and that is what this chapter aims to do.

Prices and output

Long-term price data suggest that house prices in Ireland had been falling slightly in real terms during the 1980s, and, in 1990, despite nominal increases, were back to the level of 20 years earlier in inflation-adjusted terms. Lift-off commenced in 1994 and by 2005, nominal new house prices had increased over 3.7 times (2.7 times in real terms), and nominal second-hand house prices were 4.6 times higher (3.3 times in real terms). A monthly house price index covering the recent period suggests that although house price growth had slowed in the middle of 2005 it picked up again and in 2006 amounted to 12 per cent for the year (Permanent tsb/ESRI, 2006). This was well down from the increase of 31 per cent which was recorded in 1998, the peak year of the price boom. But it was well ahead of general consumer price inflation, which by the end of 2005 was around 2.5 per cent. There are some regional differences in house prices: at the third quarter of 2005, average Dublin house prices were 27 per cent higher than the national average. However, these regional differences are not exceptionally large by UK or wider European standards, and there is no part of the country which was unaffected by the general increase in house prices.

Figure 8.1: *Trends in nominal house prices in Ireland, 1970–2005*

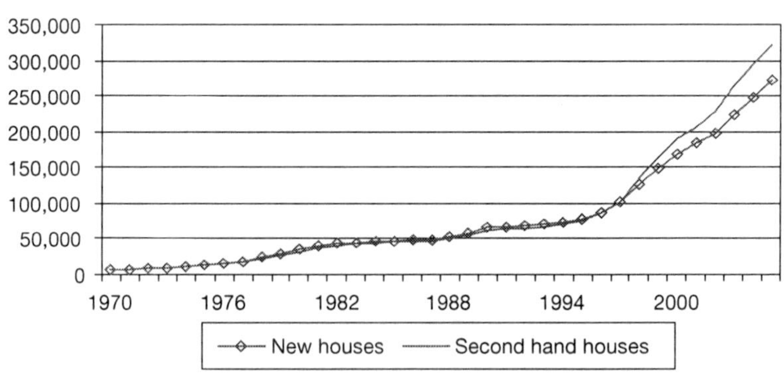

Source: Dept of the Environment and Local Government, *Annual Bulletin of Housing Statistics*

As the price rises just described would suggest, the increase in housing output has fallen short of demand. Yet the growth in the supply of housing has been spectacular. New dwelling construction amounted to little over 20,000 units per year in the early 1990s, having been in decline over the previous decade (Figure 8.2). Output rose to over 81,000 units in 2005, equivalent to over 5 per cent of the housing stock, and rose further to over 88,000 units in 2006. This is an extraordinary output performance for any country outside of wartime reconstruction conditions. It is around four times the output per head of population of most European countries today and amounted to 12 per cent of national economic output in 2005.

Figure 8.2: *New dwelling completions by sector, 1997–2005*

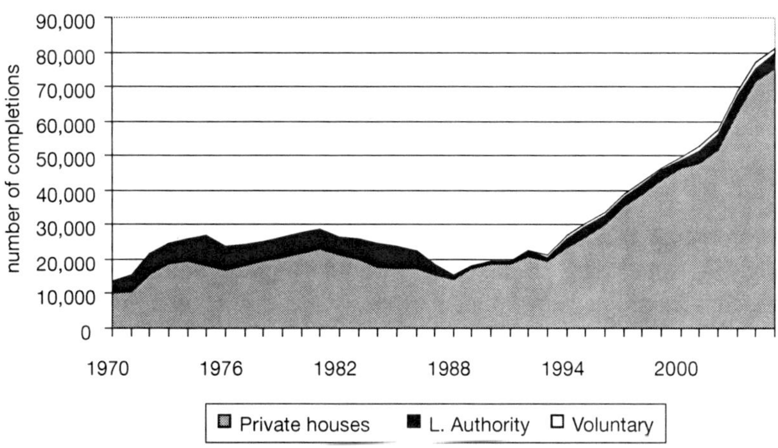

Sources: Dept. of the Environment and Local Government, *Annual Bulletin of Housing Statistics*

A feature of the housing supply is its dominance by private sector construction, a feature that had developed in advance of the Celtic Tiger period (Figure 8.2). Historically, social housing construction played a major role in Irish housing supply. In the 1970s, between one-quarter and one-third of new house construction was in the local authority (social) sector. However, social housing construction was sharply reduced during the public expenditure cuts of 1987–88 and since then has remained well below 10 per cent of total output. The total stock of social housing is also low, currently standing at about 8 per cent of the total. Thus, the housing boom has been overwhelmingly due to private sector supply and demand.

Higher wealth – a result of the economic boom – has increased the demand for second dwellings or holiday homes. A significant component of house building in recent years has been the growth in the number of dwellings that are vacant for most of the year for any number of reasons.

Using unpublished CSO census data, Fitz Gerald (2005) estimates that there were 170,000 second or vacant inhabitable dwellings (11.7 per cent of the housing stock) in 2002. Of these, some 39,000 were holiday homes, located mainly along the Atlantic seaboard from Kerry to Donegal. A further 27,000 were accounted for by temporary absence of householders. This leaves 104,000 that were vacant for other reasons, mainly, it would seem, because they were being held by investors for capital gain purposes. However, this is in the context of a very rapid rise in the number of households. The number of *second* or vacant dwellings reached over 170,000 by 2002. Furthermore, second dwellings have accounted for a significant proportion of dwellings built in recent years, contributing over one-sixth. Irish residents have also looked abroad for holiday homes or investment opportunities. It is estimated by the CSO that Irish residents spent approximately €1 billion on foreign residential property in 2005, although this is a rough estimate.

No data are available to determine the share of housing output taken up by investors. The private rental sector is small in Ireland: it had declined to 8 per cent of occupied housing stock in the early 1990s, but since then has recovered to 11 per cent. Commentary in the property press suggests that investors may take up a much larger share of new housing supply than the relatively small size of the stock would suggest, but also that many investors remain in the residential property sector only for a limited period. In addition, as already mentioned, investors may be buying dwellings for capital gain and leaving them vacant. This is because of the unattractive

Figure 8.3: *Rent index for the private rented residential sector, 1976–2005*

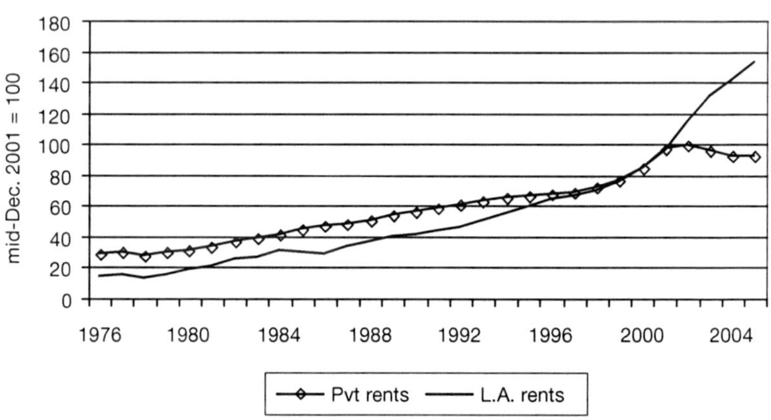

Source: CSO (special tabulation from the Consumer Price Index).

return from rents. Between 1990 and 2002, average private rents more or less doubled, thus tracking the trend in house prices. However, rents then fell quite sharply for two years and while some upward movement has reappeared since 2004, rents are no higher now than the peak reached in 2002. Relative to the current capital value of housing, rental yields in the Dublin area are said to be poor – in the region of 4 per cent gross, which, net of depreciation and management costs, amounts more or less to zero net return. Strong capital gains have more than compensated to date, but these cannot continue indefinitely. There have been many warnings that a speculative bubble has formed in the Irish housing market (see, for example, *The Economist*, 29 May 2003, OECD Ireland Economic Survey 2006) but many economists consider that a smooth transition to a slower growth path in the Irish housing market is possible (see, for example, McQuinn, 2004; Bank of Ireland, 2004; Roche, 2003).

Why the boom?

House price increases in Ireland have been greater than in any other country since the present global housing boom got underway in the 1990s, but a case can also be made that the underlying social and economic drivers of rising prices are stronger in this country than elsewhere. Thus, despite its runaway appearance, the housing market in Ireland may be less precarious than in some other countries. Three main sets of drivers of the Irish housing market can be identified (Duffy, 2002; McQuinn, 2004; Roche, 2001, 2003).

The first is demographic. Population grew at 1.3 per cent per year in the second half of the 1990s, the highest population growth rate in Europe at the time. Between 2002 and 2006, the population growth rate jumped to 2 per cent per year, the highest on record for Ireland (at that rate of growth population would double in 36 years). The impact of this growth on the housing market is greater than the already strong headline figures would suggest because the greatest rise in numbers is occurring among the young adult population and because household size in Ireland is still relatively large (see further below). Both of these factors give rise to a strong underlying pressure for new household formation and thus for increased housing demand, a pattern that is either absent or weaker in other European countries. Migration is also an important influence, not only because it is now a significant source of population growth but also because of its age patterns. The bulk of out-migration, 50 per cent in 2005, is from the 15–24-year-old age group. This age group is younger than the main household formation age groups, so emigrants are either leaving the parental home or rented accommodation. The bulk of in-migration, 53.6 per cent, is in the 25–44-year-old age group, the key age group for independent household formation. Estimates in the *Medium-Term Review* (Fitz Gerald et al., 2005) and Fitz Gerald (2005) show that having made no contribution to housing demand per annum between 1991 and 1996, migration contributed an annual average of 6,000 units between 1996 and 2002, although in reality this may well be higher. In time the rise in house prices may have negative impacts on migration (Duffy, Fitz Gerald and Kearney, 2005). Traditionally Ireland has had an infinitely elastic labour supply curve due to an extremely open labour market. However, the boom in house prices in Ireland could reduce the attractiveness of Ireland for potential immigrants. This would, in turn, reduce potential labour supply in the medium-term and act as a brake on medium-term growth in output and employment. Thus, housing emerges as an important infrastructural constraint in the labour market.

The second factor driving the housing market is rapidly rising real disposable incomes, which in turn is a consequence of three tributary influences – rising real wages, a rapid increase in the numbers at work, and large reductions in income taxes. The second of these influences is particularly important, as the numbers at work increased by almost 55 per cent between 1993 and 2004 (see Chapter 4). Much of this increase was due to the entry of married women into paid work. This made the dual-earner household the standard household type among younger couples, thus boosting the purchasing power of households in the early stages of family formation. In addition, the marginal income tax rate was reduced from 60 per cent in 1986 to 42 per cent in 2001, where it still remains. As a consequence of these influences, average household expenditure increased sharply during the 1990s. Among homeowners with a mortgage, the increase in real spending power between 1987 and 2000 was over 50 per cent (Fahey, Nolan and Maître, 2004).

The third factor driving the rise in house prices was a fall in mortgage interest rates and here there were two tributary influences – Ireland's entry into the EMU, which gave Ireland full access to European capital markets at low European interest rates, and the flexible, competitive nature of the Irish mortgage market, which made Irish retail mortgage interest rates lower than the European average. Figure 8.4 shows that real mortgage interest rates in Ireland have often been extremely low or even negative. Since 1960, it was only for a period in the late 1980s and early 1990s that rates rose above 5 per cent in real terms. In the past, however, low real interest rates were often accompanied by a shortage of funds for lending, since the supply of capital depended mainly on domestic savings, and mortgages were therefore difficult to obtain. Following Ireland's entry into the EMU, nominal as well as real interest rates fell to very low levels and, because Irish financial institutions now had full access to international capital markets, there was no scarcity of funds for lending. Mortgage lending soared as a result.

Figure 8.4: *Mortgage interest rates and inflation in Ireland, 1965–2005*

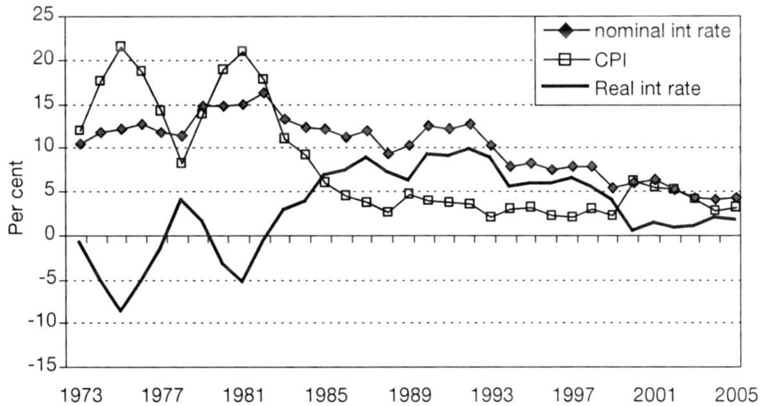

Source: Based on data from Central Statistics Office

Apart from entry into the EMU, deregulation of credit markets in Ireland has helped to push interest rates downwards. Data on retail interest rates in Europe from the European Central Bank show that Ireland is among the cheaper countries in Europe in which to borrow money for house purchase. Furthermore, non-interest charges on long-term loans in Ireland were also low. One of the concerns often voiced about mortgage borrowing in Ireland is the extensive reliance on variable rate or short-term fixed rate mortgages. In 2005, 84 per cent of new business was at variable rates (including fixed up to one year) and two-thirds of fixed-rate mortgages were fixed for terms of one to three years. This exposes households to the risk of interest rate increases, but it also enables potential house purchasers to benefit more or less immediately and completely from interest rate declines. Thus, between January and December 2003, the variable interest rate for house purchase (new business) fell from 4.08 per cent to 3.47 per cent, thus helping to account for the continued upward pressure on house prices in this period. Having remained unchanged for over two years, interest rates went through six separate increases between December 2005 and December 2006, with further rate rises expected. Irish homebuyers are therefore deeply committed to a form of borrowing that is cheap but also risky for the future.

In sum, the main proximate causes of the housing boom in Ireland were that there were very many more young adults, they had much more money to spend, and they could borrow large amounts at very low interest rates.

Effects on affordability and household formation

Public commentary on house prices in Ireland since the earliest days of the housing boom has been dominated by concerns about the affordability of house purchase for new homeowners, with concerns sometimes also being expressed about affordability for private renters (Downey, 1998; Duffy, 2004; Fahey, 2004; Downey, 2005). Some of this commentary has suggested that soaring house prices and rents made housing so inaccessible to young adults that they were hampered from forming families or moving out to independent households (Downey, 2005).

However, trends in household and family formation since the early 1990s throw doubt on such commentary since the number of households and family units grew at an unprecedented rate during this period, considerably faster than the rate of population growth. Between 1991 and 2002, the population of young adults (those aged 20–34 years) rose by 24 per cent but the number of households with a reference person in the same age bracket rose by 33 per cent (see Fahey, 2004, p. 92, for details). Population growth for the entire population in this period was 11 per cent, while total household growth was 25 per cent. There was a particularly large increase (158 per cent) in the number of households with a young *unmarried* adult as the reference person. In 2002, young single adults were less likely to live with their parents than they were in 1996 (among single 25–29 year olds, for example, 43 per cent lived with their parents in 2002 compared to 53 per cent in 1996). Growth in the formation of new families, as marked by the birth of a first child, was also very large in this period, particularly after 1995 (see Chapter 10). On the other hand, as Fitz Gerald (2005) points out, the rate of new household formation could have been even higher still had price barriers not risen so much – household size is still quite high in Ireland and has been slow to move down to average European levels. Thus, on the positive side, the housing boom could reasonably be credited with facilitating unprecedented growth in the number of households since the early 1990s and thus with helping to underpin the recent buoyancy in Ireland's demographic performance. On the less positive side, household formation has been somewhat lower than the boom in prosperity would lead one to expect, even though in absolute terms it has been impressive.

Housing affordability is a concern not only because of the effect it has on the formation of new households but also because of the impact it has on the share of household income absorbed by housing costs. There are indicators which give a factual justification to concerns on this front, though these should not always be taken at face value.

The most commonly cited such indicator is the ratio of house prices to earnings, with earnings in the Irish case usually measured by means of data on average industrial earnings. This indicator steadily worsened in Ireland during the housing boom: in the mid-1990s average house prices were three to four times average industrial earnings, but by 2003 they were eight to ten times average industrial earnings (Downey, 2005; Duffy, 2004). On that basis, it would seem self-evident that affordability should have become a problem for the *average* new entrant to the market and not just for those on low incomes.

However, the ratio of house prices to average incomes is misleading as it takes no account of the impact of falling interest rates, the doubling up of incomes in dual-earner households, or the higher incomes of young, better educated households compared to older households. Nor does it reveal anything about affordability in tenures other than homeownership. A more informative picture can be obtained by looking at actual expenditures on housing by households, taking account of both mortgage and rent payments.

Figure 8.5 provides such a picture by showing the trend in actual household outgoings on rent or mortgage payments as a percentage of total

Figure 8.5: *Weekly/rent mortgage payments as percentage of total housing expenditure, 1973–2000*

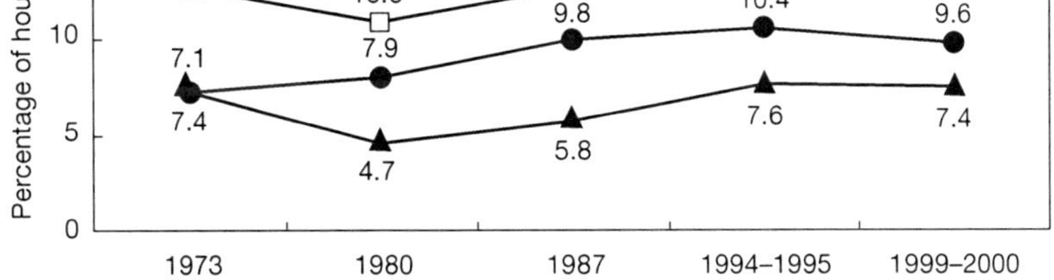

Sources: Household Budget Surveys 1973, 1980, 1987, 1994–1995, 1999–2000

household expenditure for each of the main housing tenure categories since the early 1970s. Here the only serious worsening of affordability to have occurred over this period is confined to tenants in the private rented sector. The share of private tenants' total household expenditure going on rent fell between 1973 and 1980 and rose back to the levels of 1973 by 1987. It then increased rapidly, rising from 12.5 per cent of household expenditure in 1987 to 18.9 per cent in 1994–1995 and then to 21 per cent by 1999–2000. Among owners with a mortgage, by contrast, the share of household expenditure absorbed by mortgage payments was both remarkably stable and remarkably low over the entire period. That share rose slightly from the 1970s to the end of the 1980s and peaked at 10.4 per cent in 1994–1995. Thereafter, it *fell* slightly, to 9.6 per cent by 1999–2000. For social renters the share of household expenditure accounted for by rent remained consistently low throughout the period.

The trends just looked at relate to averages within each tenure. Another way of assessing affordability pressures is to specify a threshold for the share of income going on rent and mortgage repayments, and see who is above that threshold. Here we focus on 35 per cent of household expenditure as a relevant threshold (this is the threshold used to define affordability in section 93 (1) of the Planning and Development Act, 2000). Figure 8.6 shows the proportion of owners with a mortgage and private renters whose rent or mortgage repayments were at or above 35 per

Figure 8.6: *Percentage of owners with mortgage and private renters with more than 35 per cent of household expenditure going on mortgage/rent by family cycle stage*

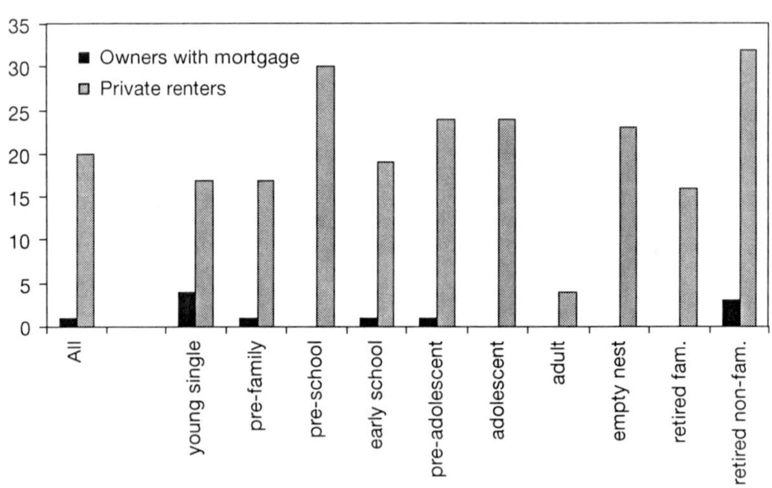

Source: Household Budget Survey 1999–2000 micro data

cent of household expenditure in 1999–2000. As might be expected from the previous section, private renters are far more likely than home purchasers to exceed the affordability threshold defined here. In 1999–2000, 20 per cent of private renters had housing expenditure above the affordability threshold, compared to 1 per cent of house purchasers. In absolute terms, this equates to approximately 20,000–25,000 private rented households above the threshold, compared to approximately 4,000–5,000 households of owners with a mortgage who were above the threshold.

Other sources tell a similar story about the relative extent of affordability problems in the private rented and home ownership sectors, although data are not available for the very recent period. Table 8.1, for example, shows a number of relevant indicators from the Irish National Survey of Housing Quality, 2001–2002 (Watson and Williams, 2003). According to these data, mortgage payments among recent first-time buyers are higher in absolute terms than rent payments among private renters, but the proportion of first-time buyers who spend more than one-third of net household income on those payments is relatively small (11 per cent) and is much lower than among private renters (28 per cent). These householders' subjective perceptions of their situation reflect the objective realities: 20 per cent of private tenants consider their housing costs to be a heavy burden compared to 11 per cent of first-time buyers and 13 per cent of all mortgage holders (for similar results from data for 2003, see Fahey, 2004, p. 84). A striking feature in these data is the high incidence of perceived affordability problems among local authority tenants.

Table 8.1: *Housing affordability indicators, Irish National Survey of Housing Quality, 2001–2002*

	Local authority tenant	Private tenant	Owners with a mortgage	Recent first-time buyers[1]
Median monthly rent/mortgage payment €	107	609	140[2] 457[3]	635
% spending more than one-third of net income on housing costs	1	28	6	11
% who perceive housing costs a heavy burden	33	20	13	11

1 Have purchased a mortgage in previous five years and are aged under 35
2 Local authority mortgage
3 Private sector mortgage
Source: Watson and Williams (2003), Tables 3.1, 3.2, 3.3, 3.4.

As we saw earlier, rents paid by local authority tenants are low, yet one in three local authority tenants perceive those rents to be a heavy burden. This reflects the high levels of income poverty among local authority tenants and the degree to which even modest rent payments can impose a strain on household finances (see, for example, the study of Dublin City Council tenants by Murray and Norris, 2002, which showed that the poverty rate among those tenants was three times higher than the national average and that two-thirds of their rent accounts were in arrears).

Other surveys have also asked respondents about their perception of the burden of mortgage debt. For example, in the Living in Ireland Surveys and EU-SILC respondents were asked how difficult they found the burden of their mortgage repayments. Overall, according to EU-SILC data for 2004, the majority of householders with a mortgage find their repayments to be somewhat of a burden, but only 17 per cent find it a heavy burden.

In considering affordability, one also has to recall how financial pressures on home buyers can ease once the earliest stages of house purchase have passed. For those who bought a house in, say, 1998 (the peak year for house price rises) or in 2002, the price and the mortgage payments at the time may have seemed large but since then will have rapidly come to seem smaller, relative both to present-day house prices and present-day disposable incomes. This positive effect of the passage of time may not always be present, especially if either interest rates rise or disposable incomes fall, but for the time being, apart from recent small upward movements in interest rates, neither of these negative trends has emerged.

To sum up the picture of affordability, two key features emerge. The first is that the affordability of mortgage payments has remained more or less stable in Ireland over the long-term and there was no particular increase in difficulties in this regard during most of the housing boom (we lack up-to-date data to complete the picture for the very recent past). Rising incomes and falling interest rates counterbalanced the rise in house prices and fuelled the demand which pushed prices up. Eventually, of course, if prices continue to rise, affordability pressures could seriously worsen, and that may have already begun to happen in the past year or two. Affordability pressures are also likely to be compounded by rising interest rates. Prior to the most recent developments, however, often expressed concerns about the worsening affordability of house purchase seem to have been overly influenced by headline house purchase prices and insufficiently attentive to the role of counterbalancing influences on affordability. The second feature is that in so far as affordability problems have emerged, they have been most severe for tenants in private rented accommodation. Relative to the capital values of properties, private rents may not be high, but they are high relative to tenants' incomes. Again, more recent developments may have changed this picture somewhat, since there has been some downward movement in private rents (see above). Yet, setting aside for the moment the situation of specific categories that we will return to later, it is unlikely that recent developments have led to any fundamental alteration in the affordability profile of housing for the majority of the population in Ireland.

Location of housing

It is sometimes said that one of the ways in which new young households cope with the price of housing is to move to remote suburbs where housing is cheaper but where quality of life is compromised because of distance from work, family and friends. Again, however, any systematic evidence we have on this issue suggests that forced locational choices of this kind are relatively uncommon. A large national survey in 2003 asked first-time buyers about their perception of the suitability of their dwellings on three counts – closeness to family and friends, closeness to work, and closeness to schools, shops and childcare – thus testing the view that high house prices have forced them to buy their homes far from their preferred locations. The responses indicate that on all three counts, the vast majority of first-time buyers perceived their dwellings as either 'very suitable' or 'suitable' (Figure 8.7). The highest incidence of perceived unsuitability arose in connection with closeness to work, but even in that case only 10 per cent of first-time buyers considered their dwellings as 'unsuitable' or 'very unsuitable'.

Housing inequalities

We have suggested so far that the housing boom in Ireland has not had some of the general *negative* social impacts often attributed to it, particularly in regard to accessibility and affordability. Even the majority of first-time house buyers – those often seen as the main losers from the boom – have fared better than is often suggested. Their circumstances would have been better still had house prices and rents remained lower, but this is not to say that their circumstances have worsened. However, matters are different when we consider some of the marginal social groups who have always run the risk of experiencing difficulties in their housing circumstances. Has the housing boom of the Celtic Tiger era made matters worse or better for them?

No clear yes or no answer is possible to this question, since developments in this area have been mixed and some of these

Figure 8.7: *Suitability of dwellings among recent[1] first-time buyers in terms of closeness to family and friends, work, and schools/shops/childcare, 2003*

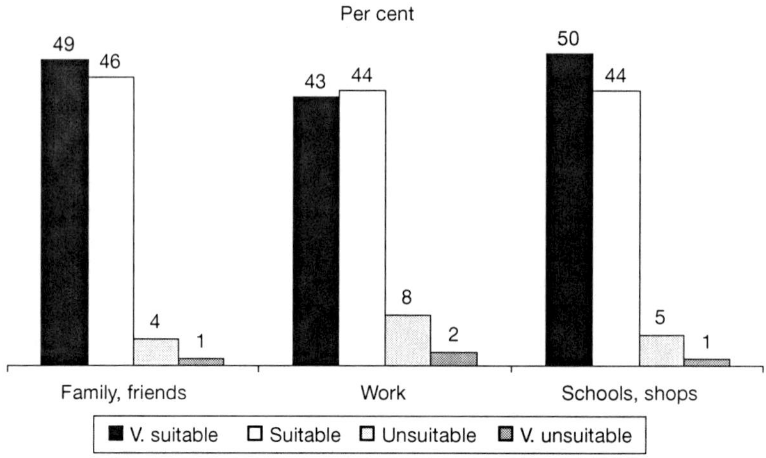

[1] Bought since 1996
Source: CSO (2003), Table 13

developments have had less to do with the Celtic Tiger than with the longer evolution of housing policy in Ireland.

The main long-term factor that has had a negative effect on the less well-off is the much reduced role of social housing in the Irish housing system, a development that had its origins before the advent of the Celtic Tiger. Prior to the 1980s, social housing output normally amounted to 20–30 per cent of new house construction. However, as part of the public expenditure cut-backs of the depressed late 1980s, social housing output was reduced to below 10 per cent of the total and fell to 6 per cent in 2000. Since then it rose marginally, reaching 10 per cent of the total in 2002, but it still left the social housing sector with a modest role in the overall system. This meant that the traditional source of housing for low-income households declined in size as the Celtic Tiger took off. This, rather than rising house prices in the home purchase sector, gave rise to a major reduction in the accessibility of housing for low-income groups and is a clear instance of supply being less adequate now than it was in the past.

The long-term reduction in social housing was in part compensated for by a massive expansion in the scheme of rent allowances provided under the Supplementary Welfare Scheme. This is a more restricted form of housing support than that provided by housing benefit in the UK as it is not available to those who are in employment. Nevertheless, it became a major form of support for low-income tenants in the private rented sector during the 1990s. This development arose as an *ad hoc* reaction to increasing demand within the social welfare system rather than as a planned aspect of housing policy. Yet, it remains for the time being a major *de facto* element of overall housing provision, particularly in the context of present high rent levels in the private rented sector. It is now estimated that at least one-third of households in the private rented sector are in receipt of supplementary rent allowances.

Although supplementary rent allowances have helped fill the gap left by the reduction in the relative size of the social housing sector, one early indication that overall supply of low-income housing was inadequate was the rise in homelessness. During the latter part of the 1990s, according to data produced by the Homeless Agency, homelessness increased. Between 2002 and 2005, however, it appears to have declined by something of the order of one-fifth, though various changes in administrative classifications and counting methods make it difficult to be precise on this question (Homeless Agency, 2005, pp. 77–8). In 2005, 1,361 households were counted as homeless.

Although recent housing trends have tended to accentuate social inequalities, they have had the opposite effect in other respects. This is particularly so when one looks at wealth distribution rather than income distribution. According to data from the Living in Ireland survey in 2000, households in the bottom 20 per cent of the income distribution received only 7.3 per cent of total national household income in that year but they owned 15.2 per cent of net housing wealth (that is, net of mortgage debt). Households in the top 20 per cent of the income distribution, on the other hand, received 40.7 per cent of household income but owned 25 per cent of net housing wealth (Fahey, Nolan and Maître, 2004, p. 70). Thus, the distribution of housing wealth across income categories, while unequal, is considerably less unequal than the distribution of income. Much of this pattern is due to the way housing wealth is distributed by age: the elderly own a lot of housing even though their incomes are low, while younger adults own less housing but have higher incomes. In 2000, for example, households headed by those aged 65–74 had 11 per cent of income compared to 15 per cent of housing wealth, while those aged 75 and over had 7 per cent of income and 11 per cent of housing wealth. Households headed by those aged under 35 years, by contrast, had 25 per cent of income but only 14 per cent of housing wealth. Housing wealth thus offsets to some degree the inequalities in current income because it is most concentrated among older people, who have low incomes, and less concentrated on younger adults, who have higher incomes.

Conclusion

In housing as in other areas, the Celtic Tiger has made many people wealthy – and not just developers, landowners and builders who have profited from the housing boom but also the thousands of ordinary households who have seen the value of their homes rise to extraordinary levels.

This new wealth may dwindle in the future if house prices fall and in the meantime it may be of little practical benefit to most people since they have no way of extracting financial benefit from the newly increased housing worth. But it has also had some real effects, particularly in the way that housing assets have enabled households to access the cheap and abundant credit now available from the financial sector. The housing system has also performed well in the sheer volume of new dwellings it has produced and the very large increase in the number of households that this has facilitated (this is apart from its economic effects as a driver of growth in economic output and employment). It may appear that those who have tried to access housing for the first time since the boom in house prices have been the losers in this process. However, the strains and blockages to housing access faced by the majority of these households can be exaggerated, at least until the recent past. Young adults in the early years of this century were more likely to form independent households than ever before, despite the cost of housing. Surveys of first-time house buyers over the past decade have consistently found that they report less difficulty with problems of affordability or other aspects of their housing than many commentators have suggested, and they do not seem to be any worse off on these fronts than previous generations of home buyers. Perhaps they are not finding things as easy on the housing front as the general economic abundance would lead one to expect, but this is a different matter from saying that they are facing unprecedented hardship, as much of present-day commentary on this question would imply. There are real problems among households who are not in the usual home ownership segments of the population, particularly those who traditionally depended on social housing or the private rented sector. It is in these areas that real inadequacies are most in evidence in the housing system. However, even among the less well-off there are those who have gained from the housing boom. This is particularly true for older people who now, as in the past, typically have low incomes but who have experienced a great increase in wealth arising from the growing value of the very large amounts of housing they own outright.

9

Changing Times, Changing Schools? Quality of Life for Students

Emer Smyth, Selina McCoy, Merike Darmody, Allison Dunne

Introduction

Public opinion of the Irish educational system is broadly positive. The vast majority of the adult population report high levels of confidence in the educational system and the public are generally satisfied with the performance of schools and teachers (Fahey Hayes and Sinnott, 2005; Kellaghan et al., 2004). In fact, the strength of the educational system has been identified as a key factor in recent economic growth (Fitz Gerald, 2000). Public discussion has focused more on academic outcomes, especially examination grades, than on young people's broader development. Perhaps paradoxically, given the level of public confidence in the system, the pursuit of academic grades would appear to be a driving force behind the increasing number of young people attending 'grind' schools and other fee-paying schools. The proportion of students going on to higher education has increasingly been used in newspaper reports as an indicator of a school's 'success'. But what impact do schools have on the actual quality of life of young people in contemporary Ireland? This question is all the more important given the significant transformation in the lives of Irish young people brought about by broader social and economic changes over the past 15 years.

Economic growth since the 1990s has led to rising living standards within families and has meant a reshaping of the boundaries between work and school for young people. Teenagers have been given more autonomy within the family and increasing freedom in their social lives. Over four-fifths of young people are now staying on in school until Leaving Certificate level. To what extent has the school system responded to these changes? The 1970s and 1980s had seen the transformation of second-level education from one serving an elite group of students to a system of mass education.

T. Fahey et al. (eds.), Quality of Life in Ireland, 139–154.

In the past decade noteworthy changes have taken place in the second-level system with the development of alternative educational programmes, but change has probably been more rapid in the third-level sector with the dramatic increase in the number of young people going on to higher education (see O'Connell, Clancy and McCoy, 2006).

Indeed, many aspects of the schooling system, in particular the organisation of the school day and the hierarchical nature of social relations within schools, have remained largely unchanged for decades. This chapter examines the extent to which school influences the quality of life among students in the context of broader social and economic change within Irish society. The focus is on second-level students, roughly 12 to 18 years of age, because this period is crucial in young people's personal, social and educational development.

School may be just one part of the day-to-day experiences of young people in Irish society. However, it is an important one in terms of both young people's current quality of life and their future life-chances. During term-time, young people in second-level education spend a minimum of 28, and sometimes up to 35, hours per week at school with additional investment of time outside school hours in school-based extracurricular activities, homework/study and paid tuition ('grinds'). Students in exam year classes spend an average of three to four hours per night on homework and study outside school time, with those in other year groups spending somewhat less time (Hannan et al., 1996; Smyth, McCoy and Darmody, 2004). This time investment has implications for participation in leisure activities, with a considerable proportion of young people, especially those at Leaving Certificate level, citing lack of time as a constraint on such activities (de Róiste and Dinneen, 2005).

The school context is, therefore, central to young people's well-being and quality of life. In Ireland, as elsewhere, school organisation and process have been found to have a significant impact on personal–social development as well as on academic progress among young people (Hannan et al., 1996; Smyth, 1999; Shiel et al., 2001).

The nature of the interaction between students and their teachers and among students themselves plays an important role in shaping their self-image. Students who have experienced positive interaction with their teachers in the form of praise and positive feedback tend to have a more positive view of themselves, in terms of their abilities and even their body-image. In contrast, students who are frequently 'given out to' by teachers have more negative self-images and higher stress levels and underperform academically. Similarly, bullying by other students tends to lead to stress, anxiety and poor self-image (Smyth, 1999; Smyth, McCoy and Darmody, 2004). On the whole, young people in Ireland tend to be broadly positive about their school experiences, though this varies over the course of their schooling career, with students becoming less positive about school and their teachers as they become older.[1] Attitudes to school also vary markedly across different groups of students in terms of social class background, academic 'ability' and gender, with greater school disaffection evident among working-class students, those with lower ability levels and male students. Even for those students who are highly engaged in school life, exam-related pressures may impact negatively on their stress levels and overall well-being (Hannan et al., 1996).

How young people fare at school, in terms of the level they reach and the grades they attain, is strongly predictive of longer-term life-chances in the Irish context. Young people who take, and do well in, the Leaving Certificate are more likely to go on to further education and training, and, when they do enter the labour market, have better employment chances along with improved access to more skilled work and higher earnings (Gorby, McCoy and Williams, 2005). Such advantages persist into adult life, with higher employment levels, better quality jobs, higher earnings and lower poverty rates among those with higher levels of educational qualifications (Layte, Nolan and Whelan, 2000; Denny, Harmon and Redmond, 2000; Smyth and Byrne, 2004).

There is evidence that educational attainment may be becoming increasingly important in the initial period after leaving school; those young people who leave school without a Leaving Certificate, especially those who leave school without any qualifications whatsoever, are increasingly marginalised in terms of access to paid employment and are especially vulnerable to any fluctuations in employment (McCoy and Smyth, 2003).

The first section of this chapter sets out the background in terms of key economic and social changes since the early 1990s. The second section examines shifts in the boundary between school and work for young people. The third section assesses the extent to which the educational system has itself undergone transformation while the fourth section explores the nature of power relations in the school context.

---

1 Young people aged 15–17 are also less likely to report feeling 'very happy' about their lives than those aged 9–11 (Friel, Nic Gabhainn and Kelleher, 1999). Among 15–17-year-olds, problems with schoolwork are the most frequently reported difficulties in day-to-day life (NSRF, 2004). A decline in positive attitudes to school as students move through the system is not unique to Ireland (see, for example, de Fraine et al., 2005).

Changing times?

Economic growth since the early 1990s has resulted in increased employment rates and rising living standards within Irish families. Household income has increased rapidly while levels of deprivation have declined (Whelan et al., 2003). Expanding employment opportunities have drawn an increasing number of second-level students into the labour market. This has happened on a part-time rather than a full-time basis, with the potential 'pull' out of school perhaps being cancelled out by policy interventions to increase student retention (see below). Among Leaving Certificate students, participation in part-time employment doubled between 1994 and 2002, with paid work outside school almost the norm among this group by the end of this period. The earnings of these working students are often substantial and, in many cases, are supplemented by pocket money from their parents. Such involvement in paid work means that young people are more financially independent and have more money to spend on their social lives but may have less time to spend on non-work activities. Indeed, there is evidence that the primary motivation for working is to finance a 'lifestyle' in terms of social activities and related consumption (McCoy and Smyth, 2004).

While such a trend may be positive in terms of promoting increased maturity and independence among young people, it may have negative effects in terms of on-going educational participation and performance, issues which are explored further in the second section of this chapter. Increased levels of disposable income may also have implications for the prevalence of drinking and smoking among young people.

Side by side with economic change, changes have taken place in the nature of the family structure and familial relations. Large families are now less prevalent than heretofore and a growing number of young people are now being brought up outside traditional nuclear family structures (with 12 per cent of children living in lone parent families in 2002). Increasing female employment rates mean that many young people live in families where both parents are in paid employment. Such changes in family life are likely to have had countervailing influences on the nature of parent–child interaction. On the one hand, smaller families may mean that parents spend more time with their children than previously; on the other hand, increasing employment rates and changing commuting patterns mean that young people are more likely to spend some time in formal care arrangements, either on a full-time basis or as part of structured after-school activities. In the absence of data on such trends in Ireland, it is difficult to say which of these effects will be stronger and whether these changes are broadly positive or negative in terms of young people's quality of life. Research in other countries (for example, Sayer, Bianchi and Robinson, 2004) indicates no evidence of a long-term decrease in the time spent by parents with their children. Any changes in the time young people spend with their parents have taken place in the context of a longer-term shift in the nature of parent–child relations away from more authoritarian to more negotiated modes of interaction, with young people now having a greater 'voice' within the family (Devine, Nic Ghiolla Phádraig and Deegan, 2004). Even in terms of choice of school, the majority of young people are consulted by their parents and have at least some input into deciding on the second-level school they will attend (Smyth, McCoy and Darmody, 2004).

Some acknowledgement of 'children's rights' has also recently become apparent in policy terms, reflecting a shift from the earlier focus on children's 'needs' (Devine, Nic Ghiolla Phádraig and Deegan, 2004). The National Children's Strategy (2000), implementing the UN Convention on the Rights of the Child (UNCRC), emerged as a cross-government response to improving children's lives and giving children a 'voice'. The strategy offers a vision of 'an Ireland where children are respected as young citizens with a valued contribution to make and a voice of their own'. The National Children's Office, established to implement the strategy, has put in place a range of initiatives to bring this about, including a national youth parliament for young people aged 12 to 18 years (Dáil na nÓg) as well as measures to encourage schools to establish student councils (see below). From 2004, there has also been an Ombudsman for Children, providing an independent mechanism to vindicate the rights of the child. This focus on the rights of children and young people is, however, at a relatively early stage in its impact on policy development.

In overall terms, recent social and economic changes in Irish society have contributed to a greater acknowledgement of young people's rights and autonomy. The following section explores in greater detail the extent to which these changes have shifted the boundary between work and school for young people.

School and part-time employment

Participation in part-time work among those in the senior cycle at school has moved from a minority to majority pursuit over the last decade; currently, over six out of ten Leaving Certificate students have a paid part-time job during term-time (McCoy and Smyth, 2004). As discussed in the introduction, such employment must be seen in the context of rapid employment growth, with growth being particularly dramatic in the market services sector, that is, in the sector which has the 'casual' and part-time jobs which better suit students. The extent to which this shift in employment drew young people into the labour market is evident among third-level students whose labour force participation increased from 7 per cent in 1991 to 40 per cent in 1999 (McCoy, Duffy and Smyth, 2000).

Despite legislative measures to curtail the employment of school-age children, part-time employment has become commonplace among second-level students, reaching a peak among fifth year and Transition Year students. Male students are particularly likely to hold jobs with longer hours and which entail weekday work, with over one-third of them working more than 15 hours per week. So what are the implications of such employment for students in both their academic and social lives and indeed in terms of the interplay between the two?

Second-level students today are earning considerable sums of money from employment, income which, in many cases, is supplemented by parental 'pocket money'.[2] For the most part, their income is spent on entertainment, clothes, CDs/music and alcohol. Having a job allows students to fund their social lives, thereby creating greater autonomy and independence. However, part-time work during term-time has a negative effect on how young people get on at school (McCoy and Smyth, 2004). Students who work long hours (that is, more than 15 hours per week) do worse in their Junior Certificate exam and are more likely to drop out of school before the Leaving Certificate than other students. At Leaving Certificate level, any amount of paid work, even for a few hours per week, is found to have a negative effect on the grades achieved. It is clear that work commitments among students are having a negative impact on students' school lives, at least in terms of their academic engagement and performance.

Despite the growth in paid employment, there are, however, few formal links between school and the workplace in Ireland. This means that the work–study balance has become a zero-sum trade-off for students; time spent on paid work detracts from time spent on schoolwork. Work experience placements have become part of the Transition Year, Leaving Certificate Applied and Leaving Certificate Vocational programmes. However, research suggests that these placements may vary in duration and quality (Department of Education, 1996; McKenna and O'Maolmhuire, 2000; Smyth, Byrne and Hannan, 2004; Department of Education and Science, 2001). In fact, work placements may have the effect of drawing

---

2 In 2001, male students working part-time received an average of 111 euro per week (from work and pocket money combined) while female students received an average of 66 euro (McCoy and Smyth, 2004).

students into paid part-time work, especially if students do not use the opportunity to explore longer-term career options. For the most part, students have little opportunity to bring their (paid) work experiences into the classroom and, unlike in certain other countries, there is no opportunity for students to be rewarded or earn 'credits' through their efforts in the labour market. This is a particularly important issue for students who are likely to enter the labour market directly after leaving school, for whom such employment experiences may well serve an important function in smoothing their integration into the labour market and maximising their success (McCoy and Smyth, 2004). Further, students have little opportunity to test out or utilise skills and knowledge acquired in the classroom in their work situation. If students had the opportunity to identify skills or competencies of use in undertaking their jobs and other activities outside of the classroom, the gains from such work might well be more than just financial.

It appears that students are faced with an increasingly paradoxical situation: increasing numbers are engaging in paid employment outside school, employment that, for the most part, gives them substantial incomes and affords them greater autonomy and an opportunity to fund their social lives. The school system, in contrast, allows students little opportunity to bring their workplace experiences into the classroom (and utilise classroom skills and competencies in the workplace) and remains largely rigid in terms of the structure and organisation of the school day and curriculum. The two sets of activities are therefore competing for students' time and efforts, having negative consequences for their academic performance. The following section further assesses the extent to which broader social and economic changes in the lives of young people have been matched by a transformation of the schooling system.

Changing schools? Recent changes in the Irish educational system

The period from the early 1990s onwards has seen significant developments in educational legislation and policy, attempting to reflect the rapid changes taking place in Irish society. Such developments have very much been based on a partnership model of change; the proceedings of the National Education Convention in 1994, for example, involved the key education stakeholders and formed the basis of the Education Act, 1998 (Coolahan, 2000). The most significant developments have centred on the introduction of new programmes and curricula and an attempt to address disadvantage and diversity within the school context. More general shifts in the relationship between the school and the family have taken place, with increased emphasis on the formal involvement of parents in school life.[3] In spite of these changes, the general public considers that parents should have a greater say in the running of schools (Kellaghan et al., 2004).

Curricular reform

The 1990s marked the beginning of a period of substantial curriculum change for schools at both primary and post-primary level. At primary level, the new curriculum introduced in 1998–9 focused on the child as an active learner and proposed the use of a variety of teaching methodologies in the primary classroom. However, it is not clear that practice has kept pace with reform, with some indications that teaching methods remain traditional and teacher-focused (Murphy, 2005). Within second-level education, the new Junior Certificate programme was first examined in 1992; this programme represented a move away from the differentiated (academic) Intermediate and (vocational) Group Certificates.

In order to cater for a small number of students whose learning needs were not adequately met by the new Junior Certificate programme, a Junior Certificate School Programme was later introduced.

The most marked changes within second-level education have occurred within senior cycle in an attempt to make schooling more relevant to the needs of students. This has involved the development (or expansion) of three programmes: Transition Year, the Leaving Certificate Vocational Programme and the Leaving Certificate Applied programme. The Transition Year programme, now taken by more than one-third of the senior-cycle cohort, is designed to promote a range of competencies and skills not usually emphasised within traditional academic education, placing an emphasis on developing personal and social skills, self-directed learning and providing young people with experience of adult and working life. Transition Year is seen in broadly positive terms by teachers and students and is found to have a generally positive influence on academic outcomes among participants (Smyth, Byrne and Hannan, 2004).

Until the 1990s, young people who stayed on to senior cycle took a single, academically oriented Leaving Certificate programme. The

[3] There is also obviously a strong informal involvement of parents in education. Young people are strongly reliant on the advice of their parents in educational decision-making (see McCoy et al., 2006), frequently discuss school-related issues with their parents, and a significant proportion receive help with their homework/study from their parents and siblings (Smyth, McCoy and Darmody, 2004). This informal involvement might be expected to become more important over time as parents themselves have a higher level of education than previously.

Leaving Certificate Vocational Programme (LCVP) was introduced in 1994 to foster in students a spirit of enterprise and initiative and to develop their interpersonal, vocational and technological skills. There is a good deal of overlap with the established Leaving Certificate but students take additional subjects that focus on enterprise education, preparation for work and work experience. A somewhat more radical innovation than the LCVP involved the introduction of the Leaving Certificate Applied Programme (LCA) in 1995. The programme was introduced to cater for less academically oriented students and those potentially at risk of school drop-out. The curriculum and approach of the LCA focus on preparing students for the transition from school to adult and working life, using more active and practical teaching and assessment methods. The upshot of these changes is that young people have a greater number of options at senior-cycle level. However, the extent to which they can avail of these options depends on the school they attend; the majority of students continue to take the traditional Leaving Certificate.

Addressing disadvantage and diversity

Per-student expenditure on education in Ireland has significantly increased since the early 1990s, especially at primary level. Additional expenditure on education has facilitated a reduction in the student-teacher ratio at both primary and post-primary levels, although class size remains a policy issue. However, spending levels at primary and second-level remain below average in international terms, at 79 per cent and 82 per cent of the respective OECD averages (OECD, 2005). Furthermore, more than twice as much is spent for each student at a third-level institution as is spent on those in the primary sector (OECD, 2005).

The 1990s saw 'educational disadvantage' emerging as a matter of policy concern. The Education Act, 1998, defined educational disadvantage in terms of the 'impediments to education arising from social or economic disadvantage which prevent students from deriving appropriate benefit from education in schools'. As a result of this policy focus, overall increases in spending levels have been supplemented by the introduction of a number of measures which involve targeting additional expenditure at 'disadvantaged' schools.[4] These measures cover early childhood education and primary and second-level schooling. These initiatives (including Breaking the Cycle, the Disadvantaged Areas Scheme, Giving Children an Even Break and the new Delivering Equality

---

4 One in ten of primary schools, and one in four of second-level schools, were designated disadvantaged prior to the new DEIS initiative.

of Opportunity in Schools initiative – DEIS) involve the provision of extra funding per pupil along with additional teacher allocation for schools that are designated 'disadvantaged' in terms of their student profile. These measures have been supplemented by the Home School Community Liaison (HSCL) scheme, aimed at facilitating communication between parents and teachers in the interest of the child's learning within designated disadvantaged schools.

Furthermore, the School Completion Programme provides schools with funds to develop appropriate intervention strategies (such as in-school and after-school supports) for young people who are at risk of leaving school early. Similarly, the recently established National Educational Welfare Board aims to address the issue of school attendance and ensure that every pupil benefits fully from education.

The rapid increase in the proportion of young people staying on to the Leaving Certificate between 1980 and 1998 (from 60 per cent to 82 per cent of the cohort[5]) means that many schools are increasingly catering for a very diverse student population in terms of academic ability. This has led to the increased provision of additional learning supports within schools, including the availability of resource teachers, additional teaching hours and special needs assistants, as well as an extension of the learning support teacher service to all primary and second-level schools. These initiatives have also been underpinned by the establishment of the National Educational Psychological Service (NEPS), which provides assessment for students with learning difficulties. There is also some evidence of increasing diversity within classrooms. In the 1980s, the majority of second-level schools used streaming, whereby students of similar assessed ability were grouped into classes, ranked from 'higher' to 'lower'. The prevalence of streaming practices has declined over time, with the majority of second-level students now in mixed-ability base classes, a trend which is positive in its impact on academic performance and school engagement among lower-ability students (Smyth, 1999; Smyth, McCoy and Darmody, 2004).

Overall, recent years have seen significant developments in the educational system, reflecting a growing awareness of the need to meet the diverse needs of the student population in the context of a rapidly changing society. What has been achieved to date?

The Transition Year programme highlights the potential for flexibility at the school and teacher level in programme design and implementation and

---

5 Rates of early school leaving remain higher in Ireland than in the Nordic countries, which have a strong equity focus, and countries (such as Austria) with a 'dual system', combining school with work.

for broadening young people's educational experience to include a broader set of competencies. While the programme is seen as having broadly positive effects, however, schools serving disadvantaged communities are less likely to provide it and the benefits tend to accrue more to young people with positive experiences of school (Smyth, Byrne and Hannan, 2004). The introduction of new programmes at senior cycle has meant quite a shift from a general to a more differentiated upper secondary system. The impact of this shift has not yet been fully evaluated. One of the motivations for the change was to increase student retention but, in spite of the new programmes and additional measures to promote school completion, overall Leaving Certificate completion rates have plateaued since the late 1990s but with some relative improvement in the position of working-class students (O'Connell, Clancy and McCoy, 2006). It may be, however, that early school leaving would have increased in response to better employment opportunities but for such measures. The net result is that almost one-fifth of the student cohort leaves school with low levels of qualification, with implications for their subsequent access to education, training and employment.

The introduction of new subjects, such as Social, Personal and Health Education (SPHE) and Civic, Social and Political Education (CSPE), has extended the school's formal role in the fostering of personal and social skills among young people. The extent to which this is carried over into greater student involvement in decision-making within the school will be discussed later in this chapter. In tandem with the introduction of these new subjects, schools have come to play a greater role in providing socio-emotional support to their students through a range of services including student mentors and designated personnel (such as class tutors) (see McCoy et al., 2006). However, the appropriate role for the school, as to whether it should provide more specialised psychological services or have a purely referral role in that respect, remains open to debate.

While the 1990s saw an increased number of initiatives targeting educational disadvantage, such measures have been subject to criticism in terms of fragmentation, lack of coverage of all 'disadvantaged' students, inadequate levels of resources and failure to take account of broader processes of school effectiveness and improvement (Educational Disadvantage Forum, 2003; Educational Disadvantage Committee, 2003; McCoy and Smyth, 2003). The new DEIS initiative changes the nature of resource allocation to schools serving disadvantaged communities and its intention to integrate previously fragmented initiatives under one umbrella is to be welcomed.

The challenge remains as to 'how to ensure that an education system originally designed to serve the needs of an elite few can be re-shaped to meet the needs of a broader, more diverse group of learners' (NCCA, 2005). The reforms proposed by the National Council for Curriculum and Assessment suggest quite a radical reshaping of senior-cycle education in Ireland.[6] They aim to make schooling a more enjoyable learning experience for a diverse student population, involving greater student choice over curriculum components, a variety of assessment methods, more active teaching methods and a better balance of knowledge and skills (NCCA, 2005). They also anticipate that such reforms would entail greater student involvement in decision-making within schools as well as a less hierarchical relationship between teacher and student (NCCA, 2003).

In sum, significant changes have taken place within the second-level educational system in recent years. However, it not clear that these reforms have adequately taken account of the diverse needs of the student population or reflected the dramatic changes within wider society. The following section explores the extent to which educational reform has reshaped the nature of day-to-day life within second-level schools in Ireland.

Power relations within Irish schools: change or continuity?

The previous sections have explored the way in which the national educational system has changed and the boundaries between school and work recast since the early 1990s. This section explores the extent to which such changes have transformed social relations within schools themselves, focusing in particular on whether young people's growing autonomy outside school has been reflected in school policy and practice.

A study of school life in the 1980s indicated that students' actions were largely determined by agencies outside of their control (Lynch, 1989). Hardly any schools involved students in determining the type of subjects on offer or the nature of disciplinary procedures. Even in terms of extra-curricular activities, students were involved in helping to organise such activities in only a minority (38 per cent) of schools and were involved in initiating new activities in only a small number (15 per cent) of cases. Lynch's (1989) study characterises the relational context within which Irish pupils are socialised in second-level schools as profoundly hierarchical; students have little control over what they do in school, when they do it or how they do it.

---

[6] The status of these proposals in terms of potential implementation is unclear at the time of writing.

The Education Act of 1998 went some way towards involving students more in terms of input into their education, by stating that a school board shall establish and maintain procedures which 'shall facilitate the involvement of the students in the operation of the school, having regard to the age and experience of the students, in association with their parents and teachers'. The Act provides for the establishment of student councils in schools and that these councils should be encouraged and facilitated. This development should be seen as part of a growing awareness of young people's rights in policy development (see above).

Student councils are a recent addition to the Irish educational landscape. By 2004, three-quarters of second-level schools had a council in place[7] (Keogh and Whyte, 2005). These student councils are seen as successful (by the councils themselves) in three out of ten schools, with four in ten seeing them as somewhat effective and three in ten as totally ineffective. There also appears to be a discrepancy between what school management and what the students themselves feel is the role of a student council. School management saw consultation as the main role of the student council, with it also having a role as a conduit of information between staff and students. Students, however, felt that their role was to make the school a better place to be in. Senior students in particular felt that the council should try to influence management decisions. There is a clear discrepancy between the consultative role envisaged by school management and the action role envisaged by students. Furthermore, student councils are currently receiving little support, either internally from school management or externally from an outside support service (Keogh and Whyte, 2005). Teachers may be fearful that a more meaningful role for students in policy formulation may lead to 'anarchy'. On the other hand, students may have little faith in the student council because they want a greater involvement in decisions and a more genuine input into the running of the school (Lynch and Lodge, 2002). Interestingly, these issues are echoed in public opinion, with the majority of adults feeling that students have too little say in what happens in the educational system (Kellaghan et al., 2004).

The existence of student councils does not appear to have transformed social relations within second-level schools. There is a growing body of international evidence suggesting that schooling practices that fail to respect the autonomy and individuality of the student may have quite negative educational consequences (see, for example, Collins, 2000; Rudduck, Chaplan and Wallace, 1996). However, within the Irish context,

[7] Interestingly, policy concern has not focused on the promotion of student consultation in primary schools (McLoughlin, 2004).

power relations between students and teachers continue to be hierarchical, a hierarchy that is taken as given (Lynch and Lodge, 2002).

The issue of power and authority emerges as the single greatest equality concern among students, over and above other equality issues such as gender, ethnicity or social class (Lynch and Lodge, 2002). Just under half of the students were concerned about the level of respect given to them as young people. A similar proportion saw unequal or perceived unfair treatment by teachers as an equality issue for them. Their understanding of unequal treatment centred on questions of power and its misuse. The students stated that the possible solutions to rebalancing these inequalities in power were based on organisational practice and attitudinal change, with almost half of students calling for greater equality of respect and improved democracy.

Outside of formal school structures, the nature of informal interaction between teachers and students on a day-to-day basis has significant implications for academic and personal development among young people (Smyth, 1999; Smyth, McCoy and Darmody, 2004). Where students report negative experiences of school, their criticisms often centre on unfair treatment by teachers and the arbitrary imposition of punishment and sanctions, a pattern which is more prevalent among students in lower-stream classes (Smyth, McCoy and Darmody, 2004). Even in areas where students are given choice (for example, in the selection of exam subjects), such choices may be constrained by school rules regarding access to subjects or by the way in which subjects are offered to students (Smyth et al., 2006; Darmody and Smyth, 2005).

It is interesting to contrast student views on unfair treatment with recent media attention to the issue of discipline in schools, with many reports suggesting that the situation has reached 'crisis' proportions. In fact, there is no systematic evidence to suggest that levels of student misbehaviour have increased over time; the Task Force Report on Student Behaviour in Second-Level Schools (2006) suggests that discipline issues in the majority of schools are amenable to correction but that, in a minority of schools, 'teaching and learning are severely curtailed by disruptive student behaviour' (p. 6). To some extent, discipline issues can be seen as resulting from the tension between hierarchical power structures within school and students' growing autonomy outside school. Especially if they feel they are treated unfairly, students can 'act out', thus perpetuating a cycle of misbehaviour on the part of students and negative sanctions from teachers (Smyth et al., 2006). Even though schools now have a greater emphasis on the provision of personal and social support for students than previously, many students may be reluctant to approach teachers for help where these teachers have both disciplinary and pastoral roles within the school

(McCoy et al., 2006; Smyth et al., 2006). When they are bullied, for example, students are much more likely to approach their friends and family for help than a teacher or other staff member (Smyth et al., 2006).

The National Council for Curriculum and Assessment has put forward proposals for the future development of the senior cycle; these entail student involvement in many aspects of schooling and learning. It proposes initiatives for 'increasing the involvement of students in the organisation and management of their learning and learning environment' (NCCA, 2005) and emphasises student choice and student involvement in their learning. Furthermore, the NCCA (2003) envisages that, under the new proposals, 'senior cycle students [will be] involved in aspects of school organisation and policy development such as the school behaviour code, the school dress code and health-promotion policies'.

In sum, there have been a number of recent attempts to give students more power and say in their education. However, change is slow and most initiatives are only in their infancy. Student councils have been established in the majority of second-level schools and students have also begun to be heard and represented through the establishment of the Union of Secondary Students in 2001. In spite of these formal structures, the extent to which students are really involved and represented is debatable. The role of student councils has mainly been one of consultation rather than policymaking. Indeed, there is a tension between involving students in decision-making while also maintaining traditional hierarchical power structures within schools.

Recent research indicates that schools continue to be hierarchical in nature, with the result that many students have little sense of ownership over school life. The proposals for the newly structured senior cycle from the NCCA go a long way in addressing this issue and their vision for the future is for a more meaningful involvement of students in the organisation and management of their education and school experience.

Conclusions

The past 15 years have seen significant changes in the nature of Irish society. Employment expansion has resulted in improved living standards for families and has drawn an increasing number of school-going young people into the labour force. At the same time, the Irish family has continued to shift towards a more negotiation-based model of parent–child interaction. These changes mean that young people now have a good deal more autonomy and freedom in terms of their work and leisure.

Significant changes have also occurred in the educational system over the same period. From a positive perspective, the expansion of the Transition Year programme has allowed for greater flexibility of coursework and teaching methods in schools while the introduction of new senior-cycle programmes caters for a greater diversity of needs and interests in the student population. Largely, however, the picture has been one of continuity rather than change. In many ways, students encounter a schooling system designed for different times. Although most older students now work on a part-time basis, the school day is very rigid and the school and work spheres remain quite separate. There is little opportunity for recognising the skills young people develop by working outside school or for applying their school-based learning in the work setting. There is no opportunity to combine part-time work with attending school on a more flexible basis. Crucially, social relations within schools remain hierarchical in nature, with students being 'told' what to do in their day-to-day lives.

In spite of the growth of student councils in recent years and a new emphasis on citizenship education within the curriculum, students have little active involvement in formulating key aspects of school policy or in influencing lesson content on a day-to-day basis. Recent proposals[8] for a reform of senior-cycle education envision a more flexible school day and increased student responsibility. To date, however, the schooling system has been slow to respond to change and developments have lagged behind those in the wider society. This has significant implications for young people's quality of life. They are caught between two worlds, increasingly treated as adults outside the school context but as children within it.

---

8 It is not clear, at the time of writing, the extent to which all aspects of these proposals will be acted upon.

10

Family and Sexuality

Tony Fahey and Richard Layte

Introduction

The referendum on divorce held in November 1995 brought more or less to a close some three decades of loud and often bitter controversy on 'moral' questions in Irish public life. Contraception was the big issue of the late 1960s and 1970s, and abortion and divorce took over in the 1980s (for a detailed account, see Hug, 1999). The final rumbles of the contraception debate passed away only when the Health (Family Planning) (Amendment) Act, 1993, introduced a fully liberalised regime on 'artificial' contraception.[1] The constitutional referendum on divorce held in 1995, which followed a previous referendum on the same subject in 1986, opened the way for the Family Law (Divorce) Act, 1996, and thereby settled the divorce question quite decisively. The triple referendum on abortion held in 1992, which followed the first referendum on abortion in 1983 and the ensuing Supreme Court decision in the 'X' case in 1992, had a less decisive effect, in that it left key issues unresolved, and a further referendum on abortion took place in 2002. Nevertheless, the 1992 referendum took most of the steam out of the abortion question and by comparison with the grand battles of that period, the referendum of ten years later was a low-key affair.[2]

1 As recently as 1991, the Irish Family Planning Association was fined £700 for selling condoms in the Virgin Megastore in Dublin, in contravention of the legislation then in force which restricted sale of contraceptives to pharmacies and other approved outlets.

2 The subdued atmosphere surrounding the abortion referendum in 2002 in part reflected weariness of the subject among voters and in part confusion about the meaning of the constitutional amendment to be decided upon (which aimed to affirm part of the Supreme Court's 'X case' judgement in 1992 but to reverse its decision to allow abortion on the basis of a risk of suicide to the mother). The pro-life and pro-choice lobbies were divided among themselves on whether to oppose or support the amendment, so that the battle lines were unclear. Turnout in the referendum was low, at 42.9 per cent of voters. The proposed amendment was narrowly rejected so that the 'X case' judgement stood in full and abortion remained legal under the circumstances it specified. However, no legislation has been enacted to regulate the area, and Irish women seeking an abortion continued to do so in Britain.

T. Fahey et al. (eds.), Quality of Life in Ireland, 155–174.

Homosexuality came to political attention in the late 1980s, but in 1993 it was decriminalised with surprisingly little controversy and quickly moved from centre stage (the quite liberal legislation was passed in the Dáil without a vote, to the applause of gay rights activists – Hug, 1999, p. 228). The legal treatment of unmarried mothers and their children was also revolutionised in this period, first by virtue of the introduction of welfare payments for unmarried mothers in 1973 – a radical symbolic as well as practical departure in its time – and then through the Status of Children Act, 1987, which outlawed discrimination against non-marital children.

By the mid-1990s, the politics of family and sexuality from which all of these measures had emerged had largely run their course, and apart from the brief re-emergence of the abortion issue in 2002, the noise and fury they had generated faded away. Public attention moved elsewhere, and over the past ten years the peace that has reigned in the politics of family and sexuality has been as striking as the controversy of earlier years.

The rise and decline of political controversy on these issues echoed the changing tempo of developments in cultural values and behaviour. The 1960s, 1970s and 1980s were decades of sexual and gender revolution and of rapid change in family patterns, while in the past ten years the pace of change has slowed and a certain degree of stabilisation has emerged in a number of areas. Beginning in the 1960s, sexuality escaped from the strictures of a repressive Catholic culture and a censorious State and gained a new freedom of expression, carried forward both by more liberal interpretations of the nature and moral value of sexuality and by commercial exploitation through advertising, the media and pornography.[3]

Women rebelled against the male-centredness of private and public life, forged new interpretations of what it meant to be female, and demanded that social institutions and male behaviour be reshaped accordingly.[4] Family life was transformed by developments such as the sharp decline in family size, the rapid increase in births outside of marriage, and the rise of marital breakdown (for a recent overview, see Kennedy, 2003).

However, by the time the economic boom arrived in the mid-1990s, these developments had arrived at what might be called a post-revolutionary phase: change had by no means come to a halt, but it had less

[3] Social research on sexuality in Ireland has been sparse (for an isolated study, see Inglis, 1998; for a more general overview, see Fahey, 1999). Systematic survey research on this area has commenced only recently (Layte et al., 2006) and is referred to further below.

[4] There is a growing body of research on the modern women's movement and its impact on Irish society (see, for example, Connolly, 2002; Finnegan and Wiles 2005; Galligan, Ward, and Wilford, 1999; Hill, 2003).

of a mould-breaking character than previously, and there were some indications of a new stability in behavioural trends. While we do not want to overstate the revolutionary/post-revolutionary dichotomy that this characterisation entails, it is nevertheless a useful way of suggesting that, amidst all the talk of how dramatic the pace of social change has been in the Celtic Tiger era, the big shifts in the realms of family and sexuality pre-dated the mid-1990s and developments since then have been modest by comparison. The economic boom of itself has undoubtedly made some contribution to change, but in some ways also it has brought a measure of stability following earlier sharp transformation. Our aim in this chapter is to outline how this is so, describe certain features of the post-revolutionary situation, assess what effects the Celtic Tiger had on recent developments, and offer some observations on the implications of change for the quality of family life in Ireland. It is not easy to make empirically based judgments as to whether Ireland at present is experiencing the best of times as far as family and sexual life is concerned. Depending on one's moral standpoint, one could argue that developments such as the sexual or gender revolutions of recent times are either unprecedented achievements for human liberty and well-being or further steps in the moral and social decay of the modern world. Here, our aim is not to offer judgment on such overarching evaluations but rather to explore some of the empirical evidence that is relevant to more modest assessments of recent trends.

A new consensus?

One feature of the recent post-revolutionary atmosphere in the arenas of family and sexuality is a considerable degree of tacit consensus on basic questions. The Catholic conservative viewpoint in these areas that had prevailed up to the 1960s disintegrated between then and the 1990s and was gradually replaced by a new secular liberal orthodoxy (though, as we shall see below, this orthodoxy was not quite as liberal on some issues, especially abortion, as in most of the rest of Europe). This is not to say that everybody agrees on all elements of the new moral regime, since marked differences persist, especially in that older people are less accepting of new attitudes and values than are younger people (Fahey, Hayes and Sinnott, 2005, pp. 114–139). Inglis suggests that by the 1990s there was widespread ambivalence among Irish people about the competing appeal of the traditional and liberal approaches to sexuality: '[m]any people want individual freedom and choice but at the same time they want the security and comfort of a traditional life in which everything, including sex, is in its proper place and proper time' (Inglis, 1998, p. 175).

However, ambivalence is not dissent and does not bring people onto the streets as did the 'moral politics' of earlier years. At the official level, orthodox Catholic teaching remains uncompromisingly opposed to new permissive standards. According to the current (1997) edition of the *Catechism of the Catholic Church*, for example, 'carnal union between an unmarried man and an unmarried woman' (which the Catechism labels 'fornication') is 'gravely contrary to the dignity of persons and of human sexuality' (para. 2353), homosexual acts 'are intrinsically disordered' and 'contrary to the natural law' (para. 2357), artificial contraception is 'intrinsically evil' (para. 2370), and 'divorce is a grave offence against the natural law' and is 'immoral' (para. 2384) (see http://www.vatican.va/archive/catechism/ccc_toc.htm). In practice, however, the institutional Church has become increasingly muted in its espousal of these doctrines, in everyday pastoral practice if not at the level of Vatican declarations. In Ireland, its moral authority to do otherwise has been severely weakened by the spate of sex scandals that has assailed it since 1992, as well as by general secularisation (Fuller, 2004).

In addition, it is evident that many of these doctrines are a dead letter for most Irish people, even among the still-numerous Catholic faithful. The near disappearance of the large Catholic family, for example, would indicate the almost total disregard now shown towards the church's teaching on contraception. Survey data collected in Ireland in 1999–2000 suggested that less than half of Catholics who attended church regularly thought that homosexuality was never justified and only one-third thought that divorce was never justified, indicating a quite high level of rejection of orthodox Catholic teaching even among active church members (Fahey, Hayes and Sinnott, 2005, p. 131). The same data indicate that only one-third of Irish people would disapprove of the idea that a woman might decide to have a child without having a stable relationship with a man, while at the same time two-thirds believed that 'a child needs a home with both a father and a mother to grow up happily' (Fahey, Hayes and Sinnott, 2005, p. 120). This again is an instance of a nuanced view, in that preference for the two-parent family as an ideal does not necessarily entail disapproval of the alternative represented by lone parenthood, even when lone parenthood is a premeditated choice.

There is, however, one area where the older morality still exerts a hold in Ireland, and this is in regard to abortion. The political campaign on abortion that commenced in the early 1980s was initiated not by pro-choice activists seeking to liberalise the law in this area but by conservative lay Catholics wishing to bolster the existing legal prohibition on abortion by adding a pro-life clause to the Constitution. It is revealing that feminists and others who opposed this move were careful to steer clear of an overt pro-choice stance, since that would have foundered on the rock of public opinion. They argued instead that a pro-life amendment would be ineffective as it would do nothing to alleviate the problems of those faced with crisis pregnancies. As Mary Robinson, a leading figure in the anti-amendment campaign, put it at the time: 'Abortion is a problem. The pro-life amendment is not a solution' (quoted in Hug, 1999, p. 147).

The 1983 pro-life amendment was carried by a two to one majority of the popular vote (66.9 per cent in favour, 33.1 per cent against), thus apparently closing the question in a decidedly anti-abortion direction. However, the solidity of public opinion on this issue was shaken in 1992 when the 'X' case, which related to a 15-year-old girl who had been raped by a neighbour, came before the Supreme Court and the Court ruled that the risk to her life posed by a threat of suicide on her part entitled her to seek an abortion.[5] Since then, Irish people have continued to strongly disapprove of abortion in general terms. The European Values Study (EVS) in 1999–2000, for example, suggested that apart from Malta, the only other population in Europe to show similar levels of opposition to abortion were the people of Northern Ireland. This indicates a conservative Protestant–Catholic consensus on this question on the island of Ireland that has no parallel elsewhere in Europe (Fahey, Hayes and Sinnott, 2005, pp. 126–137) – though it echoes the joint Protestant–Catholic activism on abortion that has recently emerged in the US. However, when it comes to abortion under particular circumstances, there is considerable ambivalence and nuance in Ireland, even among self-identified Catholics. In the 1999–2000 EVS, for example, 47 per cent of those who identified themselves as Catholics in Ireland said they would approve of abortion where the pregnancy was the result of rape and 31 per cent would approve where there was a strong chance of a serious defect in the baby. The strongest opposition was to the use of abortion for general family planning purposes – eight out of ten Catholics in Ireland voiced disapproval of abortion in the case of, for example, couples who could not afford to have more children or women who wished to avoid becoming unmarried mothers. More significantly, perhaps, even those who declared themselves to be religiously unaffiliated showed a similar unease, in that less than half would approve of abortion in these circumstances (Fahey, Hayes and Sinnott, 2005, p. 126).

---

5 The pro-life clause added to the Constitution in 1983 asserted 'the right to life of the unborn, with due regard to the right to life of the mother'. The Supreme Court ruling in the 'X' case rested on the right to life of the mother asserted here. Thus, the ironic result of the pro-life amendment was that it eventually opened the door to legal abortion in Ireland – albeit only by a crack that has not widened in the intervening years.

Thus, although there was a religious–secular dimension to the differentiation of attitudes towards abortion, these attitudes were far from being strongly and clearly polarised between religious–conservative and secular–liberal standpoints. Rather, there was a large middle ground, located (on the abortion issue at least) in a more conservative position than was common in Europe, but uncomfortable with extreme views in either direction.

Changing sexual attitudes and behaviour

If the public debate on sexual morality has become more muted in the last decade this does not mean that sexual attitudes themselves have been in stasis. Surveys of sexual attitudes in Ireland have shown a consistent trend towards a more liberal stance since the 1970s and this has continued through the years of economic growth, although change has been more pronounced on some issues than on others. The main process behind these developments is the continuing decline in the influence of the Catholic Church in Irish life, particularly in areas of private morality. For much of the twentieth century Catholic moral teaching was the dominant framework through which most Irish people learnt about and experienced sex (Fahey, 1999) and this is one of the reasons why current Irish sexual attitudes are still considerably more conservative than those in other Western European countries. Yet change continues and the dominant framework of the Catholic Church has been largely replaced by a secular moral framework based on individual responsibility (Inglis, 1998). A good example of this is the change in the last 30 years in attitudes toward premarital sex. In 1973 the Episcopal Commission for Research found that 71 per cent of Irish people surveyed believed that sex before marriage was always wrong. By 1994 the International Social Survey Project (ISSP) found that this had fallen to 32 per cent, a proportion which had fallen to just over 6 per cent by the time the Irish Study of Sexual Health and Relationships was carried out in 2004–2005. Though the Catholic Church still sees sex outside marriage as a sin it seems that the overwhelming majority of Irish Catholics now disagree.

Though older Irish people are more liberal in their views now than they were in the past, liberalism in sexual attitudes is strongest among young people. Going back to the example of sex before marriage, a negligible 2 per cent of those aged under 25 years now see this as always wrong compared to one-fifth of those aged 55 to 64 years.

Liberalism is not confined only to sexual attitudes. Results from the first Irish survey of sexual knowledge, attitudes and behaviours carried out in

2004–2005 show that there has been a significant decrease in age of first sexual intercourse across the last half century for both men and women. As shown in Figure 10.1, whereas the majority of women born in the 1940s would have had sexual intercourse for the first time after the age of 22, the same was true of most women born after 1970 by the age of 18 (the median age is the age at which 50 per cent of the group have had sex). Not only has there been a trend towards earlier age of first sex, but younger Irish people are also more likely to have a higher number of sexual partners over their lifetime. Over one-third of men and just over 10 per cent of women born after 1970 report having ten or more partners over their lifetime compared to 17 per cent of men and 1 per cent of women born in the 1940s.

Figure 10.1: *Median age of first vaginal intercourse by year of birth*

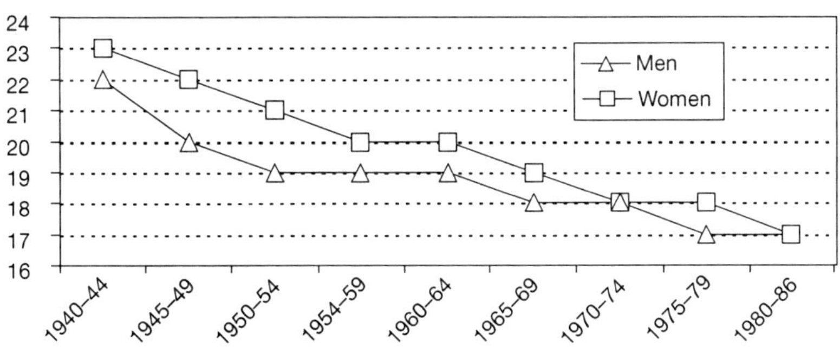

Source: Layte et al. (2006)

In many ways the weakening of the traditional Catholic framework can be seen as a positive development. Sexual behaviour was strongly associated with guilt and sin for the majority of Irish people who came to adulthood before 1990 and this made sex education and discussion problematic. It is still remarkable, for instance, that a national policy on sex education in schools was not established until 1997. Public discussion on sexual matters is now conducted in a more factual and realistic manner, although such discussions can still precipitate a vociferous reaction from some quarters. Nonetheless, it would be true to say that young people growing up in Ireland today would have trouble understanding the furore which discussions of sex education would have produced even a decade ago.

Such changes can, however, have their problems. The increase in average number of sexual partners over recent decades may be one of the reasons why there has been a very substantial increase in sexually transmitted illnesses (STIs) in the last ten years. Between 1995 and 2003 reported STIs rose from 4,781 to 11,153, with the largest increase in rates being among those under 25. For a number of reasons HIV/AIDS has not been as serious a problem in Ireland as it has been in other European countries, but the incidence of HIV infection has also increased considerably since the mid-1990s.

Stabilisation in birth rates

The most striking instance of recent stabilisation in behavioural trends in family life – and one in which rapid economic growth might plausibly be seen as having a role – is in regard to birth rates. As Figure 10.2 shows, Ireland had a baby boom in the 1970s: the annual number of births was high throughout that decade and reached a peak in 1980 at 74,100. Following that, a decline set in that continued until 1994, when births bottomed out at 47,900 for the year. Then a recovery occurred, and by 2004 annual births had risen to almost 62,000, an increase of 26 per cent since 1994. The increase was due in part to an expansion of the numbers of women in the childbearing ages, which in turn reflected the maturation of the large baby-boom generation of the 1970s. But it also reflected first a stabilisation and then a slight rise in the previously declining propensity of women to have children.

Figure 10.2: *Number of births and total fertility rate (TFR) in Ireland, 1960–2004*

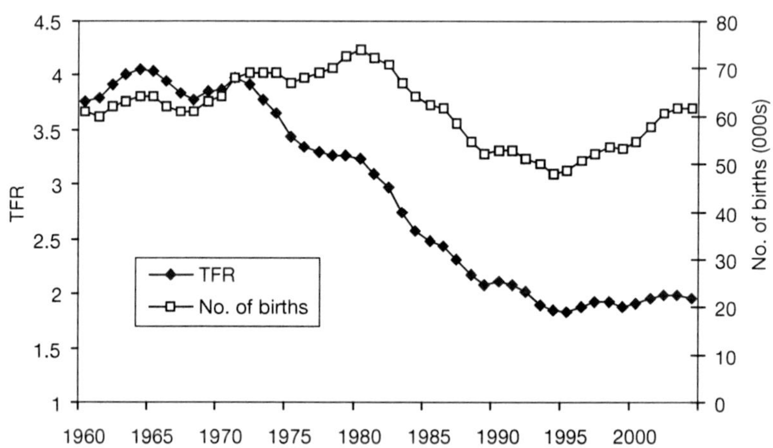

Source: CSO Vital Statistics

The long-term trend in this propensity is shown by the total fertility rate (TFR), also in Figure 10.2, which measures the number of births a woman would have if during her childbearing years she were to replicate the level of childbearing found across women of all ages in a particular year. Having hovered around 4 in the 1960s – the highest fertility rate in the developed world at the time apart from New Zealand – the TFR began to decline even as the 1970s baby boom was getting under way and continued to decrease without interruption until it reached 1.84 in 1995, a quite dramatic fall in a single generation. Then, however, the decline bottomed out and for the following decade the TFR stabilised at a level slightly above that in 1995 (in 2004, the TRF was 6 per cent higher than in 1995).

That the decline should bottom out at the level it did, which was at the top edge of the range in Europe, was a surprise. Examining fertility in the late 1980s, the demographer David Coleman raised the possibility that Ireland might be heading towards the very low fertility rates that by then were found in other Catholic countries such as Italy, Spain and Quebec (Coleman, 1992, p. 76).

By the mid-1990s, further factors emerging with the Celtic Tiger, such as the rapidly increasing cost of housing, the high cost and poor availability of childcare, and the flood of women into the labour force, would seem to have made this prediction more likely, especially as State supports for families with children remained meagre (Daly and Clavero, 2002; Fahey, 2001). The surprise, therefore, was that after 1995, instead of continuing to decline, the TFR turned slightly upwards and remained at that relatively high level since then.

Recent international research on fertility trends gives some insight into why this should have come about. The key is the role played by good educational levels and employment prospects among women in preventing fertility rates from falling to very low levels, a role that, as Castles (2003) puts it, represents a 'world turned upside down' compared to the patterns that held in the not too distant past. In the 1960s, women seemed most willing to have children in countries where their other options were limited (e.g. Ireland), while countries that offered women good education and employment opportunities had low fertility (e.g. Sweden, which in the early 1960s had the lowest fertility among Western countries). Since then, however, this pattern has inverted itself, in that lack of options for women (especially career options) now seems to be a greater deterrent to childbearing than does wide access to education and jobs. Developed countries where women have high levels of educational attainment and good job prospects (as indicated either by low female unemployment rates or high female employment rates) now have higher fertility than those developed countries where women are most confined to the home

(D'Addio and d'Ercole, 2005; Brewster and Rindfuss, 2000; Sleebos, 2003, p. 20; Ahn and Mira, 2002; Billari, 2005). In Italy, for example, where women's employment rates and levels of educational attainment are low by developed countries' standards, the present syndrome seems to be that women have one child and stay at home to mind that child.

In the US (which now has the highest fertility rate among developed countries), where women in general have high rates of participation in jobs (often having the education needed for quite a good job), those who start a family have two or three children and either stay at work full-time, go part-time or stay at home for a period to mind their children (but perhaps with the confidence that jobs will be available for them to return to if and when they want). In this high-job scenario, disincentives to childbearing that are concentrated in early childhood (such as high direct costs of childcare) or weak State supports for families with children may have some deterrent effect but it seems to be counterbalanced by women's confidence in their longer-term employment prospects.[6] Generous welfare state provision for families with children (including State-funded childcare) and strong legislative protection for women's rights, as in the Scandinavian countries, appear to work in a similar direction but the evidence now is that supportive family policies and strict gender equality provisions are less important in sustaining birth rates than is a buoyant labour market, especially in regard to jobs for women (D'Addio and d'Ercole, 2005).

Ireland seems to conform more closely to the American than the Italian scenario, or indeed to the Scandinavian model, and thus has a relatively high fertility rate. In effect, the Celtic Tiger enabled Ireland to make the transition from being a low-opportunity economy to a reasonably high-opportunity economy for women just as low economic opportunity ceased to be a positive influence on fertility rates and high economic opportunity took over that role. Ireland, in other words, managed to stay on the upside of the jobs–fertility balance even as that balance turned itself on its head – though for a time in the 1980s it seemed that Ireland might tip over into the downside of both the jobs and fertility elements of the balance, as a number of European countries have now done.

We can get a further indication of how the stabilisation of fertility rates came about by examining the changing family sizes into which children

---

6 There is a paradox here because at the individual level, women with higher education and with stronger attachment to the labour market continue to have smaller families than do less educated or stay-at-home mothers. In other words, when we look at the situation *within* countries, we find that women with weaker labour market and educational profiles have somewhat larger families, but when we compare developed countries with each other we find that those with stronger educational profiles and labour market attachment among women have higher birth rates (Castles, 2003; Billari, 2005).

were born. As Figure 10.3 shows, the recovery in births after 1995 was largely driven by increasing numbers of first-born and second-born children. The numbers of third-born children rose only slightly in the same period, thereby signalling a declining share of three-child families in the total (though in the context of shrinking family size in Europe, it is significant that third-born children in Ireland did not decline in absolute as well as relative terms). The large family became more and more exceptional, as indicated by the trend-line for fifth or higher order births: these accounted for almost one-third of births in the early 1960s but less than 3 per cent in 2003. What these figures show is that the stabilisation in birth rates after 1995 was driven by an upsurge in new family formation rather than by any reversion to larger family sizes: many more women had a first child, in most cases soon followed by a second, but fewer women had the five- or six-child families of the past. Thus, rising living standards and expanding opportunities for women seemed to have encouraged greater numbers of women to start a family and have at least one or two children, even though the same economic forces seemed to have been a deterrent to having the large numbers of children of the past. It was the cross-cutting effect of these opposing sets of influences that produced the stability in birth rates we have seen over the past decade.

Figure 10.3: *Number of births by birth order in Ireland, 1960–2003*

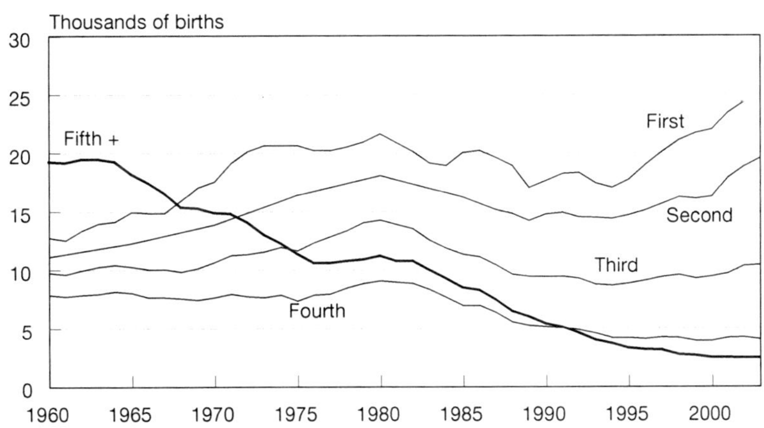

Source: CSO Vital Statistics

Non-marital births

A striking indication of the slowing down of change in family life in Ireland in recent years is provided by trends in the proportion of births taking place outside marriage. The take-off in this growth was relatively recent, getting properly underway only around 1980. Between then and the end of the next decade, however, non-marital births as a proportion of all births increased six-fold, rising from 5 per cent in 1980 to 31 per cent in 2000. At that point, however, the upward trend abruptly plateaued out and between then and the year 2005 fluctuated in the range 31–32 per cent (Figure 10.4). Whether this levelling off is temporary or not is yet too early to say, nor is it clear why it should have occurred. In the 1980s, non-marital fertility was associated with early school-leaving and poor employment prospects among young mothers, and similarly poor prospects among the young fathers who in better circumstances might have become the husbands of the mothers in question (Hannan and Ó Riain, 1993).

Figure 10.4: *Births outside of marriage, 1960–2005*

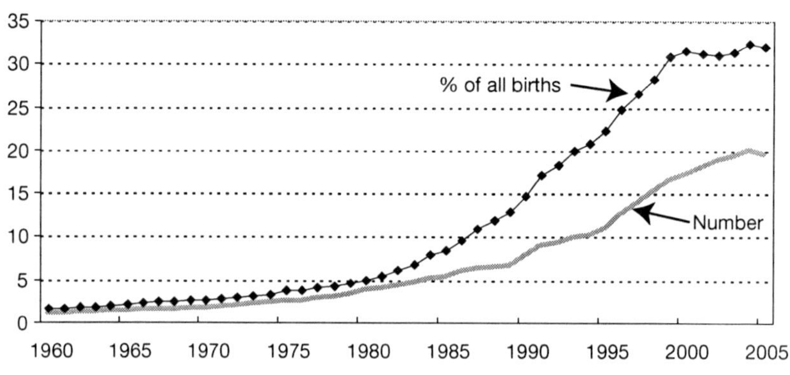

Source: CSO Vital Statistics

The decline of these factors in the 1990s (as reflected in rising educational participation and falling unemployment) did not immediately cause a corresponding slowdown in the growth of non-marital childbearing but that effect may be now becoming evident. In other words, it is possible that the levelling off in the proportion of births outside marriage is a Celtic Tiger effect, though as yet no analysis has been presented that would enable us to go beyond speculation on this question.

Recovery in marriage rates

Along with reproduction and parenthood, the further major dimension of family life is partnership between adults. There is abundant international evidence that marriage is good for both men and women – the married are happier, healthier, live longer and are materially better off than the single, divorced, separated or widowed (Layard, 2005, pp. 65–66; Waite and Gallagher, 2000). Cohabitation can have the same positive effects, but only where it has marriage-like qualities of stability and durability. How, then, has marriage fared in the Celtic Tiger years?

To set this question in context, we have to recall that Irish people in the past have sometimes shown an extraordinary reluctance to marry: they either married late or never married at all, a pattern usually interpreted as a reaction to poor economic conditions (Guinnane, 1997). This pattern reached an extreme in the 1930s, at which time over half of 30–34-year-olds in Ireland were single and 27 per cent of 50–54-year-olds were single. The average age of marriage around this time was also exceptionally old – 33 years of age for men and 28 for women. The popularity of marriage improved steadily for four decades after the 1930s and reached its apex in the 1970s. The highest number of marriages of the twentieth century was recorded in 1974 (Figure 10.5) and marriages occurred at their most youthful age at around the same time (on average at just over 26 years of age for men and 24 years of age for women). The peak of the 1970s was followed by a two-decade decline in the number of marriages and a rise in the age at which people married. As with births, however, the 1990s brought decline to a halt and turned it into recovery. By 2004, there were

Figure 10.5: *Annual number of marriages in Ireland and size of 20–29-year-old cohort, 1960–2004*

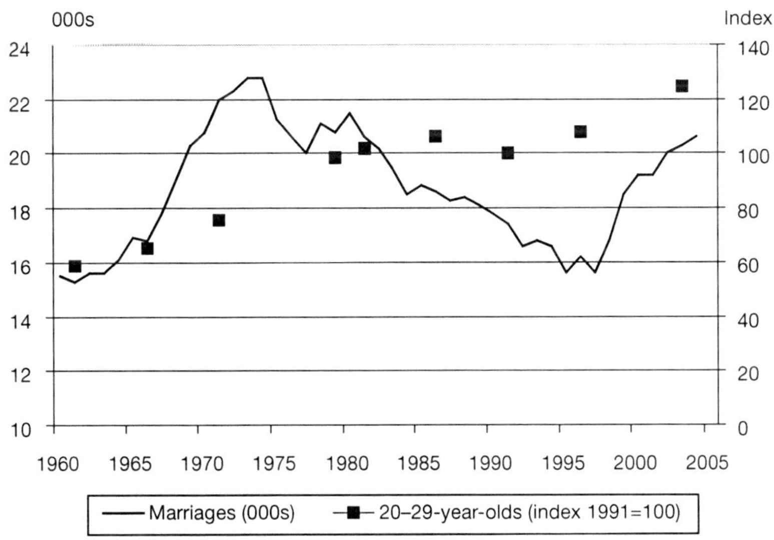

Sources: CSO Vital Statistics, Census of Population

32 per cent more marriages per year than in 1995. Again, as with trends in births in the 1990s, some of this increase was caused by a rise in the size of the relevant age-cohort. But there was also some rise in the propensity of people to marry – the marriage rate among those aged 16–49 rose from 17.7 per 1,000 persons in 1996 to 19.7 in 2002 in the case of males and from 17.8 to 20.2 in the case of females. The rise in marriage rates followed hard on the heels of economic boom and makes it hard to avoid the conclusion that the latter was a major cause of the former.

A number of factors complicate the interpretation of the recent upward trend in marriage. One is the introduction of divorce in 1997, which means that marriages registered after that year could include second marriages (that is, where at least one of the spouses has been married previously). From census data, it would appear that 14,000 people entered second marriages between 1996 and 2002 (see further below). This represents an annual average of some 2,300 marriages of this kind. These marriages amounted to about 12 per cent of the marriages occurring each year over this period, compared to the increase of 30 per cent in the annual number of marriages by 2004 mentioned earlier. It would appear, therefore, that some, but by no means all, of the increase in marriages after 1997 arose from second marriages.

A further feature of the recent increase in marriages is that it is accompanied by a sharp rise in the age of marriage, in contrast to the growing youthfulness of marriage that occurred in the marriage boom of 1965–1974. Average age at marriage rose by about two years in the 1980s but jumped by a further four years between 1990 and 2002, rising to 32.5 years for men and 30 years for women.

Average ages of marriage as high as this had not been seen among men since the 1940s and had never before been recorded among women. This outcome reflected a sharp backing away from marriage among those aged under 30 years during this period: by 2005, as Figure 10.6 shows, 81 per cent of 25–29-year olds were single, which was double the proportion single in that age group in the late 1970s. However, marriages among those aged over 30 increased – for example, the marriage rate among those aged 30–34 almost doubled between 1991 and 2002. This is probably best interpreted as a consequence of catch-up among those who deferred marriage during the 1980s and early 1990s and then crowded into marriage from the mid-1990s onwards. The catch-up achieved was not complete since, as is evident from Figure 10.6, it did not prevent the proportion single among those aged in their 20s and early 30s, which had started to rise in the early 1980s, to continue to rise throughout the 1990s. However, between 2002 and 2005, the increase in singlehood began to slow down and among those aged over 35 actually turned into a decline.

Figure 10.6: *Percentage single* in selected age groups, 1926–2005*

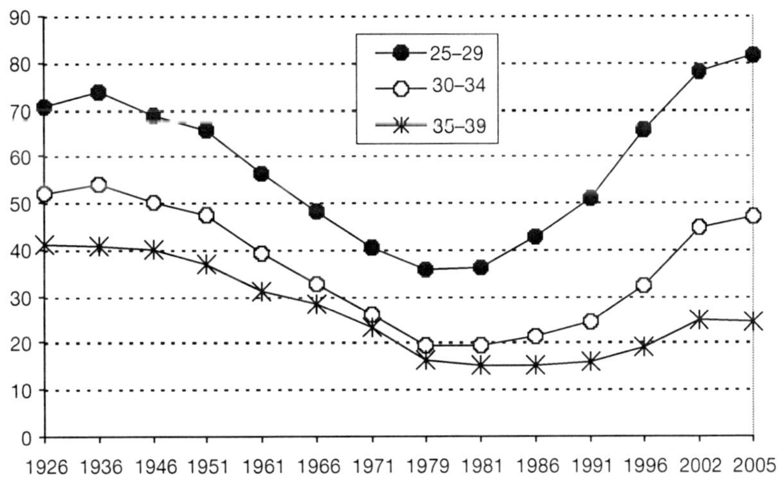

*includes cohabitees who have never been married.
Sources: Censuses of Population 1926–2002, Population and Migration Estimates 2005

Although marriage avoidance among young adults today is as common as it was in the 1930s, it has little of the significance for family formation that it had in the past. Marriage was once the gateway to sex and childbearing but now sexual activity before marriage is accepted as commonplace and, as we saw earlier, almost one-third of births take place outside of marriage. Furthermore, cohabitation has also become an option for young people. The number of cohabiting couples rose from 31,300 in 1996 to 77,600 in 2002, by which time they accounted for 8.4 per cent of all family units. Halpin and O'Donoghue (2004) examined patterns of cohabitation in more detail using panel data for Ireland from the European Community Household Panel Survey. They found that for all the increase in cohabitation, it does not appear to be developing as a long-term alternative to marriage but is most often a temporary arrangement found mainly among young urban adults that either dissolves after a relatively short period or leads on to marriage.

Marital breakdown

If the rate of entry into marriage showed some increase over the past decade, so too did the rate of exit from marriage. The divorce legislation enacted in 1996 is an obvious factor to consider here. In other Western countries, the wave of liberalisation of divorce law that took place in the

1960s and 1970s had been immediately followed by a spike in divorce rates, as the accumulated backlog of broken marriages was cleared, while in the longer-term, rates of marital breakdown moved upwards for an extended period (Goode, 1993). The new provision for divorce in Ireland is on the somewhat restrictive end of the spectrum of what is now available in most Western countries, in that it allows for divorce only after four years of marital breakdown. Yet it is a no-fault system which is part of the general Western pattern of reasonably 'easy' divorce. Consequently, echoing earlier patterns in other countries, one would have expected the arrival of divorce in 1996 to have been followed by a sharp surge in applications for divorce as pent-up demand was released, possibly within a longer trend of rising rates of marital breakdown.

As there was no system of registration of marital breakdowns prior to the advent of divorce, it is not possible to quantify long-term trends in rates of marital breakdown precisely. However, the available evidence suggests that marital breakdown had been increasing slowly in Ireland prior to the introduction of divorce, though on the eve of the advent of divorce those rates would appear to have been relatively low, similar to the levels found in the low-divorce countries of Southern Europe (Fahey and Lyons, 1995). The most informative data on marital breakdown for the pre-divorce era are those provided by census counts of the number of people who are separated, presented either in absolute terms or as a percentage of the ever-married population, and these can be combined with census counts in 2002 to get an impression of the extent of marital breakdown before and after the introduction of divorce (Figures 10.7 and 10.8).

Figure 10.7: *Numbers of divorced, separated and those who re-married following dissolution of marriage, 1986–2002*

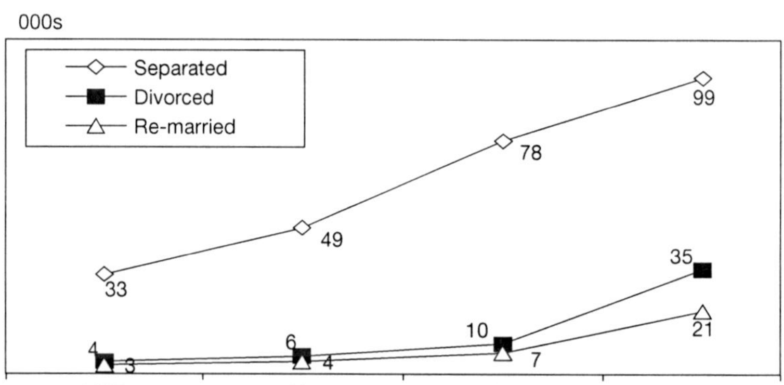

Source: Census of Population

Figure 10.8: *Separated/divorced as a percentage of the ever-married population*

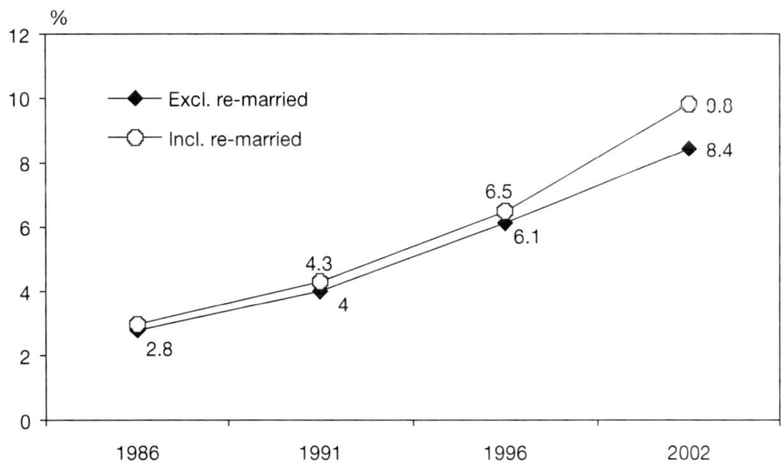

Source: Census of Population

These figures suggest that the numbers who were separated and divorced increased between 1996 and 2002 but not to a degree that would suggest that the introduction of divorce in 1997 had a major impact on trends. The increase in *separated* persons between 1996 and 2002 was of a similar order to that which had occurred in the decade prior to the advent of divorce. The numbers *divorced* showed a bigger relative increase (from 10,000 in 1996 to 35,000 in 2002), but the increase was modest in view of the numbers who were already separated in 1996 (78,000) and would have qualified for divorce by 2002 under the four-year rule. Thus, there was no post-liberalisation spike in the incidence of divorce of the kind found in the liberalisation phases of divorce in other countries. The numbers who had remarried following a previous dissolution of marriage increased by 14,000 between 1996 and 2002, which amounted to an annual average of some 2,300 over the six-year period.

Expressed as a proportion of the ever-married population, the separated and divorced trebled between 1986 and 2002 – rising from 2.8 per cent in 1986 to 8.4 per cent in 2002 when the divorced who remarried are excluded from the count, and from 3 per cent to 9.8 per cent when the latter are included (Figure 10.8). Again however, the rate of increase between 1996 and 2002 was more or less the same as it had been in the previous decade. It should be recalled that these data measure the *stock* of persons whose marriages had dissolved, not the *rate* of marital breakdown.

Since the rate of exit from the stock was modest (as indicated by what appears to be a low rate of remarriage following divorce), much of the increase in the stock can be considered the consequence of an accumulation of people whose marriages had dissolved rather than of an increase in the rate of marital breakdown. Thus, while some increase in the rate of marital breakdown may have occurred, it was likely to be far less than might be inferred from the tripling of the accumulated stock of separated and divorce people that occurred over the period 1986–2002.

A further indication of how the introduction of divorce had less of an impact than might have been expected was the lack of any dramatic shift towards divorce as a way of resolving broken marriages. In the pre-divorce era, judicial separation orders could be obtained from the Circuit Court by separating couples who were able to undertake the slow and costly procedures involved. However, the more common solution was to seek the simpler, quicker and cheaper remedies available in the District Court, such as orders for maintenance, child custody or access to children. There was also a heavy reliance on applications relating to domestic violence, which were the most heavily used family law proceedings of all (Fahey and Lyons, 1995).

Since the advent of divorce, the resources and efficiency of the family courts appear to have improved under the aegis of the Courts Service, an independent State agency set up in 1999 to administer the courts (Courts Service, 2004). However, as Table 10.1 shows, the distribution of family law applications between the District Court and Circuit Court changed little: in 2003, as in 1994, the former exceeded the latter by a ratio of four or five to one. In addition, applications relating to domestic violence continued to be numerically the largest element of the system, though at a somewhat lower percentage of all family law applications in 2003 (34 per cent) compared to 1994 (44 per cent). By 2003, in sum, divorce had acquired an important but in numerical terms still far from dominant place in the system. This adds to the sense that the arrival of divorce in 1996 was not the transformational event that both its proponents and detractors had suggested it would be.

Conclusion

There is a common tendency to marvel at the pace of social change underway in the present, irrespective of how fast or slow it might prove to be in a rigorous comparison with previous experience. This chapter has suggested that the realm of family and sexuality is a case in point: far from being in unprecedented flux, it can reasonably be portrayed as having

Table 10.1: *Family law applications in 1994 and 2003**

	1994	*2003*
District Court	14,274	23,316
Domestic violence**	7,548	9,881
Circuit Court		
Judicial separation	2,806	1,802
Divorce		3,733
Total	17,080	28,851

*Refers to legal years 1993–1994 and 2002–2003
** Barring and protection orders in 1993; barring, protection and safety orders in 2003.
Source: Fahey and Lyons (1995); Courts Service (2004)

settled down somewhat over the past decade, following a period of turmoil and transformation that had extended over the previous three decades. Political controversy on the big 'moral' questions of contraception, divorce and abortion had loomed large in the 1970s, 1980s and early 1990s but faded after the mid-1990s, with the divorce referendum of 1995 marking something of a turning point in this regard. Public opinion largely came to accept a new liberal regime on these and related issues, even though some people were more accepting than others, and on abortion the consensus was less liberal than almost everywhere else in Europe.

Behaviour also continued to evolve in this period but when compared with the lurches of the preceding three decades it too seemed to attain a condition of almost post-revolutionary stability.

The sharp decline in birth rates of the 1980s bottomed out in the early 1990s and stabilised over the following ten years at a level that was low by historical standards but high by comparison with the rest of Europe. A similar decline in marriage rates also bottomed out at around the same time and turned sharply upward, in part caused by catch-up among people who had deferred marriage in the insecure economic conditions of the previous decade. While people in their 20s became increasingly reluctant to marry in this period, in statistical terms echoing patterns last seen in the 1930s and 1940s, they compensated by becoming more likely to marry after the age of 30. They also had access to pre-marital sex, cohabitation and child-bearing outside of marriage to a degree unknown in previous generations. Exits from marriage through separation or divorce also continued to rise but it is striking how moderate the pace of change was. The advent of divorce in 1997 was not followed by a surge of divorce applications and there was a great deal of continuity with the pre-divorce era in the way that couples in conflict made use of family law.

These outcomes suggest, then, that the Celtic Tiger era was less transformational for family and sexual life than the decades that preceded it. What effect it did have seems to have been benign in important ways – economic growth encouraged more marriage, more children and thus, simply, more family, the mirror image of how economic stagnation in the 1980s had done the opposite. These were important benefits of the Celtic Tiger, not just because societies need children but also because most people benefit from the intimacy and security that family life provides. Many have wondered whether the *quality* of family life increased with its quantity, and have pointed to growing marital breakdown and lone parenthood as signs that it did not. However, one can read too much into such signs. Marital breakdown can be interpreted as a consequence of rising expectations for intimacy and affection in marriage – a good thing in itself – rather than as a symptom of decay. Lone parenthood certainly brings certain vulnerabilities, especially if the family income is low, but the increase in this family type has to be set against the decline at the same time of other equally vulnerable family types, such as the poor, two-parent family with six or seven children that was common in the past.

In general, for every new problem in family life that has emerged in recent years one can point to old ones that have faded away. These counterbalancing elements are not easy to weigh against each other, and one cannot definitively say whether the scale is rising or falling. But positive trends are certainly present and make for a strong case that the Celtic Tiger, on balance, was good for family life.

11

Ties that Bind? The Social Fabric of Daily Life in New Suburbs[1]

Mary P. Corcoran, Jane Gray and Michel Peillon

Introduction

The greater Dublin conurbation has now reached the 1.5 million mark. Over the last 15 years, most urban growth has taken place not at the core of the city, but on its periphery. The word 'suburbs' refers to those residential areas that are found around the periphery of urban centres. Suburban residents were previously thought to depend upon the urban core for work, shopping, and recreational and cultural pursuits. But this dependence on a centre is no longer seen as a crucial feature of suburbs. As Figure 11.1 clearly illustrates, Dublin has been characterised by peripheral urban development since the early 1990s. While the Dublin urban core grew only minimally between 1991 and 2002, the city expanded into the hinterland creating new suburban neighbourhoods. The further one travels from the city centre, the more marked this suburban growth.

A negative view of the suburbs infuses the sociological literature and the public imagination. The suburbs are frequently represented as places of homogeneity and uniformity, of stifling conformity, of social atomisation and isolation, of withdrawal from public life into the privacy of domestic life. Indeed, although people move to the suburbs in order to enhance the quality of family life, sociologists and other commentators have portrayed suburbs as negative environments for the family, due to the isolation of the nuclear family from the support that wider kinship networks provide, both in inner city and rural environments. This portrayal of suburban life is found in some of the specialised literature on the subject (for instance, Baumgartner, 1988; Fishman, 1987, and, less directly, Sennett, 1970), but

[1] This chapter is based on data collected for the New Urban Living study which was funded by the Royal Irish Academy, the Katherine Howard Foundation and was facilitated by the granting of consecutive research breaks to the investigators by the National Institute of Regional and Spatial Analysis (NIRSA) NUI Maynooth.

T. Fahey et al. (eds.), Quality of Life in Ireland, 175–197.

Figure 11.1: *Percentage growth of the Dublin population according to mileage radius from city centre, 1991–2002*

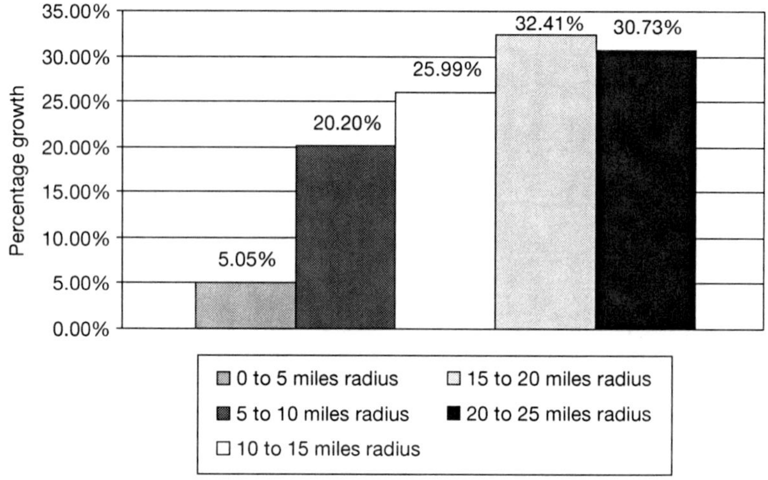

Source: Based on Small Area Population Statistics from the Census of Population 2002 and Ordnance Survey Ireland ED (Electoral Division) boundaries.[2]

this characterisation of suburbs prevails mainly in a range of journal articles and books that touch the topic without engaging with it.

The specialised literature is often more cautious and qualified. Gans' study of the Levittowners (1967) in a sense debunked this portrayal of suburban living, as do essays that query the negative image of suburbs and link it with a rather elitist ideology (Oliver, Davis and Bentley, 1981; Clapson, 2000). Nevertheless, the dominant discourse about suburbs remains negative.

The media have developed an interest in the forms of urban and suburban growth in Dublin, but also in all major Irish cities. They have pointed to the unregulated nature of this suburban sprawl, which seems to run counter to the policy set out in various official documents (e.g. Office of Strategic Planning Guidelines 1999; Department of the Environment

---

2 We wish to thank Mary O'Brien, from the National Institute for Regional and Spatial Analysis at NUI Maynooth, for providing this information. The procedure she devised for making these calculations is as follows: distance buffers were created around a point in the centre of Dublin (approximately the location of O'Connell Bridge) at intervals of 5, 10, 15, 20 and 25 miles. This distance is along straight lines. Population data for the Electoral Divisions whose centroid lies within the buffers were summed to show approximate population within these distances from Dublin city in 1991 and 2002. Any error in the use of the information which was produced in this way is entirely our own responsibility.

and Local Government, 2002). Furthermore, they have highlighted the plight of commuters, who face a long and arduous journey to work every day, which seriously undermines the quality of their lives. Interestingly, Church leaders have also highlighted this theme. Recently, for example, the former Church of Ireland Primate, Dr Robin Eames, expressed misgivings about changing family lives:

> For many people, their recent experiences of 'progress' in Irish society is both dehumanising and demeaning. Too many families struggle with the daily commute to jobs in distant cities. Children are dropped with minders as early as six or seven o'clock in the morning and may not be reunited with parents until 12 hours later. I hear of young mothers whose only waking time with the baby is when the little one wakes crying during the night before a working mother has to stagger back out on the commuter trail at an astonishingly early hour next morning ... [The] last three decades have almost eradicated the old reality of parents, children, grandparents and close relatives all living in sufficient proximity to offer support to one another ... Economic development frequently drives young parents to live at a considerable distance from the family support network as they seek employment or affordable housing. (Eames, 2005, pp. 1–2)

Yet, media reports have recorded the satisfaction that many residents in these distant locations express about their move out of the city and how, despite the many problems and shortcomings encountered, they feel that they belong in the places where they have elected to reside.

This unresolved tension between a denunciation of soulless and alienating suburban locations and an acknowledgement of residents' satisfaction is found, for instance, in the Commuter Counties series, published in *The Irish Times* (from 26 April 2003 to 9 May 2003). Once again, the media have put across a rather negative image of suburbs, even when, in the best of cases, they had to qualify it.

The aim of the New Urban Living study reported on here was to investigate social and civic life in suburban locations across three domains: sense of place and the construction of social identity; family life, including household work strategies and networks of social support in the community; and local participation in social and civic life. Our research strategy was based on a comparative analysis of four different suburbs at contrasting stages of development, and located at different points in relation to the metropolitan core. Ratoath in county Meath provided a good example of a totally new peripheral growth, in a previously rural setting. The new electoral division of Lucan-Esker, sited to the south of Lucan village in South Dublin county, has grown at a staggering rate, in a locality which was already heavily suburbanised. Leixlip offered a counter-case of a suburban neighbourhood that has now aged and stabilised. New estates on the periphery of Mullingar pointed to a new situation, one in which the suburbs of a provincial town may also function as a suburb of the distant metropolis of Dublin.

The study used a range of research methods that combined quantitative and qualitative data. The survey of a representative sample of local residents was conducted in selected estates in each location between summer 2002 and spring 2004, and 200 questionnaires were filled in each place.[3]

Focus groups were organised in each locality involving various categories of local residents: older people's groups, Mother and Toddler groups, sixth-class primary school pupils who were also asked to write an essay on 'The place where I live'. A focus group was also organised in Lucan with an intercultural group. A series of in-depth interviews were conducted as a follow-up to the survey, focusing on selected respondents who actively participated in the collective life of the locality.

Figure 11.2 provides an overview of the profile of the four suburban locations. Around two-thirds of the respondents were aged between 26 and 39 years, with the exception of Leixlip where the large majority of respondents were over 40 years old. While manual workers constituted a small minority in all locations, a majority of respondents were engaged in professional, managerial and technical occupation in Ratoath and to a lesser extent Lucan, with Mullingar following slightly behind. Leixlip once more formed the exception, with a lower class profile.

The vast majority of respondents were married or living as married, but not necessarily in the conventional type of household of two parents with dependent children. Around 76 per cent of respondents did so in Ratoath but only 50 per cent in Lucan (and, not surprisingly, only a minority of 38 per cent in Leixlip). One-third of the respondents lived in a dual-income family in Lucan (28 per cent in Mullingar, 20 per cent in Leixlip and Ratoath). Finally, women's participation to the labour force, both full-time and part-time, was always higher than the national average: marginally so

[3] In each location it was necessary to identify clear parameters for the drawing of the sample. In Ratoath, all new estates in and around the village were included in the sample, but not single homes on outlying access routes to the village. In Leixlip, the village bisects two relatively large suburban settlements known locally as 'The Hill' (Confey) and 'The Far Side'. Our sample was drawn from amongst the estates located on the Far Side, which are located to the west of Leixlip Main Street. In Lucan-Esker, the sample was drawn from a large cluster of recently built estates, on the south of the village immediately beyond the by-pass. In Mullingar, the sample was based on all newly developed estates on the periphery of the town centre.

Figure 11.2: *Age, class and family profile of respondents in the four suburban locations (% in each category)*

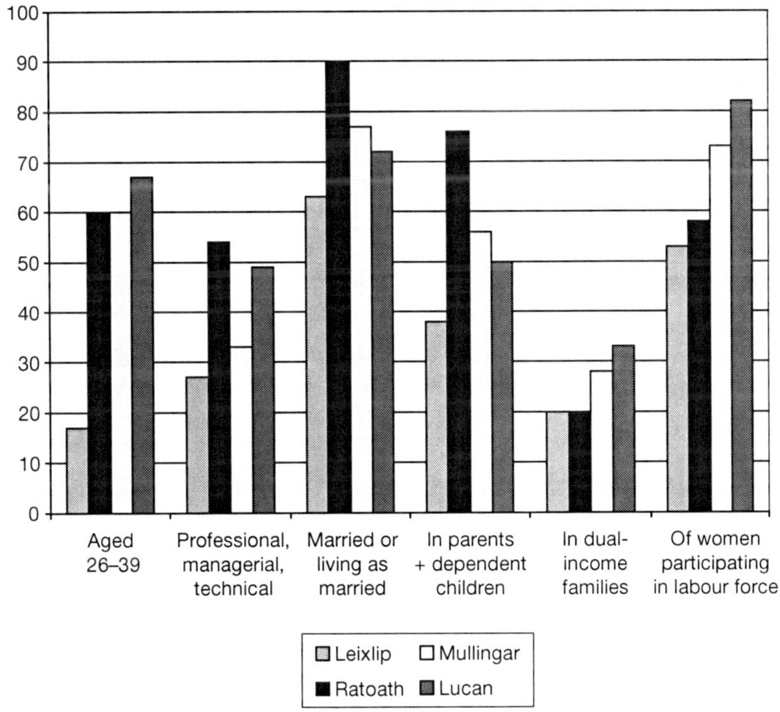

in Leixlip (53 per cent) and Ratoath (58 per cent), but dramatically so in Mullingar (73 per cent) and Lucan (82 per cent). On the whole, Lucan and Mullingar display a rather similar age, class and family profile, which differs significantly from Ratoath (slightly older, higher class, more conventional family pattern) and Leixlip (considerably older, lower class and a more varied family pattern).

The analysis focuses in the first place on the idea of place attachment, and examines the mechanisms that help to generate a sense of belonging among members of a community. It then addresses the issue of whether (or not) suburbs can be deemed to be family-friendly places. It also examines social participation and activism in suburban communities: to what extent has the increasing suburbanisation of Irish society enhanced or diminished the quality of family and civic life?

Against the main thrust of the relevant literature, the study highlights the social embeddedness of suburban residents. Social embeddedness refers to the extent to which residents are anchored in the locality. They are, for instance, inserted in networks of personal support which are locally centred and may participate in the public life of the locality in which they feel they have a stake. The sense of attachment to place depends to a large extent on the presence of friends, kin and good neighbours in the locality. The personal networks of social support are predominantly local and are mobilised in the daily life of suburban families. Social participation too depends on the 'connectedness' between suburban residents, and it enhances it. It is largely through this embeddedness that the quality of life in suburbs is upheld; that residents feel positively about the place where they live; that families find the locality supportive; and that a wide range of services are provided and local concerns addressed.

Suburbanites, however, face many challenges and have only a limited capacity to deal with the issues and problems that confront them. This is not because of a seriously deficient social fabric, but has rather to do with locally weak forms of governance.

Neighbourhood, markers of identity and quality of life

Places that undergo suburbanisation are frequently assumed to lose their distinctiveness, their unique sense of place. Suburbanisation is equated with homogenisation and the destruction of traditional village life and its surrounding countryside. When country fields are redeveloped as up-market suburban outposts; when country villages hum to the sound of juggernauts trundling through; when a provincial town becomes, in the words of the locals, 'a dormitory suburb of Dublin,' the locally rooted sense of place becomes destabilised. People fear that the place is losing something of its character, popular memory and tradition. And yet, the majority of residents who participated in the New Urban Living study across the four different localities felt attached to the place where they lived: 53 per cent of Lucan respondents indicated such an attachment, but the figure rose to 64 per cent in Mullingar, 72 per cent in Leixlip and 79 per cent Ratoath. Suburban living does not preclude the persistence of local attachments based on nurturing personal social relations and familiarity with place.

A number of key themes emerge from the literature as being crucial in establishing a basis for a sense of place or place attachment. These can be summarised as follows: the backdrop of the built and natural environment, the culture of place, 'elective belonging' and associational life. In this section, we examine the extent to which these factors resonate for suburban dwellers in contemporary Ireland, and impact on the quality of their life.

Built and natural environment

Nature, as Molotch, Freudenburg and Paulsen (2000, p. 794) point out, 'both influences and takes on different reality depending on how, as a continuous matter, it lashes up with the other aspects of the local milieu'. Environmental backdrops, both natural and constructed, come to be inscribed in our place consciousness and offer important markers of local identity. In Ratoath respondents identified very specific features that had attracted them to Ratoath as a place to live. The most commonly cited features included the village character, country feel, friendliness and sense of community. This finding was borne out in the qualitative responses in the survey and in the focus group discussions. Ratoath's greenery – the hedges, fields and trees – acted as important signifiers of the countryside and rurality for focus group participants, both young and old. Children remarked that despite all the development, and the fact that a lot of people do not know each other, Ratoath had not lost 'its country look.' Such comments suggest that it is the *aesthetic of rurality* to which people are attached, rather than to the countryside itself. For the reality is that the countryside around Ratoath is under threat from development and that the very reasons that attracted people in the first place are fast disappearing.

Leixlip, a much bigger and longer established suburb, continues to constitute itself as a 'country place.' A number of natural boundaries in the area reinforce the rural village character: the canal, two rivers, a lake and picnic area. One interviewee identified Leixlip as a safe area and 'not just another suburb of Dublin'. The idea of 'the country' exerts a powerful hold over residents in Leixlip as it does in Ratoath. People respond to 'country' signifiers in a very positive way, and associate them with good quality of life. Interestingly, the picture in Mullingar and Lucan where we recorded somewhat lower levels of place attachment, is more nuanced. When thinking about Mullingar as a place to live, 48 per cent of respondents in the new housing estates cited its character as a provincial town, while almost the same proportion (43 per cent) identified it as a modernising town. The town's rural aspect was alluded to by 37 per cent of respondents.

As in Mullingar, the features that people called to mind when thinking about Lucan were somewhat contradictory. Thirty-five per cent of respondents mentioned its 'built-up' character, while 34 per cent also identified the place with 'quietness'. When asked what they most liked about Lucan, survey respondents mentioned its convenience and closeness to Dublin more frequently than any features that inhere in the place itself. In the focus group discussions conducted in Mullingar and Lucan, participants had greater difficulty identifying key features of the physical and social environment which they saw as defining their place. This suggests that the absence of clear environmental signifiers that give definition to place, explains, in some part, the lower levels of place attachment recorded in both Mullingar and Lucan.

The culture of place

Molotch, Freudenburg and Paulsen (2000, p. 792) approached the comparative analysis of localities in Southern California by focusing on the twin notions of character and tradition as ways of accessing the idea of place distinctiveness. Our unique, human responses to places and the associations they carry in terms of memories and fantasies, are at the roots of attachment. We found evidence of an embedded 'structure of feeling' in our study of suburbia in Ratoath and Leixlip, the places where we recorded the highest levels of place attachment. Here we give two examples of how this structure of feeling comes into being. The first example demonstrates the importance of 'local character' to place definition, and the second demonstrates the legacy of 'tradition' which allows the past to resonate in the present.

According to one informant, the character and tradition of Leixlip are based around the old nucleus of the village which provides the common ground for the communities that have grown up around it, Leixlip and Confey. Identity is derived from the history and old structures of the place as well as the newer initiatives, such as the GAA and other activity-based clubs. The Leixlip festival, held in June every year since 1990, provides an important focal point that mobilises the entire community. History walks organised by a local historian 'attract a lot of people who have come to consciously seek out identity markers' (key informant interview).

In the case of Ratoath, older residents reported that the proximity of Fairyhouse to the village has historically been an important symbol for the area. The racecourse is an important source of identity and pride for the community generally. Historically, Grand National Day (Easter Sunday) was known as 'the day of the year'. People would whitewash their houses in acknowledgement of, and participation in, the event. They conceded that the frequency of race meetings at Fairyhouse has lessened their significance as a major day of celebration and pride for the local community today (Active Age focus group, Ratoath). Nevertheless, the 'Fairyhouse factor' continues to have currency locally.

Elective belonging

In three of our four case studies (Mullingar being the exception), the majority of people interviewed had moved from the Dublin metropolitan area to the suburb. Respondents living in the community for even a relatively short period of time felt a strong identification with place. The vast majority of respondents intended to live there for the foreseeable future. They are neither locals nor transients who remain disinterested and detached. They know what they like about the place where they live, and equally they know what they dislike. Our findings seem to suggest that the process of becoming attached to place is bound up with what Savage, Bagnall and Longhurst (2005) have termed 'elective belonging', whereby individuals *choose* to live in a particular locale. The aggregate effect of many individual families choosing to live in a place like Ratoath reinforces a strong sense of place attachment and contributes to a feeling that the place offers good quality of life. On the other hand, in Lucan, where the decision to locate is more connected to affordability than place signifiers per se, there is a weaker sense of place attachment. Our findings are commensurate with those of Savage, Bagnall and Longhurst (2005, p. 45) who conclude that 'those who have an account of why they live in a place, and can relate their residence to their choices and circumstances, are the most "at home"'.

Informal associational life

It has been argued that the existence of associational life in the form of interactions, personal relations and institutional practices at the level of locality are crucial to place attachment (Simonsen, 1997, p. 172). Furthermore, the existence of community voluntary associations are significant not only as integrating mechanisms that cover a range of fields of activity, but because 'they harbour "memory traces" through which something like a social structure can transpose itself from one time or institutional realm to the next' (Molotch, Freudenburg and Paulsen, 2000, p. 794).

In all four localities, the extent to which residents are socially embedded is suggested by the range and nature of the personal networks of social support. We asked our respondents to indicate those people they turn to when they need some help or face a range of personal problems. We generated in that way a list of people who matter personally to them. Respondents were allowed to list up to 12 people. The size of such networks does not vary greatly on average between the four locations, with just over five ties per respondent. But the networks display considerable variation in relation to their composition. Work colleagues never figure prominently in such networks, while the relative importance of kin, friends and neighbours is subject to significant variations.

Kin predominates in the personal networks in two of the locations investigated (Lucan and Mullingar), while neighbours represent the dominant element in the other two suburbs (Leixlip and Ratoath). Friends are never the predominant element, but they figure in second place in three cases. Such networks may also vary according to the extent to which the

Figure 11.3: *Distribution of types of network ties*

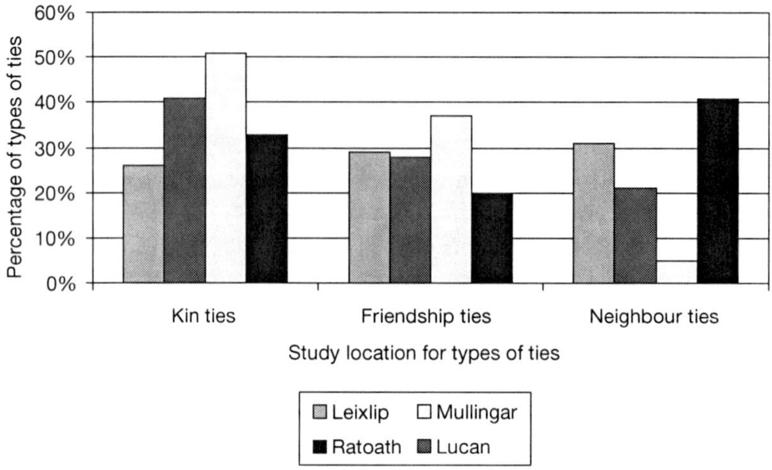

'ties' live locally. Personal networks of social support are highly localised in Leixlip and Mullingar (with around three-quarters of the ties residing in the locality), and less so in Ratoath and Lucan. Generally speaking, we found a significant relationship between having local and neighbourly ties, and feeling a sense of attachment and belonging to place.

The survey findings were confirmed in our analysis of focus group transcripts. Children, adults and older people consulted in each locality were generally able to provide many and varied testimonies of neighbourliness. We recognise, however, that neighbourliness is not uniformly distributed across the four localities. Furthermore, many people with whom we spoke worried about the impact of time, or the lack of time, on the quality of life in their neighbourhoods. In Mullingar, some respondents regretted that 'Nobody stops to talk after mass' (Mullingar 1428 Club). Another respondent in Lucan could see that the kind of neighbourliness that was second nature to her in her well-established estate, was patently absent from the new estate on which her daughter lives:

> There's the old Lucan and then there's the new Lucan. I have a daughter living in the new Lucan and she doesn't know her neighbours and we know her neighbours because we cut her grass. We know about three or four of her neighbours. I'd say to her in the evenings, you should get out to cut the grass, there's a lovely chap next door and he works in Baggot Street and he's an accountant and you should get to know him but she

> just doesn't. It's a new estate, but she just doesn't seem to have any interest in getting to know the neighbours (University of the Third Age focus group, Lucan).

Attachment to place appears, at least in part, to be a function of the particular qualities of a place as well as the strength of ties that have developed in the locality and how long a person has lived there. The picture presented in the four localities under investigation is suggestive not of anomie and alienation but of supportive ties and bonds. While the overall portrait of associational life is a dynamic and vibrant one, we cannot discount the expressions of concern by several respondents about its long-term sustainability. The possibility of disengagement or of withdrawal from locally based associational networks – through, for example, difficulties in renewing the leadership of local voluntary associations – could affect sense of place and quality of life.

Family-friendly communities?

Two-parent families with young children comprised 50 per cent or more of all households in the samples from the three suburban localities characterised by rapid growth (or continued growth) during the Celtic Tiger years, namely, Ratoath, Lucan-Esker and the new estates around Mullingar town. Leixlip, by contrast, is a well-established suburb, and two-parent families with young children make up only a small proportion (16 per cent) of all households in our sample. Because of this distinct family life-stage profile, discussion of Leixlip is omitted from this section of the chapter.

Historical and sociological research has linked suburbanisation to the emergence of the conjugal family ideal in the first half of the twentieth century, and to its democratisation in the period following the Second World War (Clapson, 2000, pp. 157–9; Miller, 1995). This ideal emphasised close and companionate relationships amongst married couples and their children, and the liberation of the nuclear family unit from obligations towards the wider kinship group (Goode, 1963). It was also strongly associated with the 'breadwinner' ideal whereby men, through their participation in the labour market, met the family's 'instrumental' needs and women, as full-time homemakers, met its 'expressive' needs (Parsons and Bales, 1955). Similar to British studies from the same period, Humphries' (1966) ethnographic account of 'New Dubliners' in the 1950s associated urban living with a more democratic pattern of family life, and with a 'breadwinner' household strategy.

Despite the increased labour force participation of married women with young children in Ireland, our research indicates that providing a better environment for family life still governs people's decision to move to the suburbs. As one of our Ratoath respondents put it:

> [C]ity living is wonderful at a particular stage in life for me. Like, once we had the children we reckoned that we needed more space. We needed companionship for them. You couldn't let them out. You couldn't, like … nothing like that. You just needed a little bit more … ehm … family life, if that's what you want to term it. (In-depth personal interview)

Even though people move to the suburbs in order to enhance the quality of family life, sociologists – and other commentators – have often portrayed suburbs as negative environments for families, due to the isolation of the conjugal unit from the social support networks – rooted in extended kinship ties – that were found in both inner-city and rural environments.[4] Consistent with this image, Humphries found that those 'New Dubliners' living in more recently developed housing estates in then suburban areas like Drimnagh, Kilmainham and Inchicore, had more formal and less frequent interactions with their neighbours than those living in older, inner-city neighbourhoods. Neighbours were considerably less likely to assist one another in times of crisis. The greater social distance between families in the new neighbourhoods was attributed by Humphries' respondents to their newness, size and, interestingly, to the diversity of people's social backgrounds.

Somewhat different findings emerged from Gordon's (1977) research in two Cork districts – one an urban working-class area and the other a middle-class suburb – carried out in the early 1970s. He found that while respondents in lower occupational prestige groups did report larger numbers of primary kin living in Cork, respondents in higher occupational prestige groups (presumably living in the middle-class suburb) drew greater numbers of non-kin into the circle of people to whom they felt close, irrespective of the number of primary kin available to them. This finding is consistent with other research showing that, over time, suburban residents develop networks of social support amongst friends and neighbours that compensate for their reduced access to extended kin (Wilmott and Young, 1960; see also Phillipson et al., 1999). However, recent scholarship on the theme of 'social capital' has reinvigorated the negative sociological depiction of suburbs, arguing that the growing

---

4 Young and Wilmott (1957) provided a classic account.

prevalence of time-poor dual-earner families leads to reduced levels of interaction amongst neighbours and less civic engagement in suburban communities (Coleman, 1987; Putnam, 2000). According to Miller (1995, p. 413) this trend is further reinforced by the lack of public spaces in suburbs, and by the ubiquitousness of the car.

To what extent are young families in growing Irish suburbs embedded in networks of social support beyond the conjugal family household? In our study, married respondents with children named an average of just over five ties in each study area.[5] Figure 11.4 shows the average number of local ties named, by type of support received. (Note that each tie named could provide more than one type of support.) Respondents in the Mullingar estates named significantly more local ties than did respondents in either Ratoath or Lucan. In relation to practical forms of everyday support, such as helping with childcare, and at times of sickness, the greater number of local ties available to Mullingar respondents is statistically significant when compared to Lucan. Lucan respondents can call on fewer local people for lending or borrowing an item compared to respondents in either Mullingar or Ratoath.

Figure 11.4: *Number of local ties, by support provided (married respondents with children)*

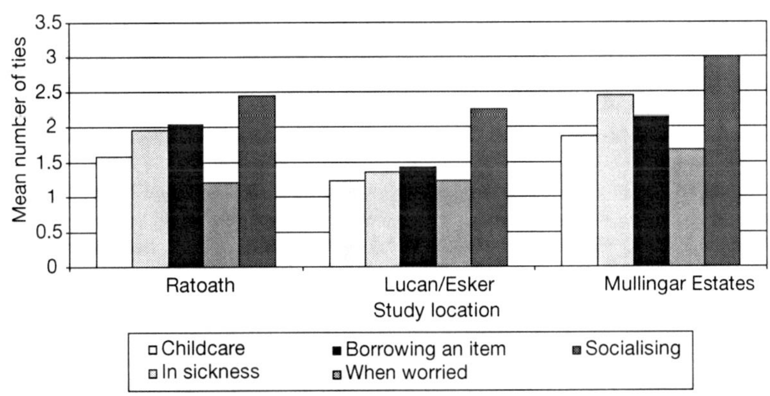

The three suburban locations also differed in terms of the composition of respondents' networks. This can be examined by distinguishing between four main types of tie: local friends and neighbours; not local friends; local family; not local family.[6] Figure 11.5 shows that contrary to the most

---

[5] Throughout this section, the findings refer to married (or living-as-married) respondents with children, unless otherwise stated.

[6] The number of other ties mentioned, such as work colleagues, was negligible.

negative depictions of suburban life, local friends and neighbours constituted the single largest category of ties in both Ratoath and Lucan. Amongst married respondents with children, they comprised 50 per cent of all ties, and 59 per cent of frequently visited ties in Ratoath. They comprised 39 per cent of all ties, and 42 per cent of all frequently visited ties in Lucan-Esker. In the Mullingar estates, local family comprised the largest proportion of ties named (39 per cent), but local friends and neighbours comprised the greatest proportion of frequently visited ties (45 per cent). There is evidence, therefore, that in each of our three suburban localities, couples with young children are embedded in local networks of everyday social support.

Figure 11.5: *Number of ties, by type of relationship (married respondents with children)*

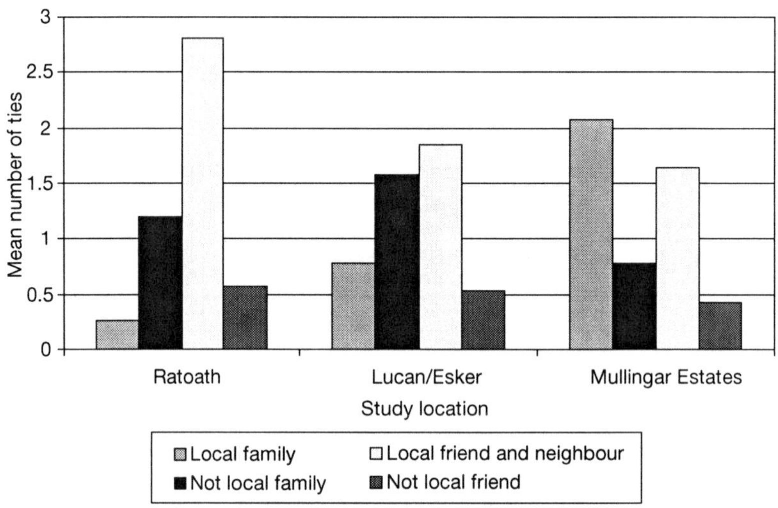

Some of the differences between our three suburban cases can be explained by differences in their demographic composition. Amongst married couples, those with primary school age children predominate in Ratoath, in contrast to Lucan-Esker and the Mullingar estates, where couples without children are more prevalent. When we examine variation in the composition of ties by family life stage, we find that, in all three cases, there is a statistically significant difference in the number of non-local friends named by those whose youngest child is of preschool age, compared to those whose youngest child is of primary school age.

As Figure 11.6 illustrates, local friends and neighbours comprise a greater proportion of all network ties amongst those married parents whose youngest child is of primary school age in all three cases, although the difference is not statistically significant in the case of Lucan. Nonetheless, there does appear to be a general tendency for people to increase their reliance on local non-family ties as their children grow older. As one Ratoath resident commented in a focus group discussion: 'Kids make you settle in more.' This finding is consistent with international research on social networks across the family life course (Ishii-Kuntz and Seccombe, 1989).

Figure 11.6: *Local friends and neighbours as a percentage of all social ties, by family life stage (married respondents with children)*

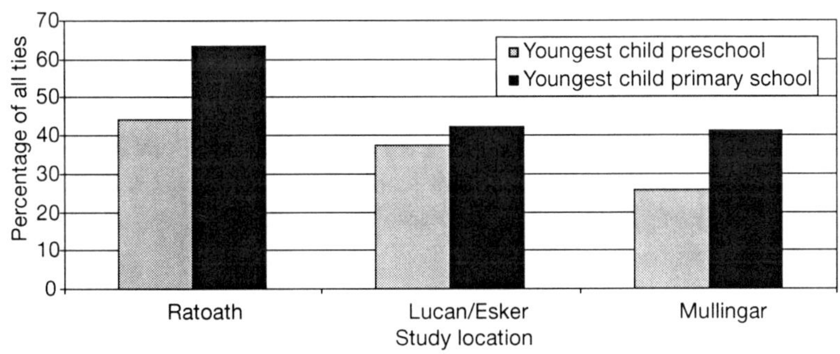

While some of the differences between the three locations are attributable to their demographic composition, this cannot explain all of the variation. Respondents in Ratoath named a greater proportion of local friends and neighbours in their networks of social support at each family life stage. When we examine variations by family life stage in the composition of frequently visited ties, the differences between our suburban cases are highlighted further. There is a pronounced increase in the intensity of interaction with local friends and neighbours in Ratoath, as children reach primary school age: they comprise 74 per cent of all frequently visited ties, compared to just over half amongst those married respondents whose youngest children are of preschool age. In Lucan, by contrast, the increased share of friends and neighbours amongst the frequently visited ties of parents of primary school children is not statistically significant, but the reduced share of both non-local friends and non-local family is significant. This suggests that, on average, in Lucan-Esker married parents reduce their contact with non-local ties as children grow older, but do not significantly increase the intensity of their interaction with local friends and neighbours. In Mullingar, strikingly, there is no significant difference in the intensity of interaction with local friends and neighbours by family life stage. The new Mullingar estates are distinctive in the extent to which many residents who live there are able to draw on continued support from family ties in the local area. This means that while they develop more ties with friends and neighbours as their children grow older, these relationships are probably not as significant from the perspective of social support as those in Ratoath and Lucan-Esker.

In both Ratoath and Lucan-Esker, parents of very young children – those whose main sources of social support lie outside the locality – are less likely to say they are 'attached' or 'very attached' to the suburb where they live than those who have children that have reached primary school age (see Table 11.1). For residents of Ratoath and Lucan-Esker at this life stage, Dr Eames' depiction of economic development separating young families from the social support provided by wider kin might have some resonance. However, our research suggests that, as children grow older, their parents develop local support networks with friends and neighbours. Nonetheless, close examination of the composition of social networks by family life stage has shown that there are differences between Ratoath and Lucan that cannot be attributed solely to variations at the level of individuals and households.

Table 11.1: *Married (or living as married) respondents who were 'attached' or 'very attached' to the place where they live, by family life stage*

	Ratoath		*Lucan-Esker*		*Mullingar*	
	N	*% attached*	*N*	*% attached*	*N*	*% attached*
No kids	35	74	46	67	47	64
Preschool only	43	65	40	43	40	65
Primary and below	66	88	40	63	36	69
Secondary and below	34	79	13	77	24	79
Total	178	78	139	59	147	68

Research from the US suggests that residents are more likely to describe their communities as 'family-friendly' or 'caring' when there is a high proportion of families at a similar life stage (Swisher, Sweet and Moen, 2004), or when there are high proportions of homemakers (Bould, 2003). Both characteristics seem to improve the quality of interaction amongst friends and neighbours in the community.

We have already seen that Ratoath has a high proportion of families with primary school age children. While there is evidence that, in all three locations, married women 'scale back' their work commitments – becoming part-time employees or full-time homemakers – as children reach primary school age, in Ratoath more women scale back earlier and to a greater extent. Given its demographic composition, this means that fully one-third of households in our Ratoath sample have a 'breadwinner–homemaker' arrangement, compared to 16 per cent of all households in Lucan-Esker, and 17 per cent in the Mullingar estates. Thus it seems likely that certain characteristics of Ratoath as a suburb – including 'life stage community fit' and the greater presence of homemakers in the community – explain the greater degree of attachment to place and local social embeddedness of married parents in this suburban locality.

So, are the new Irish suburbs 'family-friendly' in terms of the availability of social support to couples with young children? Our research suggests that it depends, both on family life stage, and the social composition of the suburb itself. Those factors that appear to make Ratoath the most 'family-friendly' suburb of the three cases considered here might not be either replicable across other suburbs, or necessarily desirable. It seems likely that the high proportions of professional and managerial occupations in Ratoath facilitate the extent of 'scaling back' of married couples with children. Moreover, as Bould (2003) observed, high proportions of homemakers may have positive consequences for social capital in the community, but negative consequences for the human capital of the individual women involved. Our study suggests that negative sociological depictions of family life in the suburbs are unwarranted, in the main.

However, in the absence of social supports to replace distant family members, some suburbs, such as Lucan-Esker, may be relatively unfriendly places for couples with very young children. Paradoxically, the availability of family support nearby, as in the Mullingar estates, may inhibit the development of dense networks of friends and neighbours amongst families with young children.

Social participation

'A successful city neighbourhood is a place that keeps sufficiently abreast of its problems so it is not destroyed by them. An unsuccessful neighbourhood is a place that is overwhelmed by its defects and problems and is progressively more helpless before them' (Jacobs, 1993, p. 146). This statement by Jane Jacobs points to a central element of what can be termed the sustainability of a 'neighbourhood', and it applies to suburban localities as well as urban districts. The extent of social participation gives an indication of the capacity of local residents to come together and address the problems they face. In the absence of prior relevant studies, we are not in a position to determine if new suburbs generate more or less social participation than rural or urban areas. Nevertheless, against the dominant perception of suburbs as soulless sprawls where residents lead a thoroughly privatised and isolated life, our study of four suburban locations should help us determine if the suburbs that are emerging around the major cities in Ireland can sustain a significant level of social participation.

An indication of the extent of social participation is often given by the propensity of individuals to engage in voluntary activity and also by membership in voluntary organisations. The Survey of Social Capital, 2002, recorded an overall 17.1 per cent rate of volunteering (National and Social Economic Forum 2002). The National College of Ireland survey registered a decline in volunteering from 39 per cent in 1992 (Ruddle and O'Connor, 1993) to 33 per cent in 1998 (Ruddle, 1999). By contrast, the European Values Study found an increase in the number of individuals doing unpaid work for an organisation: from 27 per cent in 1990 to 33 per cent in 1999. Furthermore, in 1999, 57 per cent of Irish respondents were members of at least one voluntary association; this figure represented a significant increase from 1990, when 49 per cent of respondents in the representative sample had stated such a membership (Fahey, Hayes and Sinnott, 2005, p. 182).

These figures provide a rough point of comparison for our study of the four suburban locations. We did not seek information about volunteering as such and the extent of social participation was measured in our study by the level of membership in local voluntary associations. The emphasis was placed on membership of local organisations, or at least associations operating in the locality. This implies that our figures cannot be compared with the findings of the other surveys mentioned. Keeping this point in mind, the figures for the four suburban locations appear significantly lower than those recorded in national surveys. They range from 31 per cent of Lucan respondents claiming membership of local voluntary associations, to 34 per cent in Ratoath, 40 per cent in Mullingar and 48 per cent in Leixlip. In the four locations, a majority of respondents stated no membership; but the level of social participation varies greatly. Such a result signals that suburbs are not uniform, and different new suburbs experience different levels of social participation.

Respondents were asked to indicate the organisations to which they belonged and state the main purpose of such associations (sport, quality of local life, leisure, local problems, etc.). These organisations were then assigned to two broad categories: those involved in providing a service (leisure, sport, personal support, etc.) and those dealing with local civic issues (e.g. Lucan Together for Quality of Life, Tidy Towns, Ratoath Combined Residents' Association). Figure 11.7 gives an overview of the distribution of this membership.

Figure 11.7: *Membership by types of voluntary associations*

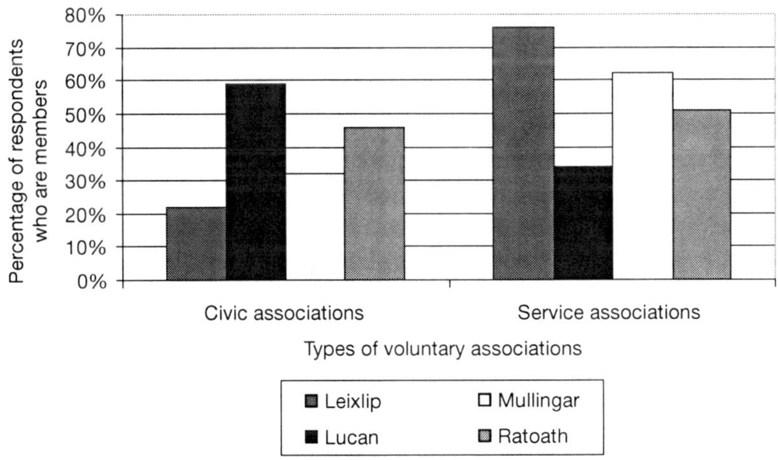

Figure 11.7 registers the fact that the type of membership in local organisations also varies greatly. The full scope of this variation is actually hidden by these figures, and it came to the fore mainly through in-depth interviews. In Ratoath, membership in sport–leisure associations predominates and it involves residents performing a range of services: for instance, the GAA and soccer clubs, mainly meant for children, are thriving. Parents take turns to drive the children to various events. One finds a similar preponderance of membership in recreational and service-oriented associations in Mullingar, as residents in the new suburbs continue to join the established local clubs and associations that have long provided a range of services and leisure activities. In Leixlip, the GAA club is also thriving and enjoys a very high membership. However, many respondents indicated that their GAA membership applied only to bar-membership. It turned out that around 3,000 Leixlip residents have availed of such bar-membership of the GAA club, which in this context becomes a meeting point and a place of sociability. Lucan residents display a low level of membership in local voluntary organisations and, quite crucially, they are more inclined to join organisations that address the many issues faced by the locality.

The variation in the level of membership of voluntary associations has long been debated in terms of the very nature of urban/suburban life. Two models of interpretation compete in this context. One, which derives more or less directly from Wirth's early characterisation of urban life, asserts that urban residents join voluntary organisations in order to overcome the loneliness and general alienation of urban life: they compensate for the loss of primary ties by multiplying secondary ties (Wirth, 1938). As opposed to such a perspective, analysts working in a social network perspective emphasise that joining local organisations and volunteering for various activities is firmly rooted in social networks (for example, Gould, 1993; McAdam and Paulsen, 1993; Oliver, 1984). Residents who are already part of networks join voluntary organisations, not those who are isolated. In Ratoath, social participation is clearly associated with the inclusion of residents within social networks, particularly networks which are locally centred. Inclusion in networks of personal support, and particularly local ties within them, also greatly matters for membership in voluntary associations in Leixlip and Mullingar. Social embedding emerges as the main explanation accounting for the level of membership in local voluntary organisations and of social participation in general.

Social participation is generally seen as closely associated with the quality of life in the neighbourhood. For some, voluntary organisations emerge when concern arises about the state of the neighbourhood (Crenson, 1978), and local residents come together to address the problem. Membership of voluntary associations constitutes the main mechanism through which individuals become integrated in the local neighbourhood (McPherson, 1981). Social participation also produces a sense of empowerment, a collective capacity to deal effectively with problems (Taub et al., 1977). The well-being of the group, and of individuals within it, is not only served through the civic engagement of local residents pursuing a shared goal. In most of the suburban locations we surveyed, the link between social participation and quality of life appears more direct. Many of the voluntary associations, and much of the membership registered in these locations, are involved in the production of services, mainly, but not exclusively, services which are directed at children and, more generally, services which relate to recreation, leisure and sociability, and personal support. The availability of such services is crucial to the quality of life of residents.

Another aspect of social participation, perhaps more significant when it comes to assessing if a suburban neighbourhood can be deemed sustainable or successful, relates to the extent to which it can in some way address the problems it faces. Do suburbs generate and sustain a sufficient level of activism? Most respondents in our surveys clearly identified the main problems facing the locality. They were also asked if they had done anything in the locality to address these local problems. Even minimal action, such as talking to a local politician, was deemed to constitute activity, and consequently 'activism'. The latter could of course cover a wide range of activities: signing a petition, supporting a media campaign, participating in a protest rally, etc. The proportion of respondents who had engaged at any time in a form of action relating to local issues varies quite considerably: 18 per cent in Mullingar, 25 per cent in Leixlip, 47 per cent in Lucan and 51 per cent in Ratoath.

These figures are surprisingly high, if one compares them to the findings of the NESF Survey of Social Capital (2003) which recorded that 21.7 per cent of respondents in their representative sample had been actively involved in the locality. The difference may be accounted for in terms of the context in which the set of relevant questions was asked. In our study, the question was raised at the end of a progressive build-up. It came after questions focusing on local issues and problems, the awareness of respondents of what had been done to address such problems and, then, the query about what they themselves had done, if anything at all. Very minimal level of activity (such as mentioning it to canvassing local politicians) was coded as activity.

Local activism in the four locations we studied rarely took the form of public protests; nonetheless, local action has become an important source of protest in Ireland today. Local residents did not constitute a central category of protesters in the early 1970s: about 10 per cent of recorded protests originated in this category (while employees were involved in half the total number of protests). By the mid-1990s, local residents were the instigators of around 30 per cent of all protests and formed, by far, the largest category of protesters. In 2002, close to 20 per cent of protests were initiated by local residents and were mostly triggered by what was perceived as neglect from relevant authorities (state of roads, condition of schools), threats to the quality of life in the locality, protection of local heritage and also action to keep undesirable groups or services out.

Local activism, as we have defined it, is usually of a limited nature and rarely requires membership of voluntary associations or sustained engagement. Nevertheless, some residents are involved in the public life of the locality in a more sustained way, and this usually implies membership and active participation in voluntary associations. They volunteer for positions within associations and commit some of their time and energy to help these organisations perform their function. But even this kind of local activism appears to be quite a complex and varied phenomenon. A series of in-depth interviews was conducted with some actively engaged respondents. They revealed the diversity and complexity of local activism. Suburban local life is animated by very different kinds of local activists. Suburbs continue to exhibit the kinds of activism (political, GAA) that have long been a feature of public life in Ireland, but they also uphold types of activism (such as activism oriented toward the provision of services or the maintenance of the estate) that help to shape the social fabric of the new suburban neighbourhoods.

Conclusion

The accelerated suburbanisation of Ireland is one of the key legacies of the Celtic Tiger. Population growth and a robust economy have contributed to an unprecedented demand for housing. Suburban expansion, particularly on the periphery of large cities, has been largely developer-driven, leading to concerns about the viability and sustainability of these communities in the long term. Our investigation of four such suburban localities presents a picture that is much less bleak than that which fuels the popular imagination. Generally speaking, our respondents 'electively belonged' to their communities – they felt attached to the place where they lived. People still saw the suburbs as good places to raise children. They derived sustenance from close relations with others, particularly those who were at similar stages of family formation. Finally, our research suggests relatively modest but not negligible levels of social and civic participation. In all these respects, local residents are socially embedded in their respective localities. Such a conclusion goes against the dominant perception of suburbs.

The findings from the four suburban locations did not register a fundamentally deficient social fabric. Nonetheless, the very intensity of suburban development creates its own difficulties. The built and natural environment, which acts as an important signifier of place, may be obliterated by development that proceeds unabated, and attachment to place may be undermined. The family-friendliness of suburbs appears to be linked to a pattern of demographic homogeneity that marginalises those at different family stages, while reinforcing traditional gender roles. Furthermore, such suburbs face immediate and pressing problems that have a negative effect on the quality of life of local residents. The latter clearly identified the main problems they faced in the locality: these related mainly to the unregulated nature of development, the lack of a range of basic amenities, the school situation, heavy traffic on inadequate roads, etc. Although many residents stated that they had done something to address these problems, they were also aware of the ineffectiveness of their action. Local residents in the suburbs found it difficult to deal collectively with the many problems they faced. The lack of institutions of local government at neighbourhood level meant that they were struggling in their efforts at managing their own local affairs. Local residents encountered an institutional void, which they found difficult to overcome despite their best efforts (Peillon, Corcoran and Gray, 2006). So, while there are many ties that bind in suburbia, those ties are in danger of being eroded by the intensification of development and its attendant problems on the one hand, and the absence of locally embedded institutional structures for responding to community needs on the other.

12

Gender, Work–Life Balance and Quality of Life

Frances McGinnity, Helen Russell and Emer Smyth

Introduction

The past 15 years have seen dramatic changes in women's lives, with much greater numbers in paid work, often combining this work with childcare and other responsibilities. Undoubtedly, having jobs has improved women's lives in many ways, raising their living standards and giving them greater economic independence. However, there may be a downside to these gains: women's quality of life may be under pressure and they may be subject to new forms of gender inequality. If more work for women outside the home is not accompanied by a fairer share-out of work within the home, women can end up with a double burden of paid and unpaid work. If adequate childcare and other family supports are not provided, family life can come under stress and conflicts can arise between the demands of work and home. This chapter examines the extent to which the increasing involvement of women in paid work has created new tensions for families and assesses whether these new conflicts cancel out the advantages for women of increased employment opportunities.

The first section of this chapter explores recent trends in labour market behaviour among both women and men. It outlines changes in the level of employment, and the quality of employment in terms of pay, job characteristics and occupational segregation by gender. Such changes are placed in the context of parallel trends in gender role attitudes. The second section examines the time allocation of men and women within households to paid work, unpaid work and leisure. The third section examines the consequences of labour market changes and the gender division of labour for quality of life among women and men. Quality of life is assessed in relation to two main dimensions: work–life tensions and life satisfaction. We explore whether these dimensions are affected by different working arrangements (e.g. dual v. single earner) and differing degrees of involvement of women in paid employment.

T. Fahey et al. (eds.), Quality of Life in Ireland, 199–215.

Trends in labour market behaviour among women and men

Changes in the level of employment

The period since the early 1990s has seen dramatic changes in the nature of women's labour force participation in the Irish context.[1] Between 1993 and 2004, the proportion of women aged 15 to 64 in paid employment increased from 39 to 57 per cent (see Chapter 4, Table 4.1), while the proportion of women at work increased from 38 per cent to 56 per cent over the same period. This represents an extra 352,000 women in paid work by 2004. Changes in labour force participation rates were much more marked among women than men, although male rates also increased somewhat. Reflecting the reduction in unemployment rates, however, the proportion of men actually at work increased significantly, from 64 per cent in 1993 to 76 per cent in 2004. By 2004, male employment rates were higher in Ireland than for the EU as a whole, while female rates were around the EU average. Overall, the gender gap in participation and employment in Ireland narrowed markedly from the early 1990s onwards, though significant differences remain.

Changes in the level of women's involvement in paid employment have not reduced the gender gap in the intensity of such involvement, that is, in the hours of work entailed. Among women, part-time employment grew somewhat faster than full-time employment over the period 1997 to 2005, and by 2005, almost one-third of all women in employment held part-time jobs (CSO, 2005a). On average, women tend to work shorter hours than their male counterparts, 31.7 hours per week compared with 41.1 for men in 2005, although there has been a long-term decline in average hours for both men and women (CSO, 2005a). Women are more likely than men to work fewer than 30 hours per week, a difference that applies controlling for marital status: 22 per cent of single women work fewer than 30 hours per week compared with 8 per cent of single men, while 42 per cent of married women do so compared with only 4 per cent of married men.

Increased employment has not occurred equally for all groups of women but varies by age group and marital status. Participation is highest among women aged 25 to 34 years of age (at 77 per cent) but a majority of women aged 20 to 54 are in the labour force. Around half of all married women are in the labour force compared to 60 per cent of single and separated/divorced women. Involvement in paid work also varies significantly by childcare responsibilities. Among women aged 20–44, those without children are the group most likely to be in employment (at

---

[1] A broader discussion of labour market trends is given in Chapter 4.

85 per cent) and those with a pre-school child are least likely to be in paid employment (at 55 per cent). However, it is worth noting that the majority of mothers are now working outside the home (CSO, 2005a), which represents a very different pattern from that of 15 years ago, though maternal employment rates are lower than in many other European countries. Looking at the dynamics of moving from full-time home duties to paid employment in the late 1990s, certain groups of women were more likely to make this transition than others. In particular, younger women with higher levels of education, those without pre-school children and those who had more recently been in employment were more likely to go back to work after being out of the labour market than other groups of women (Russell et al., 2002).

Rising employment levels among both women and men have had a number of consequences for quality of life among households. They have directly contributed to rising income and material living standards within families as well as providing greater financial independence for women. Data from 1996 indicated that the average contribution of the female partner to household income was 39 per cent for full-time workers and 20 per cent for part-time workers. The contribution of women to household income varies across different kinds of families, being highest for younger couples, those with no children, and those with higher levels of education and income. Although women contribute less to household income than men on average, their income can be crucial in determining the overall living standards of households; 30 per cent of households were found to be below the relative income poverty line before taking account of women's income but this dropped to 13 per cent when the female contribution was taken into account (Maître, Whelan and Nolan, 2003). While no more recent data are available, rising female employment levels mean that the female contribution to household income is likely to have increased since the mid-1990s.

Labour market trends have also had implications for the extent to which paid employment is concentrated in certain kinds of households. Between 1994 and 2000, the proportion of workless households (that is, those with no adults in paid employment) among working age households declined while the share of households where all adults work grew significantly. By 2000, half of all couples were both in paid employment (dual earners) (see Figure 12.1). This trend was evident across different types of households but the changes were particularly marked for households with dependent children; by 2000, just under half of households with dependent children (both couples and lone parents) had all adults in paid employment.

These trends resulted in a transformation of the division of paid labour within households; in 1994, the single breadwinner model predominated

Figure 12.1: *The employment status of couples under 65, 1994–2000*

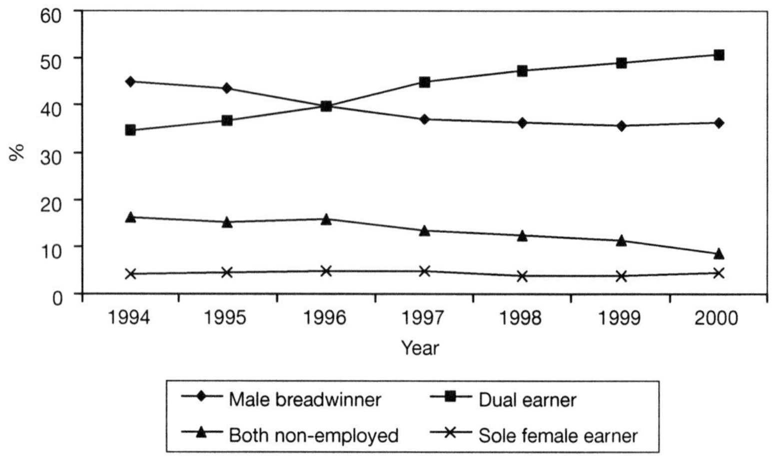

Source: Derived from Russell et al. (2004)

for couples with dependent children but by 2000, this model applied to only 38 per cent of such households.

Changes in the 'quality' of employment

There is no necessary relationship between an increase in the level of female employment and the quality of female employment. On the one hand, if the growth in female employment is confined to low-paid occupational niches, it will increase inequality among those in the labour market. On the other hand, if women have increased their share of high-quality employment, such gender-based inequalities will diminish.

In terms of hourly pay levels, some narrowing of gender differentials was evident between 1987 and 2000, from a gap of 20 per cent to 15 per cent (Russell and Gannon, 2002). More recent estimates indicate that female hourly pay has stabilised at around 85 per cent of male levels (CSO, 2005a).[2] The gender pay gap is greatest for older age groups and for women with lower levels of education. However, even among recent graduates, women tend to earn less per week than their male counterparts, with a gap in hourly pay rates between male and female graduates in the private sector (Russell, Smyth and O'Connell, 2005). Evidence suggests

---

2 Provisional figures from EU-SILC suggest that the gender wage gap declined from 14 per cent to 11 per cent between 2003 and 2004. This would be an unprecedented drop in such a short space of time.

that the overall gender pay gap is relatively wide in Ireland compared with other European countries (Barrett et al., 2000; Plasman et al., 2002; Simon and Russell, 2004).

Men in employment are more likely to be able to determine or plan their own work and working time schedules than their female counterparts (CSO, 2001). Furthermore, women are less likely to have control and autonomy in relation to their day-to-day work, reflecting their over-representation in the lower levels of the occupational hierarchy (O'Connell et al., 2004).

Men are slightly more likely to have participated in employer-provided training in the past two years (O'Connell et al., 2004), although when all forms of education and training are considered (both within and outside the workplace), rates of participation by employed women are higher than those for men (O'Connell, 2005).

The period since the early 1990s has been characterised by some change but a remarkable degree of continuity in the kinds of jobs held by women and men. Women continue to be over-represented in clerical and, to some extent, sales and personal service occupations (see Chapter 4). In contrast, they are under-represented in craft and machine operative jobs. Similarly, in terms of the types of industries in which women work, they continue to be over-represented in the education and health sector and under-represented in construction (CSO, 2005a). In spite of this continuity in the gender-typing of certain occupational and industrial spheres, there is some evidence of change. In the early 1990s, the level of occupational segregation by gender, that is, the extent to which women and men work in different occupations, declined somewhat with indications of a continuation of this trend in subsequent years (Hughes, 2002). Between 1998 and 2004, women increased their share of employment in a range of occupations, particularly in the traditionally female personal service occupations but also in the more male-dominated managerial occupations; women also increased their share of professional occupations.

Trends in attitudes towards female employment

Changes in the actual behaviour patterns of women and men in the labour market have been accompanied by shifts in general attitudes towards 'appropriate' gender roles. Since the late 1980s, there has been some reduction in the prevalence of 'traditional' attitudes and greater support for women engaging in paid employment (Scott, Braun and Alwin, 1998; Fahey, Hayes and Sinnott, 2005; Lück, 2005; Lück and Hofäcker, 2003). By the late 1990s, the vast majority (81 per cent) of adults felt that both husband and wife should contribute to household income and a minority (35 per cent) felt that pre-school children suffer if their mother works.

Side by side with this shift in attitudes, however, is a continuing high value placed on the role of housewife, with the majority (60 per cent) seeing it as just as fulfilling as working for pay. To some extent, men hold more traditional attitudes than women, at least on some items (such as the negative impact of mothers working on pre-school children), but these differences do not occur across the board. As might be expected, adults currently in the labour force have less traditional attitudes than those who are not (Fahey, Hayes and Sinnott, 2005). However, it is not clear the extent to which a shift in attitudes was a response to, rather than a driving factor in, rising female employment levels over the same period.

For couples with pre-school children, there is some evidence of a mismatch between actual and preferred employment patterns at the aggregate level. In 1998, the male breadwinner appears to be more common than was desired. Over one-third of couples were in households where the man worked full-time and woman was not in paid employment, but this option was preferred by under one-tenth of couples. More couples preferred that the man would work full-time and the woman part-time than were actually able to put this into reality (42 per cent compared with 19 per cent). Contrary to many media reports, there was no evidence that couples in dual-earner arrangements did so out of necessity rather than preference (Jaumotte, 2003).

Changes are not only evident within the Irish context but the Irish pattern has shifted compared to other European countries. At the beginning of the period, those in Ireland tended to be much less supportive of working mothers than those in other countries like Sweden and Britain (Scott, Braun and Alwin, 1998). More recently, attitudes (at least among working-age women) have moved closer to those in many other European countries; by 2002, there was somewhat less support for the male breadwinner model (that is, a sole male earner) in Ireland than in Britain (Lück, 2005). In spite of increasing approval of women working, the cultural value placed on home and family still remains high in Ireland compared to other European countries (Lück, 2005; Lück and Hofäcker, 2003).

In sum, there have been quite dramatic changes in recent years in the involvement of women in paid work, changes which have been paralleled by a shift in attitudes in support of female employment in the Irish context. However, there remain significant gender inequalities in employment, both in occupational positions and rewards. The extent to which these trends in employment have consequences for the division of unpaid labour within households and for the quality of life among women and men is explored in the remainder of this chapter.

Gender differences in paid work, unpaid work, caring and leisure

The previous section focused on gender differences in labour market participation but this is only part of the story. What about gender differences in unpaid work, caring and leisure? These have important implications not only for the nature and extent of women's labour market participation, but also for gender inequality more generally.

A body of international literature has explored unpaid household work, caring work and the gender division of labour (see Shelton and John, 1996, for a review), and how unpaid work affects the nature and supply of paid work (see, for example, Kalleberg and Rosenfeld, 1990). There has been particular interest in whether the division of household work has changed over time and whether patterns of caring and time spent with children have altered. The main finding from other countries is that the dramatic rise in female labour market participation has not been associated with a major shift in the domestic division of labour: women still tend to do more housework, regardless of how much they work outside the home (Bianchi et al., 2000; Shelton and John, 1996). Has the increase in paid work by women in Ireland affected the gender division of labour in the home? There has been almost no previous research on this topic in Ireland.[3]

Recently collected time-use data allow us to analyse current gender differences in time spent in paid employment, unpaid domestic work, caring and leisure for the first time. The Irish National Time-Use Survey 2005 asked respondents to supply a complete record of their daily activities over one weekday and one weekend day. Results reported below are based on just over 1,000 respondents who filled out time-use diaries in the period April–June 2005.[4] The initial 26 categories are collapsed into the following groups: care (comprising childcare supervision, childcare play and adult care); employment and study; household work, including DIY, gardening and shopping; travel; personal care and eating; leisure (including all active and passive leisure and resting, voluntary activity and religious activity); sleep and time-use unspecified.[5]

---

3 Fahey (1992) examines housework but does not examine who does it; Leonard (2004) looks at the gender division of housework among teenagers.

4 For further details on how the survey was conducted and details of the categories see McGinnity et al., 2005.

5 Note that the grouping of activities follows normal conventions. For example, gardening, DIY and shopping are counted as household tasks, whereas, in some instances and/or for some people, these might be seen as leisure activities.

Table 12.1: Average time (hours: minutes) spent on main activities, weekdays and weekends[1]

	Care	*Employment and study*	*Household work*	*Travel*	*Personal care and eating*	*Leisure and vol./relig. activity*	*Sleep*	*Unspecified time use*	*Total*
					Weekday				
All	1:33	4:14	1:53	1:07	1:47	4:58	8:05	0:22	24:00
Male	0:34	5:46	1:08	1:18	1:49	5:09	7:57	0:19	24:00
Female	2:31	2:44	2:36	0:57	1:45	4:48	8:13	0:25	24:00
					Weekend				
All	1:40	1:23	2:05	0:56	2:00	6:57	8:38	0:20	24:00
Male	0:53	1:52	1:31	1:03	1:60	7:41	8:39	0:20	24:00
Female	2:24	0:56	2:36	0:50	2:01	6:15	8:37	0:20	24:00

[1] Figures are based on weighted data for all adults, 18 and over. For further details see McGinnity et al., 2005.

Table 12.1 indicates the time spent by women and men on different forms of labour, that is, paid employment, household work and caring activities. Women spend somewhat longer on 'work', broadly defined, than men on weekdays and substantially more time on labour at weekends. What is even more remarkable is the gender difference in time spent on different forms of labour. Women spend almost five times longer on caring activities during the week than men. Domestic labour is also significantly higher for women than men. In contrast, time spent on employment/study is significantly higher for men. Similar gender patterns emerge for the weekend. Men continue to spend longer in paid employment/study (almost one hour more), while women spend twice as much time on caring and household work (5 hours versus 2 hours 24 minutes).

Gender differences are also evident when one considers the proportion of women and men participating in activities during the diary day. For example, 71 per cent of Irish men do no cooking/food preparation and 81 per cent do no cleaning/laundry on a weekday, and these figures change little at the weekend. In contrast, over two-thirds of women spent time on these activities on weekends and weekdays (McGinnity et al., 2005). Further analysis reveals that women spend, on average, just over three hours 'multi-tasking' (doing more than one activity at once); for men, this figure is closer to two hours.

To what extent does workload vary by hours of paid work? Women working full-time do more caring and housework, but considerably less paid work, than full-time men. Women working part-time (less than 30 hours per week) do much more caring and housework than full-time men or women. Total time on paid work, caring and domestic work on weekdays is highest for part-time women (9 hours, 39 minutes). It is lower for full-time women (8 hours, 56 minutes) and full-time men (9 hours, 9 minutes). This compares to, for example, 7 hours 38 minutes for those engaged in home duties (McGinnity et al., 2005).

The finding that there is a substantial difference in the gender division of gainful work and domestic work is found throughout Europe, though the extent of the difference in Ireland is higher than many European countries (Eurostat, 2004). Part of this may be due to the relatively recent rise in paid work by women, and time use may change in the next decades.

And what of gender differences in leisure? The 'leisure gap' between men and women has been shown to vary cross-nationally (Bittman and Wajcman, 2004). Travel time is sometimes added to paid work, unpaid work and caring time to calculate total committed time (the remainder of activities comprising free-time or uncommitted time). Combining these four categories, there is no gender difference in average committed time on weekdays. At weekends, women and men's employment time declines but women's unpaid work and caring time remains virtually unchanged.

This leads to a significant leisure gap between women and men at the weekends: men on average have almost one and a half hours more leisure time than women (7 hours 41 minutes leisure per weekend day for men versus 6 hours 15 minutes for women; see Table 12.1).

Some commentators have suggested that there has been an increasing concentration of work within certain households (Jacobs and Gerson, 2004) and that this has led to feelings of increased time pressures and work–life tensions. For this reason, we examine the levels of total committed time amongst couple households with different work patterns (Figure 12.2). We do find some evidence that dual-earner households have high levels of committed time and little free time. On weekdays, women in dual-earner households have the highest level of committed time of all, followed by men in male breadwinner households. The fact that women in dual-earner couples have a significantly higher total work burden than women in male breadwinner couples suggests that the recent substantial increase in paid employment among women has increased their total work burden. Combining the mean scores of men and women in these households at the aggregate level, we find that dual-earner households have an hour and ten minutes more committed time on weekdays than male breadwinner couples (the next busiest household type). At weekends, men and women in dual-earner and male breadwinner households have very similar total workloads. Further analyses of the characteristics of those with little free time (McGinnity and Russell, 2006) show that, apart from employment status, the presence of young children has the biggest impact on being 'time poor'.

Figure 12.2: *Time-use in couple households by household employment: total committed time (hours: minutes)*

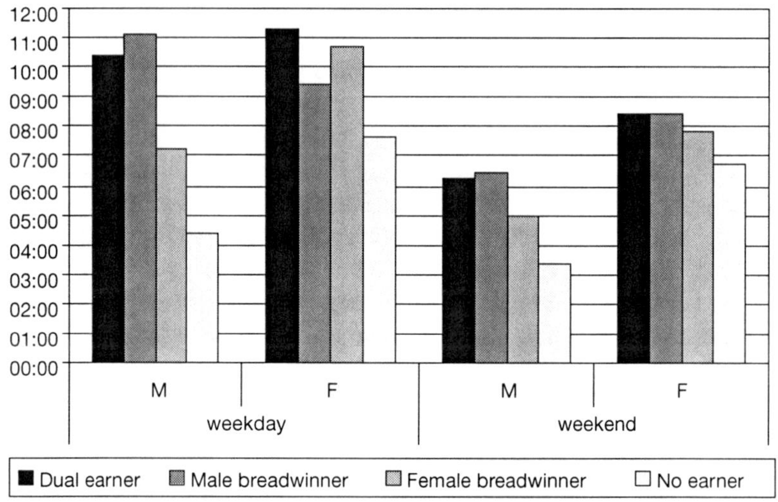

Source: Irish National Time-Use Survey 2005
Committed time = employment, study, housework, caring and travel

Irish evidence from time-use data shows limited evidence of a 'double burden' for women, whereby increases in paid employment are simply added to undiminished hours of unpaid work. In fact, total work time on weekdays is rather similar for men and women. However, the findings do point to a significant difference in total work at the weekend, and, more importantly, substantial differences remain in the division of paid and unpaid work; this is salient precisely because the work women do is unpaid and carries less status than paid work in Irish society. The results also suggest that some groups such as those with young children and dual-earner households are most likely to experience time pressures and, potentially, the work–life tensions discussed in many popular accounts of the Celtic Tiger; we turn to these quality-of-life issues next.

Quality-of-life outcomes and work–life tensions

The opening section of this chapter explored how the Celtic Tiger transformed the extent of households' engagement in the labour market. By 2005, 58 per cent of women were in employment and dual earning had become the norm among couples. So what are the consequences of these rapid changes in female employment for quality of life? Has the increased financial well-being and economic independence for women been gained at the cost of increasingly stressed-out individuals and families who struggle to meet the competing demands on their time? The previous section showed that some people are combining both high levels of paid and unpaid work with little free time, a pattern which may well result in increased stress and poorer quality of life.

Here we consider a range of measures of well-being over the last ten to fifteen years drawn from Eurobarometer data and a recent survey of employees. We start with a measure of work–life tension, which deals directly with the issue of whether work is increasingly intruding upon family life or life more generally.[6] Despite rapid increases in employment over the period, there is no evidence of increasing levels of work–life tensions among the employed (Figure 12.3). In contrast, the proportion of respondents who say their job often or always takes family time or that they are always or often too tired to enjoy things after work has decreased over the period. While these tensions have not increased over time, they are likely to impact on the quality of life of the minority of workers who experience these tensions.

Figure 12.3: *Work–life tensions, 1996–2003*

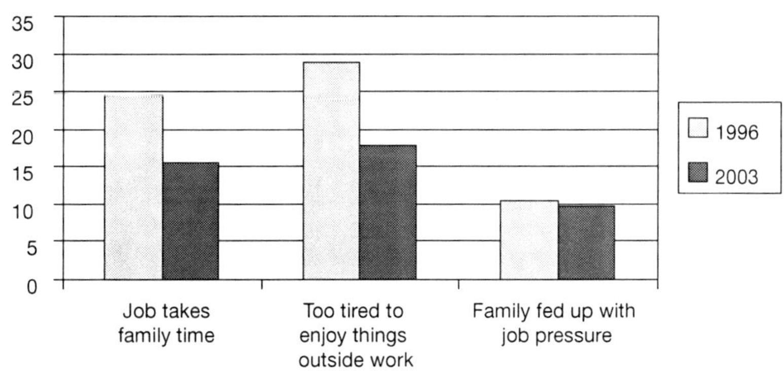

Source: 1996 Eurobarometer 44.3; 2003 ESRI/NCPP Changing Workplace Survey

Further analysis of these issues (O'Connell and Russell, 2005) shows that in 2003 work–family tension was higher among those with young children and among women (when job characteristics and other factors are controlled).

6 It should be noted that the number of respondents in the Eurobarometer survey (1996) is relatively small.

Questions on the experience of work–life tensions can only be asked of those in employment. Therefore it is impossible to compare the well-being of those with and without employment. In order to provide a broader picture, we examine more general measures of well-being: psychological distress; satisfaction with work/main activity, leisure, and life in general; and feeling rushed and stressed.

We look first at psychological distress as measured by the General Health Questionnaire (GHQ) over the period 1994–2000. The GHQ is a short, well-validated measure of psychological distress (Goldberg, 1972). We have calculated the proportion of each employment group who score above the threshold, which has been established as indicating an abnormally high level of distress. The results in Figure 12.4 show that the level of psychological distress declined for men and women between 1994 and 2000. In both periods, employed women and men are less likely to experience psychological distress than those who are unemployed or non-employed (home duties, retired, in education, etc.). These patterns are consistent with international research. It is interesting that by 2000 it is non-employed rather than unemployed women who exhibit the highest risk of psychological distress.

Figure 12.4: *GHQ psychological distress by employment status, 1994–2000*

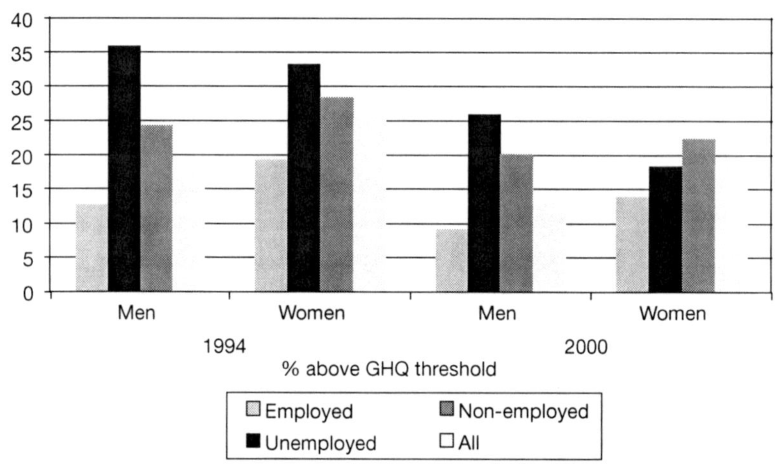

Data Source: Living in Ireland Surveys 1994 and 2000

Similar results emerge if we examine levels of satisfaction with work or main daily activity. Employed women show significantly higher levels of satisfaction than any other group of women and indeed men. Levels of satisfaction with work/main activity were relatively stable over the period for both men and women. Satisfaction with leisure time taps into the issue of whether increasing employment has had a detrimental impact on people's leisure time. Those in employment are less satisfied with their leisure time than the non-employed and, in most cases, the unemployed. However, there is no evidence that satisfaction with leisure time declined between 1994 and 2000 for either men or women. These results suggest that the changing composition of the population in terms of the numbers at work and the numbers combining work and caring has not led to any downward trend in satisfaction at the societal level.

It might be argued that the real time-crunch and potentially greatest challenges to quality of life occur within households where both partners are working. We find that this is not the case: both men and women in dual-earner households show the lowest level of psychological distress and greatest satisfaction with their work/main activity (Figures 12.5 and 12.6). Again it is the non-employed who have lower well-being/satisfaction scores. However, there is evidence that women and men in dual-earner households are somewhat less satisfied with their leisure time than other groups: 45 per cent report that they are very satisfied compared to 50 per cent of all women and 48 per cent of all men. This suggests some hint of the strain mentioned in many accounts of recent societal change, but the difference is modest. It is interesting to note that men and women in female breadwinner couples have the highest level of psychological distress; however, there are relatively few households where this reversal of roles has occurred. Comparing these results with those for 1994 shows that, if anything, those in dual-earner households have become slightly more satisfied with their leisure time over time between 1994 and 2000 (Russell et al., 2004, p. 55).

The relationship between the well-being of individuals and their own and partner's employment situation outlined in the preceding graphs does not control for the number of hours worked. While, in general, employment is associated with better psychological well-being and greater satisfaction with main activity, this does not preclude the possibility that excessive workloads (of paid or unpaid work) are linked to reduced well-being. To test this, we return to the time-use data and examine the impact of total workload on feeling 'rushed and stressed' and overall life satisfaction.

The time-use survey is a question which asks respondents 'Did you feel rushed and stressed during the diary day?' On weekdays, 8 per cent of respondents reported feeling rushed most of the day, 38 per cent reported feeling rushed some of the day, leaving 54 per cent not feeling rushed. Feelings of time pressure are highest among those who are solo

Figure 12.5: *Psychological distress by household work situation 2000: percentage above GHQ threshold*

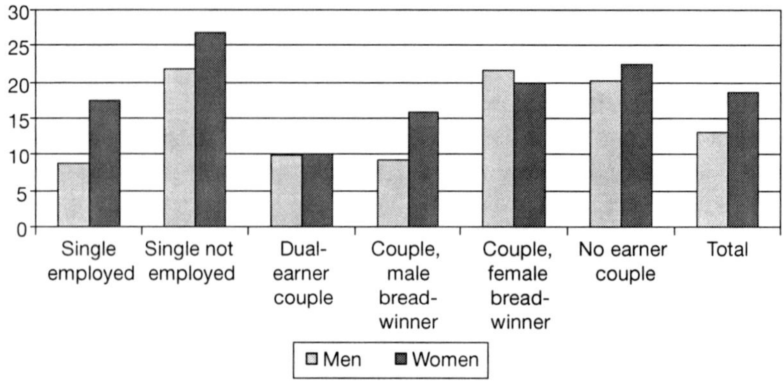

Data Source: Living in Ireland Survey 2000

Figure 12.6 *Satisfaction with work/main activity by household situation*

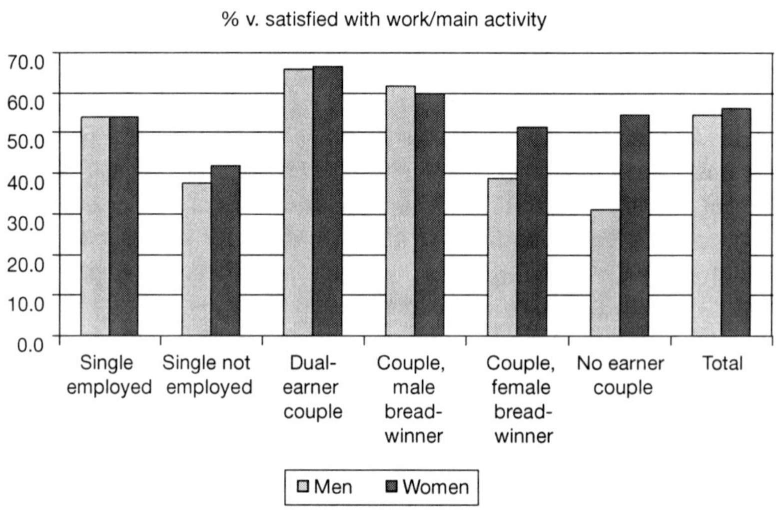

Data Source: Living in Ireland Survey 2000

breadwinners and those in dual-earner households (Figure 12.7). Distinguishing those who felt rushed some or most of the day from those who did not feel rushed, we examine the impact of total work on this measure (McGinnity and Russell, 2006). We find that, other things being equal, those with high volumes of total paid and unpaid work are more rushed than those with low total hours of work. Separating the effect of paid work and unpaid work, both contribute to feeling rushed, but the effect of paid work on feeling rushed is stronger. Those in higher-income households are also more rushed, as are the employed and those with a partner. Older people feel less rushed. Both men and women with high total work, the 'time poor', are more likely to feel rushed than those with low total work.

Figure 12.7: *Percentage feeling rushed and stressed during diary day*

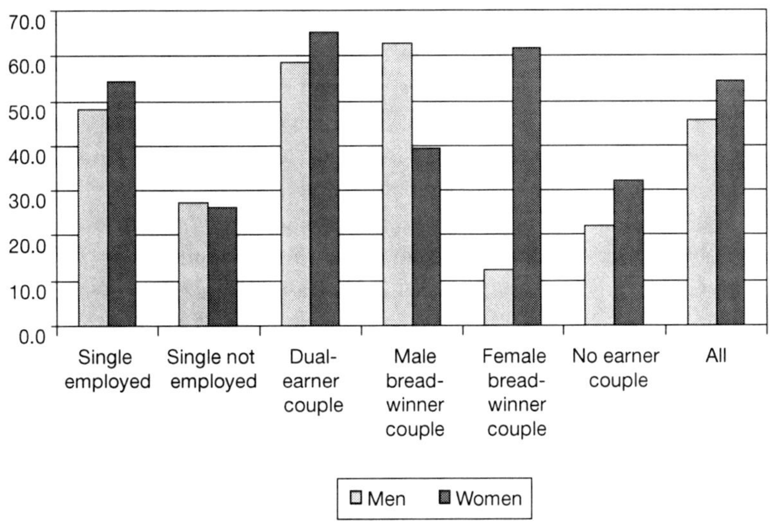

Source: Irish National Time-Use Survey 2005
Note: Single people do not necessarily live alone.

A more general measure of quality of life is overall life satisfaction.[7] If we examine the effect of having a high level of total work on overall life satisfaction, we find a significant negative effect: those with high volumes of work are less satisfied with their life in general, other things being equal (McGinnity and Russell, 2006).

Feeling rushed leads to lower levels of life satisfaction, over and above the effects of the amount of paid and unpaid work.[8] Interestingly, looking at the patterns for men and women separately, we find it is only women who experience lower satisfaction if they are time poor or feel rushed: this effect does not hold for men.

---

[7] In answer to the question 'How satisfied are you with your present situation in your life in general?', respondents mark their response on a scale of 1 to 6, with 1 being not satisfied at all and 6 being fully satisfied.

[8] The effect of feeling rushed on life satisfaction is roughly the equivalent of an extra 30 minutes of work per day.

These results should be placed in the context of the effects of other factors: unemployment has a much greater negative impact on life satisfaction than high hours of work, as do health problems. Being overworked clearly matters for life satisfaction and the quality of life, but other things matter too.

Conclusions

The past 15 years have seen significant changes in the labour market behaviour of women and men in Ireland, changes which have been particularly dramatic for women, with rapidly growing labour force participation and employment rates. Such changes have raised living standards and increased financial independence for women. They have also transformed the way in which employment is distributed across households. Dual-earner arrangements are now the predominant model for working-age couples, even those with dependent children.

This chapter set out to examine the consequences of these changes from both a quality-of-life and a gender equality perspective. We have focused in particular on the question of whether the increase in female employment has led to a double burden of paid and unpaid work for women and new stresses for households trying to juggle work and family life.

From a gender equality perspective, the dramatic influx of women into the labour market has had less of an impact on the quality of women's employment than might have been anticipated. Women continue to have lower average pay levels than men, have less access to employer training than men and are strongly clustered in traditionally female occupational niches (although women have made their way into higher-level occupations in greater numbers). In addition, increased female employment has not led to a renegotiation of the allocation of paid and unpaid work between women and men. Time-use data show that a traditional division of labour persists within the household, with women (even those in full-time employment) spending more time on caring and household work than men. There is some evidence of a double burden for women in that they have much less free time than men at weekends. And the fact that women in dual-earner couples have a significantly higher total work burden than women in male breadwinner couples suggests that the recent substantial increase in paid employment among women has increased their total work burden. Further improvements to quality of life would involve addressing these fundamental gender inequalities and adjusting employment structures and support systems to recognise both women's and men's family and life interests.

On the whole, the evidence presented here does not support the view that women's increased employment has been detrimental to the quality of life of Irish adults.[9] Women (and men) in employment have much lower levels of psychological distress than the unemployed, full-time homemakers and other non-employed groups. Employed women also express higher levels of satisfaction with their work or main activity than women outside the labour force. Furthermore, men and women in dual-earner households are the most satisfied with their main activity and have the lowest psychological distress of all types of households. The available trend data provide no evidence that the increasing involvement of women in paid employment has led to increasing work–life tension or declining levels of life satisfaction over time. On the contrary, general levels of psychological distress in the population decreased between 1994 and 2000 and fewer respondents reported work–family tensions in 2003 than in 1996. Certainly, there are some stress points; a significant proportion of the population reports feeling rushed and stressed, particularly those with high volumes of paid and unpaid work. High workloads are also linked to lower life satisfaction. However, these do not cancel out the positive impact of employment on well-being. At a societal level, the problems arising from too little work appear to far outweigh the problems arising from too much work, so that the greater engagement with work that has emerged in the Celtic Tiger era has yielded a net improvement to quality of life in Ireland.

---

9 Our data do not include children so we cannot examine the impact of change on that group.

13

The Impact of Immigration

Gerard Hughes, Frances McGinnity, Philip O'Connell and Emma Quinn

Introduction

Migration has been important for Ireland since the nineteenth century. For most of that time, migratory flows have been outward but occasional bouts of return migration have also occurred. It is only since the exceptional economic growth of the past decade that we have seen large and sustained inflows and that non-Irish immigrants have come to outnumber returning Irish migrants. Our purpose in this chapter is to assess the significance of this new era of inward migration. People are now clamouring to get into Ireland rather than rushing to leave it and that in itself is a powerful indicator of how much more attractive a society Ireland now is compared to the past. However, if we look deeper, a number of questions arise about what new migration patterns mean and what their impact will be. These questions concern the economic and social impact of immigration as well as the challenge of integrating the new Irish.

The chapter begins with a review of recent trends in migration, and tracks the change from a pattern of emigration to one of immigration. A notable feature of present immigration is that it comes primarily from within the EU and so is less racially, culturally and religiously heterogeneous than that experienced by other immigrant societies. We then turn to the economic impact of immigration on the economy, focusing in particular on the labour market. This is followed by a discussion of the social impact of immigration, focusing on public services as well as the attitudes of the indigenous population towards immigrants. We then examine new survey data on immigrants' experiences of racism and discrimination in Ireland. The conclusion discusses the need for a coherent policy for integration of migrants into Irish society as an essential requirement for the successful management of immigration.

T. Fahey et al. (eds.), Quality of Life in Ireland, 217–244.

Recent migration experience

From emigration to immigration

The economic boom resulted in an increase in employment of 650,000, or 55 per cent, between 1993 and 2004 and the emergence of widespread labour shortages. This attracted large numbers of migrants.

Figure 13.1 shows the change from net emigration in the late 1980s to net immigration from the mid-1990s onwards. In 1987, 23,000 more people left than entered the country (40,000 left while 17,000 came in). In the early 1990s the outflows and inflows were almost in balance. However, from 1996 onwards net migration has made a positive contribution to Ireland's population growth. The net inflow of immigrants increased from 8,000 per annum in 1996 to 53,000 per annum in 2005. In 2005 over 6 per cent of the population, or 259,000 people, were foreign nationals (see Table 13.1). Of these, 165,000 were nationals of other EU countries and 95,000 came from outside the EU25. This compares to 126,000 non-Irish nationals in 2000, of which 92,000 came from other EU countries and 34,000 from outside the EU15.

Figure 13.1: *Emigration, immigration and net migration, 1987–2005*

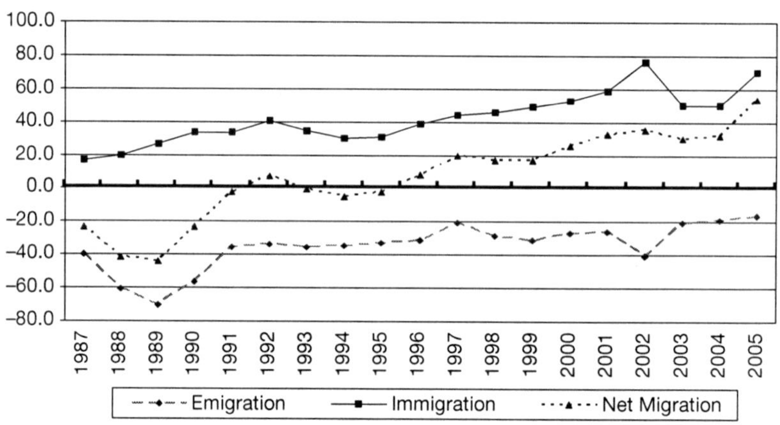

National groups migrating to Ireland

In recent years, migratory flows to Ireland have become less dominated by return Irish migration and more dominated by migration from the new EU Member States. In 1991 about two-thirds of immigrants, 22,600 out of 33,300, were Irish people returning home. By 1996 returning Irish migrants accounted for less than half of the gross inflow of 39,200, and by 2005 they had fallen to 19,000 or about one-quarter of the gross inflow of 70,000.

Table 13.1: Total population in 2000 and 2005 classified by nationality (000s)

Nationality	*2000**	*2005*
Irish	3,660.4	3,871.3
UK	66.9	74.8
Other EU	25.3	90.0
Non EU	34.3	94.6
USA	8.0	11.5
Other	26.3	83.1
Total population	3,786.9	4,130.7
Foreign population	126.5	259.4
Per cent foreign	3.3%	6.3%

*Note: The CSO has revised total immigration figures for 2000 but not nationality data. Consequently, the unrevised figures are supplied here.
Source: Hughes and Doyle (2006), Sexton (2001)

Figure 13.2 compares the composition of migration flows to Ireland in 2000 and in 2005 and shows the dominance of migration from the ten new EU Member States in 2005. Nationals from the new EU Member States enjoy almost full EU rights in Ireland, since along with Sweden and the UK this country was one of just three EU–15 countries to allow them full access to the labour market.

Figure 13.2: *Estimated immigration flows classified by nationality, 2000 and 2005*

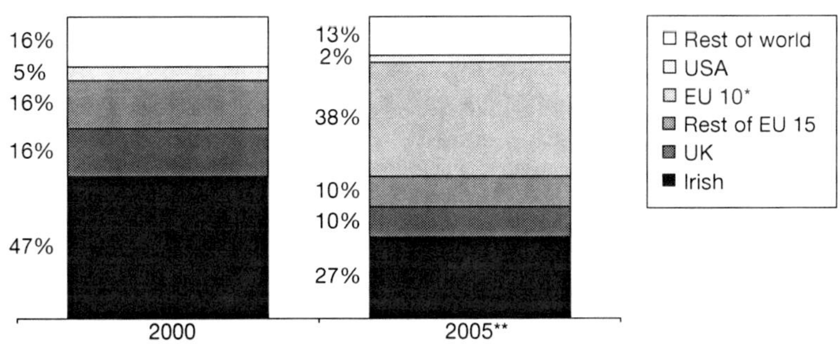

*Prior to 2005, data for EU–10 were included in the 'rest of world' category.
**Data for 2005 are preliminary.
Source: CSO (2005b), Population and Migration Estimates[1]

[1] The principal source of information for this publication is the Quarterly National Household Survey. Other migration indicators used include the continuous Country of Residence Inquiry of passengers, conducted at airports and seaports; the number of visas granted; the number of work permits issued/renewed; and the number of asylum applications. The flow data therefore covers all immigrants other than those who enter illegally.

This accessibility appears to have given rise to a great deal of short-term movement between Ireland and the new EU states. Between May 2004 and November 2005, for example, 160,853 Personal Public Service (PPS) numbers were issued to EU–10 nationals in Ireland.[2] The Department of Social and Family Affairs has cross-referenced the PPS number allocations with income tax data from the Revenue Commissioners and have concluded that a substantial proportion of recipients come for a short period only and that many are likely to be students who work during their holidays.[3]

Non-EU immigrants

Compared to movements from within the EU, immigration from outside the EU is modest (excluding immigration from the US, 'rest of world' immigration to Ireland in 2005 accounted for only 13 per cent of the gross inflow). Figure 13.3 outlines the legal routes into Ireland for non-EU citizens. Employment-led immigrants include work-permit holders, visa/authorisation holders,[4] intra-company transfers/trainees and business permit holders. Non-employment related immigrants include asylum applicants, students, family members and dependents of both Irish and EEA (European Economic Area) nationals as well as non-Irish and non-EEA nationals.[5] It is reasonable to assume that most illegal immigrants come to Ireland with an intention to work.[6]

The majority of non-EEA nationals coming to Ireland to take up work are work-permit holders. The total number of work permits issued (new permits and renewals) increased nearly eightfold from around 6,000 in 1999 to 48,000 in 2003. However, as Figure 13.4 shows there was a substantial fall in the number issued in 2004 as nationals of the new EU Member States no longer required work permits after 1 May 2004. Government policy now strongly favours employers sourcing their migrant workers from within the enlarged EU. In 2005 27,000 work permits were issued, including almost 19,000 renewals.

---

[2] Communication from the Commission to the Council, the European Parliament, the European Economic and Social Committee and the Committee of the Regions. 'Report on the Functioning of the Transitional Arrangements set out in the 2003 Accession Treaty (period 1 May 2004 to 30 April 2006)'.

[3] Contribution by Brian O'Raghallaigh (Department of Social and Family Affairs) to the Joint Committee on European Affairs on 26 October 2005.

[4] This category is now obsolete with the implementation of the new employment permits legislation (see below).

[5] The EEA comprises all EU States plus Iceland, Lichtenstein, Norway and Switzerland.

[6] Note that although a person may enter on non-economically active grounds this may change with time. For example, an asylum seeker may be granted refugee status or the spouse of a work-permit holder may secure a work permit of his or her own.

Figure 13.3: *Channels of legal immigration into Ireland for non-EU nationals*

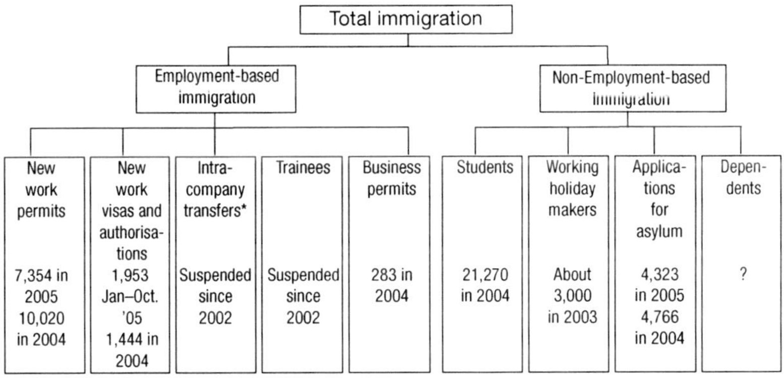

* Issued on a concessionary basis.

Notes: (a) This diagram is adapted from Ruhs (2005); (b) Short-term immigration for tourist purposes is excluded; (c) ? indicates that data are not available.

Source: Ruhs (2005), Department of Justice, Equality and Law Reform and Department of Enterprise, Trade and Employment.

Figure 13.4: *Work permits issued and renewed, 1998–2005*

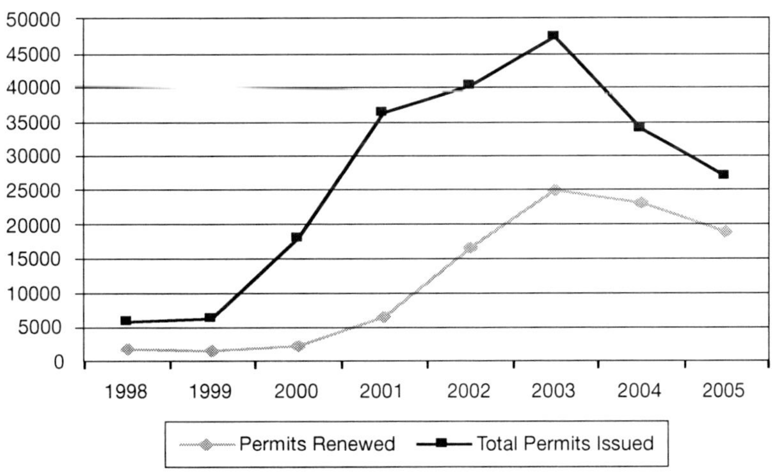

Source: Department of Enterprise, Trade and Employment

In order to facilitate the recruitment of suitably qualified persons from non-EEA countries a working visa/authorisation scheme was introduced. Visa/authorisations are issued for two years, may be renewed for another two years and are issued directly to the employee rather than the employer. In 2005, 2,585 such visas/authorisations were issued. In recent years the number of immigrants entering the country on intra-company transfers/trainees programs[7] or as business permit holders has been relatively small. There were 752 permits for intra-company transfers issued on a concessionary basis during 2003 and 2004 despite the suspension of the scheme in 2002.

In 2004 there were an estimated 21,270 registered non-EEA students in Ireland and approximately half of these came from China (Ruhs, 2005). Until April 2005 all non-EEA students could access the Irish labour market. Now only students who are pursuing courses which are of at least one year's duration and which lead to a 'recognised qualification' may enter the Irish labour market.

No estimates are available of the number of dependents of non-EU nationals who come to Ireland to join family members. Data from the QNHS, Quarter 4 2005, on the economic status of immigrants show that the proportion of immigrants aged 15 and over who are dependents, 28 per cent, is substantially less than the proportion of Irish nationals, 39 per cent, who are dependents. Family members of non-EEA residents in Ireland may not freely take up employment.

Asylum seekers

Applications for asylum began to build up from a very low base of 39 in 1992 to around 8,000 by the end of the decade. The increase in the number of applications continued into the new century and reached a peak of 11,600 in 2002. The number of asylum applications made in Ireland fell by almost two-thirds to around 4,300 in 2005 (see Figure 13.5). Asylum applicants may not take up work in Ireland and they must reside in direct provision centres where all food and board costs are met by the State.

Immigrants are sometimes allowed to reside in Ireland on other exceptional grounds, for example, an unsuccessful asylum applicant may be granted humanitarian leave to remain by the Minister for Justice, Equality and Law Reform. During 2005 the Department of Justice, Equality and Law Reform processed almost 18,000 applications for permission to remain in Ireland based on the parentage of an Irish citizen child; of these, 16,700 applications were approved.

Illegal residents

The number of illegally resident non-Irish nationals in Ireland is not known. Almost no statistics exist on stocks of illegally resident immigrants

---

7 The intra-company transfer scheme was suspended in 2002 due to abuses.

Figure 13.5: *Number of asylum applications, 1992–2005*

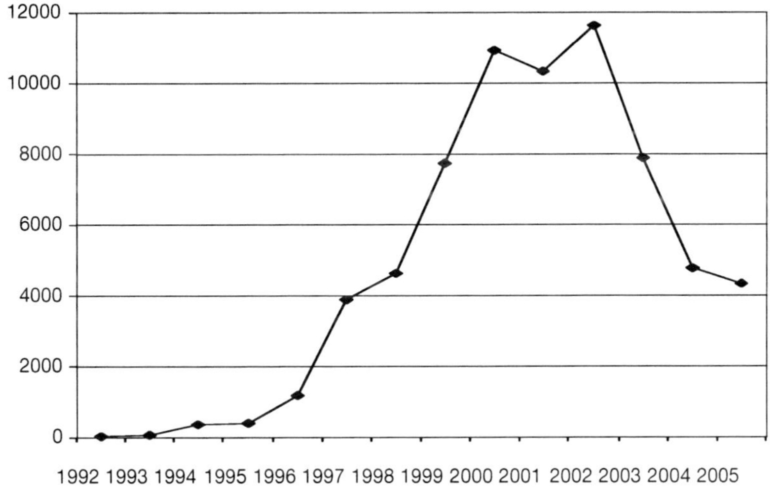

Source: Office of the Refugee Applications Commissioner

beyond the number of outstanding deportation orders (8,902). Data on the number of persons refused leave to land (4,893 in 2005) may be indicative of flows of illegal immigrants to Ireland, however it should be noted that permission to enter Ireland may be refused for a range of reasons. There are two categories of illegal immigrant: persons who enter the State illegally and continue to reside illegally and persons who enter legally and whose residence status later becomes irregular[8] (Quinn and Hughes, 2005). Illegal immigrants have no legal entitlements. However, any person in Ireland can expect to have their basic human rights protected by the Irish courts. As will be discussed below Irish equality and human rights legislation is relatively strong.

Legislative change

Until recently the basic legislation governing entry and residence of non-Irish nationals in Ireland was the Aliens Act, 1935, and the Aliens Order, 1946, as amended. The rapid increase in the immigration of non-Irish nationals since the mid-1990s led to substantial new legislation. The most urgent challenge to policymakers in the 1990s was to establish a structure

[8] Data supplied by the Immigrant Council of Ireland show that of the illegally resident migrants it deals with the breakdown between these two categories is approximately 23 and 77 per cent, respectively.

for processing asylum applications. The 1996 Refugee Act was introduced to codify the provisions for dealing with asylum applications. Other legislative developments to date regarding immigration have been somewhat piecemeal, responding to specific issues as they arise. The heads of a proposed Immigration, Residence and Citizenship Bill were published in 2006. The scope of this legislation is broad and it should help draw together currently disparate instruments. An Employment Permits Act (2006), which forms the basis of a new employment permits system, was passed in June 2006.

Among the most significant legislative changes in recent years has been that relating the acquisition of citizenship. Perceptions that large numbers of immigrants, particularly asylum seekers, were migrating in order to acquire Irish citizenship for their children led to a public debate which culminated in the redefinition of the concept of Irish citizenship through constitutional change.

Until mid-2004 Ireland was the only country in the EU to grant citizenship based on the principle of *jus soli* (place of birth) alone. Concerns about abuse of that system led to a referendum on a constitutional amendment that passed by a large majority in June 2004, reinstating the power of the Oireachtas (Parliament) to legislate on the acquisition of citizenship. Now only children who are born in Ireland before January 2005, or children born after that date with an Irish parent, have a constitutional entitlement to Irish citizenship.

The accession of ten new EU Member States occurred one month before the referendum and may have influenced the result, as the Irish electorate reassessed their position within a now much larger European Union. Despite the fact that Ireland is not a Schengen signatory,[9] domestic immigration and asylum policy must take account of developments at EU level. The constitutional referendum and the European Court of Justice case Chen v. UK[10] underlined how closely Irish citizenship is now linked to residence in other EU countries.

The evolution of Irish migration

Arguably, migration policy in the last ten years has been driven mainly by economic necessity, with the work-permit system primarily oriented

---

[9] The Schengen system involves the abolition of border controls between participating States and the strengthening of external borders and addresses participants' security concerns. All EU Member States, with the exception of Ireland and the UK, are full participants in the system, as are Iceland and Norway.

[10] The European Court of Justice ruled that Ms Chen, a Chinese national, has the right to reside anywhere in the EU with her Irish citizen child (C-200/02).

towards the needs of employers to meet short-term labour shortages but on a time-limited basis and linked to one employer. The work-permit system assumed that permit holders would leave Ireland when their skills were no longer required.

EU enlargement, entailing a dramatic increase in labour supply from within the borders of the European Union, as well as a decline in the inflow of asylum seekers, heralds a new phase in Irish migration.

Since 2004, nationals of the new Member States have enjoyed broadly the same rights as EU citizens. In particular, they are free to move in and out of Ireland at will, to be accompanied by their families, and to settle here. This is in contrast to work-permit holders whose residence is time-limited and linked explicitly to an employer. Since May 2004, an ever-increasing number of jobs have been filled by nationals of new Member States, and it is government policy that EU nationals will fill most of Ireland's future skills and labour deficits, and the number of work-permit holders has fallen.

The evolution of Irish migration can be characterised in terms of three phases: 1. Substantial outward migration from before the Famine to the early-1990s; 2. A dramatic increase in inward migration from the mid-1990s to 2004, linked to the economic boom and eliciting *ad hoc* State policies; 3. Since 2004, a phase of more secure, stable and perhaps permanent immigration in which the majority of migrants are likely to be entitled to a more comprehensive package of economic and civil rights than in the previous phase.

These characteristics of the new phase apply most particularly to EU nationals, but may also be reflected in other recent changes in Irish immigration policy. The new Immigration, Residence and Protection Bill is expected to codify issues such as family reunification, visitor visas, etc. In addition, a new body, the Irish Naturalisation and Immigration Service (INIS) has recently been established within the Department of Justice, Equality and Law Reform to streamline the provision of asylum, immigration and visa functions formerly spread across the Department of Justice, Equality and Law Reform, the Department of Foreign Affairs, and the Reception and Integration Agency. There is also a commitment to include in INIS an Immigrant Integration Unit.

The Employment Permits Act (2006) introduces a new employment permits system that seeks to shift the balance of economic migrants towards the highly skilled by introducing more selective migration, and to extend the rights of these migrants by issuing permissions akin to green cards for selected high-skilled occupations with salaries above set thresholds. Holders of these permissions will be entitled to change employers at their own discretion, to bring spouses and families and to apply for long-term residence after two years. Both nationals of the enlarged EU and 'green card' holders thus have a more extensive set of rights than work-permit holders. Their status in Ireland will be more permanent and more secure.

While highly skilled non-EU labour migration has been facilitated, the new employment permits system makes it more difficult for lower skilled non-EU nationals to travel to Ireland to work. A revised work-permit scheme has been introduced for a restricted list of occupations with an annual salary of €30,000 to €60,000, and in exceptional cases, permits may be issued for positions with an annual salary below €30,000. A work permit may be issued to a non-EU worker only after the position has been advertised without success for four weeks within the EU. The policy of sourcing most labour from within the EU–25 has already clearly impacted on the composition of flows shown in Figure 13.2. Employees may now change employers after twelve months. This should somewhat increase the potential mobility of work-permit holders and thus provide some degree of protection against exploitation.

A final relevant policy development has been the establishment of the National Employment Rights Authority on a statutory footing and the expansion of the labour inspectorate to underpin employment rights and labour standards throughout the labour market, with a particular concern for the rights of migrant workers.

The impact of immigration on the economy and society

Economic impact of immigration

The economic and social impact of immigration has recently been reviewed by Hughes and Quinn (2004). The main thrust of available evidence is that the economic impact was favourable up to that time. For example, Barrett, Bergin and Duffy (2006) show that the educational qualifications of immigrants in the labour force in 2003 were considerably higher than the native labour force. Just over 54 per cent of immigrants had third-level qualifications: twice that of the native population. It would be expected, therefore, that immigrants would be more heavily concentrated in high-skill occupations than the native workforce, but the data do not reflect this. Controlling for the effects of education and age on occupational attainment shows that immigrants were less likely to be in the top three occupational categories, with the exception of immigrants from the UK or the US. The over-concentration of immigrants from non-English speaking countries in relatively low-skill occupations suggests that weak English language skills may be a contributory factor. Difficulties for employers in recognising foreign qualifications may also result in a gap between qualifications and occupations.

Despite the difficulties that some immigrants encounter in integrating into the labour market, the economic impact of immigration in Ireland is judged to be positive. Barrett, Bergin and Duffy (2006) estimate that the immigrant inflow in the five years up to 2003 increased GNP by 2.6 per cent and GNP per head by 0.4 per cent. If all of the immigrants had been employed in occupations appropriate to their levels of qualification both figures would have been about a half percentage point higher. In addition, the increase in the supply of highly qualified immigrants up to that time helped to reduce earnings inequality. Overall, therefore, Ireland gained significant economic benefits from the inflow of immigrants that occurred up to May 2004. There is some evidence that many of the immigrants who have come from Central and Eastern European countries since then are working in unskilled jobs that only pay around the minimum wage. This could mean that the reduction in inequality that occurred following the earlier immigrations may be reversed in the future.

The economic benefits that accrued up to 2004 occurred in a policy environment in which work permits were issued to overcome skill and labour shortages and to maintain economic growth. The latest population and migration projections made by the CSO (2004a) indicate that if net inward migration continues to run at a high level up to 2030, the foreign-born population could exceed 1,000,000, or 18 per cent, by 2030 compared with 400,000, or 10 per cent, in 2002.[11] Continuing high net inward migration would accentuate existing problems in the housing market and put increasing pressure on the transport system and other infrastructure (Clinch, Convery and Walsh, 2002).

In view of these considerations, a number of issues relating to migration policy need to be addressed. Should Ireland continue to operate a liberal immigration policy to maximise growth or should it aim to increase per capita income by upskilling the labour force and relying more on domestic sources of labour supply? How can migration policy be developed in a way that is fairer and more transparent? The new employment permits system can be characterised as a very liberal migration regime in relation to nationals of the 25–EU Member States and to highly qualified labour migrants from the rest of the world, with a highly restrictive regime in respect of lower-skilled workers from beyond the borders of the EU–25 states. It follows, however, that as regular channels of non-EU labour migration become more restricted there is a risk that would-be migrants

[11] The foreign-born population includes foreign nationals as well as the children of Irish nationals who have returned to Ireland.

might attempt other routes to enter the state, for example, via the asylum system or illegally.

Labour market issues

One of the key challenges arising from increased immigration is to find a balance between protection of migrant workers and the need for a flexible migration system. The Irish work-permit system is employer-driven. The permit is issued for up to one year, with the possibility of renewal, for a specific job, for a named individual and for posts that cannot be filled by Irish or other EEA nationals. This type of system can leave work-permit holders vulnerable to exploitation by unscrupulous employers. The Employment Permits Act 2006 has introduced measures to protect migrant workers but the proposed system remains employer-led, enabling the government to respond quickly to changing labour market conditions.

The work-permit system is just one element of the problem however. Nationals of the ten new EU Member States who joined the EU in May 2004 have been allowed unrestricted access to the Irish labour market. This has resulted in a substantial increase in the number of immigrants from these countries. It has also led to a number of cases where employers have sought to replace Irish workers with lower paid workers from the new Central and Eastern European states. In three high-profile cases, Irish Ferries, Moneypoint and Gama, for example, Irish workers were replaced by more poorly paid immigrant workers or by subcontract work to companies registered in Central and Eastern Europe who pay their immigrant workers significantly less than the hourly pay rates agreed in legally binding collective agreements.[12]

The scale of the displacement problem is unclear. A recent analysis of QNHS data suggests that there is no evidence that the very rapid growth in the employment of non-Irish nationals has led to a rise in unemployment among Irish workers (Beggs and Pollock, 2006). That study did identify three sectors (manufacturing, hotels and agriculture) where employment of Irish workers fell while that of non-Irish nationals increased. While this suggests some displacement in certain sectors, there is no indication of whether Irish workers are moving to other employment with equal or better employment conditions. However, as the National Economic and Social

---

[12] The Gama case involved a Turkish company allegedly exploiting Turkish construction workers by paying them less than the collectively agreed rates of pay. In the Irish Ferries case the employer used special international legislation governing the employment of seamen to replace a significant number of Irish workers with workers from Latvia. In the Moneypoint case it was alleged that a Polish subcontractor on a construction project for the Electricity Supply Board was paying its Polish workers less than the minimum wage and less than one-third of the legally enforceable registered employment rate for the construction sector.

Council (NESC) (2005, p. 138) notes, 'Many of those who experience Ireland's social deficits most acutely are not in the labour force and, therefore, migrants are not in direct competition with them for jobs.' Doyle, Hughes and Wadensjö (2006) show that demand for labour remained strong after enlargement: the percentage of firms reporting vacancies increased between May 2004 and February 2005, and the unemployment rate has remained at around 4 per cent of the labour force.

Nevertheless, public concern about exploitation of migrants and the potential undermining of standards throughout the labour market have increased. The trade union movement delayed entering into social partnership talks at the beginning of 2006 until they received an undertaking from the government that issues relating to the enforcement of pay and employment conditions through the labour inspectorate would be addressed in the talks before the social partners negotiated on pay.

Discrimination in the workplace has emerged as a particular concern in public debate. Survey results discussed later in this chapter support the view that immigrants are frequently at risk of racism and discrimination at work. Almost 20 per cent of all cases taken by The Equality Authority in 2005 under the Employment Equality Acts related to allegations of discrimination on the basis of race. Ireland has relatively robust legislative provisions around racism and discrimination. Measures such as the Equality Act, 2004, the Equal Status Act, 2000, and the Employment Equality Act, 1998, provide important protections for immigrants in the labour market and in accessing goods and services. Adequate enforcement of legislation is essential. As discussed above, a new National Employment Rights Authority has been established. It remains to be seen whether the substantial increase in the number of labour inspectors in this Authority is sufficient to ensure adequate protection of Irish workers or immigrants in the workplace, particularly in labour market sectors with low rates of unionisation (shops, restaurants, agriculture).

Social impact of immigration

In general, Irish social welfare legislation does not distinguish between nationals and legally resident non-Irish nationals. This situation was reviewed ahead of the accession of ten new EU Member States in 2004 and a Habitual Residence Condition (HRC) was introduced to protect the Irish welfare system in the event of large-scale migration from the accession states. The basic requirement for a person to be deemed 'habitually resident' is to have been resident in Ireland or the UK for a continuous period of two years before making an application for social welfare. The implementation of the HRC has been problematic, however, and the European Commission initiated an 'infringement procedure' over the extent to which benefits were being denied to EU citizens.[13] There was a relaxation in the implementation of the HRC towards the end of 2005, with the effect that EEA nationals with a work history in the State could access benefits under the Supplementary Welfare Allowance scheme.

Restrictions on Child Benefit and the One-Parent Family Allowance were also lifted, with the effect that all workers, whether EEA or third-country nationals, may now apply for Child Benefit, and all EEA workers may apply for the One-Parent Family Allowance.[14] This policy shift gave rise to some concerns about the impact of migrant workers from the new EU–10 states on the Irish welfare state, with widely varying estimates of the expected costs.[15] Illegally resident non-Irish nationals have no entitlements to public services. However, lack of formal arrangements for sharing information between the immigration authorities and those responsible for running hospitals, schools and other public services means that illegal residents could access public services (Quinn and Hughes, 2005).

The impact of immigration on health has received much media attention in recent years, particularly centred on the pressure put on maternity services by large numbers of non-EU nationals arriving in Ireland to give birth at short notice. Immigrants in Ireland are providers as well as users of the Irish health service and the Irish health sector is dependent on continued immigration to function effectively. In December 2005 there were almost 14,700 doctors holding full registration with the Medical Council in Ireland; of these 20 per cent had overseas addresses.[16] QNHS data indicate that the total number of nurses increased by over 13,000 between 1998 and 2004 to 50,200.[17] The proportion of non-Irish nurses in the workforce increased from 2 per cent to 8 per cent in the same period.[18]

Immigration has affected the education system in a variety of ways. Increasing diversity enriches the school environment but it also requires increased resources, particularly for the teaching of English. Research has shown that students from non-Irish national backgrounds are significantly more likely to report having been bullied than other students. Non-Irish

---

[13] *The Irish Times*, 'State queried on welfare for EU immigrants', 23 September 2005

[14] Nationals of EU Member States working in Ireland may claim Child Benefit even if their children are not resident in the State with them. However, third-country nationals may only claim Child Benefit if their children are residing in the State with them.

[15] *The Irish Times*, 1 February 2006, 'Migrant childcare cost just €1m, says Taoiseach'; *The Irish Times*, 31 January 2006, 'FG claims migrant child payment to cost €150m'.

[16] These figures exclude doctors who currently hold temporary registration.

[17] Annual averages supplied by Skills and Labour Market Research Unit, FÁS

[18] Quarterly National Household Survey Q2 1998–2004, CSO; Skills and Labour Market Research Unit, FÁS

national students are more likely to report feeling isolated in school and are much less likely to see themselves as popular (see Smyth, McCoy and Darmody, 2004; Smyth et al., 2006).

Immigration of overseas students has brought significant revenue to the third-level and English as a Foreign Language (EFL) sectors in Ireland. An inter-departmental working group (Department of Education, 2004) recently reported that total earnings from overseas third-level students in 2001/2002 is estimated to be approximately €140 million, of which fees accounted for €68 million. The English as a Foreign Language (EFL) sector brought almost 200,000 visitors to Ireland in 2003 and the sector is estimated to account for around €300 million in foreign earnings annually.

The occupational gap found in research by Barrett, Bergin and Duffy (2006), discussed above, suggests that migrant workers may be experiencing problems with English language skills and with the recognition of foreign qualifications. There have been some new initiatives developed recently to address this problem. English language classes are provided for economic migrants by the Vocational Education Colleges. The recently launched 'Know before you go' information DVD produced by FÁS and distributed through employment services throughout the EU, provides some information on how to access English language training in Ireland.

Other impacts

There are indications that a significant number of immigrants are purchasing houses in Ireland. The latest *Medium Term Review 2005–2012* (Fitz Gerald et al., 2005) observes that a large proportion of immigrants are in the key household-forming age groups between 25 and 44 years old. It estimates that migration contributed an annual average of 6,000 units to housing demand between 1997 and 2002, 8,300 between 2003 and 2006 and is projected to contribute an annual average of 12,300 units to housing demand between 2007 and 2011.

The impact of immigration on politics is just beginning to become apparent. All resident non-Irish nationals may vote in local elections or stand for local office in Ireland. Press reports indicate that 19 non-Irish national candidates contested the local elections in June 2004. Research commissioned by Amnesty International in 2001 on the views of black and ethnic minorities (including Irish persons and Travellers) showed that 60 per cent stated that local political representatives do not represent them or their community (see Loyal and Mulcahy, 2001).

Attitudes of the indigenous population

While Ireland was traditionally an ethnically homogeneous country, migration into the country has increased rapidly in the last decade, and a range of new policy challenges concerning migration have arisen. People may be concerned about the arrival of immigrants for a number of reasons. These may be economic in nature, such as fear of wage competition or job loss, or concern over the cost of social welfare programmes, or they may be more cultural, relating to fears that immigrants may undermine traditional religions, culture, and way of life or language of an indigenous population. These fears are often expected to intensify if there is a sharp increase in immigration or if immigrants come to represent a substantial proportion of the total population (Card, Dustmann and Preston, 2005).

Apart from anecdotal evidence, relatively little is known about the attitudes of the population in Ireland towards migrants and migration. One survey of Dublin residents suggested high levels of hostility toward refugees (Curry, 2000). However, there was no evidence relating to other migrants, including those from other EU countries and work-permit holders, and it is difficult to interpret survey findings in the absence of comparative data.

The European Social Survey (ESS) 2003, a nationally representative sample survey conducted in Ireland as well as 21 other European countries using a harmonised questionnaire, offers an opportunity to examine the attitudes of the indigenous population to migrants in a comparative framework. Migrants are defined as people who have come to Ireland from other countries – for work, education, to join family or for political reasons (asylum seekers).

Figure 13.6 shows several indices of attitudes to migrants across Europe. With regard to the measure of resistance to immigrants, Ireland ranked eighteenth out of 19 countries, suggesting a generally low level of resistance to immigrants of different races and from different countries.[19] However, Ireland ranked in the middle of the distribution (ninth out of 18) with regard to attitudes to ethnic distance, tapping into preferences regarding becoming related to, or working with, an immigrant or someone of a different race. Ireland ranked in twelfth position on the extent to which

---

[19] 'Resistance to immigrants' is based on an index combining agreement/disagreement with three statements relating to allowing more or less immigrants of different race/ethnic group from majority, from poorer countries in Europe and from poorer countries outside Europe. 'Perceived collective ethnic threat' is based on an index combining agreement/disagreement with six statements relating to whether immigrants take jobs away or create new jobs; take out more in taxes and services than they put in; are bad or good for the economy; undermine or enrich cultural life; make the country a worse or better place to live; make crime problems worse or better. 'Favouring ethnic distance' is based on an index combining agreement/disagreement with a series of statements relating to whether the respondent minds if the boss is an immigrant of same or different group as the majority and if a close relative is married to an immigrant of same or different group as the majority.

Figure 13.6: *Comparative indices of attitudes to migrants, ESS 2003*

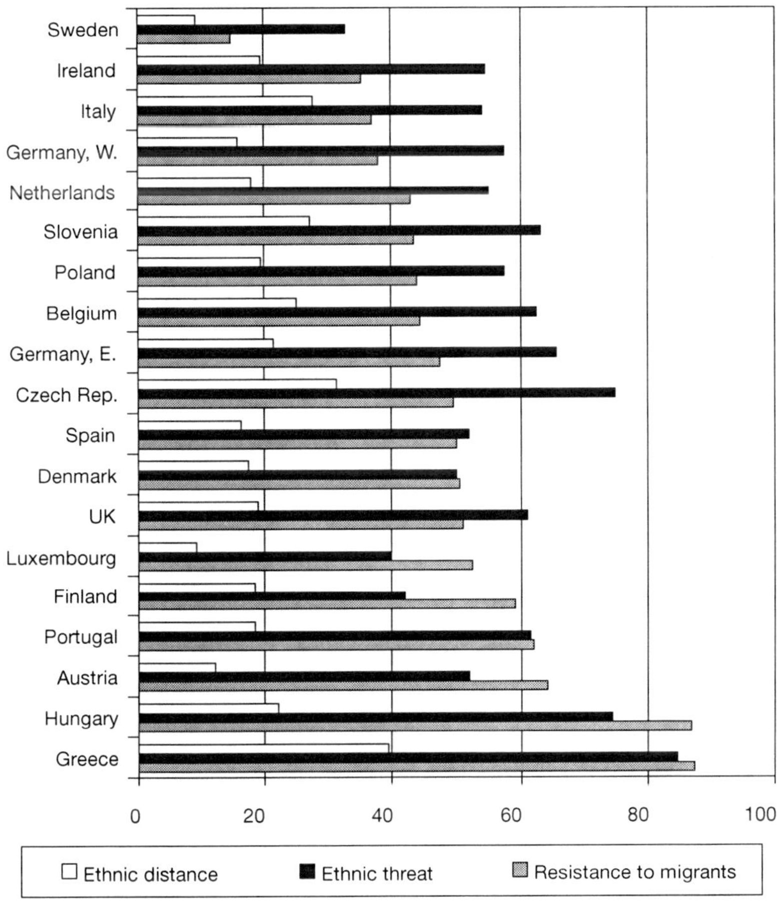

Source: EUMC, 2005

immigrants are perceived as a threat – in relation to employment, taxation and social services, the economy and cultural identity.

On balance, these indicators would suggest that, by comparison with other European countries, the indigenous population in Ireland is reasonably open to, and tolerant of, immigrants. It should of course be noted that these averages conceal important differences between sub-populations, and that in Ireland, as elsewhere, more highly educated people, and younger people, are more likely to exhibit more tolerant attitudes to migrants.

As we have already seen, the influx of the 'New Irish' has been a relatively recent and fast-growing phenomenon, so it is interesting to see

Table 13.2: *Changes in indexes of resistance to immigrants, Ireland and the EU*

		1997	*2000*	*2003*
1 Resistance to multicultural society • It is a good thing for any society to be made up of people from different races, religions or cultures. • Ireland's diversity in terms of race, religion or culture adds to its strengths.	Ireland EU av.	.223 .355	.374 .381	.257 .366
2 Limits to multicultural society • There is a limit to how many people of other races, religions or cultures a society can accept. • Ireland has reached its limits; if there were to be more people belonging to these minority groups we would have problems	Ireland EU av.	.579 .659	.766 .683	.805 .702
3 Opposition to civil rights for legal immigrants • Legally established immigrants from outside the European Union should have the same social rights as Irish citizens. • Legally established immigrants from outside the European Union should have the right to bring members of their immediate family to Ireland • Legally established immigrants from outside the European Union should be able to become naturalised easily.	Ireland EU av.	.309 .423	.344 .443	.325 .409
4 Repatriation policies for legal migrants • Legally established immigrants from outside the European Union should be sent back to their country of origin if they are unemployed. • Legally established immigrants from outside the European Union should all be sent back to their country of origin.	Ireland EU av.	.171 .293	.254 .311	.410 .352
5 Insistence on conformity to law • In order to be fully accepted members of Irish society, people belonging to these minority groups must give up such parts of their religion or culture which may be in conflict with Irish law.	Ireland EU av.	.390 .621	.518 .675	.684 .726

Higher scores indicate greater resistance to immigrants
Source: Coenders, Lubbers and Scheepers (2005)

whether the increase in immigration has led to changes in attitudes among the indigenous population. To answer this question we can draw on successive waves of the Eurobarometer survey carried out in 1997, 2000 and 2003 (Table 13.2) – a period that coincides with increased immigration to Ireland. On average, Irish respondents to the Eurobarometer survey have been well below the European average with respect to generalised resistance to a multicultural society, which relates to the evaluation of whether ethnic and cultural diversity are beneficial for society. This index increased between 1997 and 2000, but fell back to previous levels in 2003.

In 1997, before the surge in immigration, the Irish population was well below the European average with respect to the perceived need to maintain limits to cultural and ethnic diversity, to the need for repatriation policies that would require legal migrants to be sent back to their countries of origin, for example, in the case of unemployment, and in their insistence that people belonging to minority groups should give up parts of their religion or culture if these were in conflict with Irish law. However, the Irish scores on each of these indices increased substantially over the following six years.

By 2003 Ireland had converged with the rest of Europe in insisting on conformity to national laws, and exceeded the EU average in terms of perceived limits to multicultural society and in terms of favouring repatriation policies for legal migrants. Notwithstanding these increases in expressed reservations about the potential impact of increased migration, Irish responses have been quite nuanced in terms of how migrants should be treated. In particular, opposition to according civil rights to migrants has been lower in Ireland than the EU average, and there was no significant increase in this index over time.

The experience of migrants: racism and discrimination

The preceding section reports the response of the population in Ireland to migration; but what of migrants themselves? What is their experience of coming to live in Ireland? In the absence of systematic research on the topic, in summer 2005 the ESRI conducted the first nationally representative survey of migrants to investigate their experience of racism and discrimination in Ireland.[20] The survey was a postal survey based on administrative records of work-permit holders and asylum seekers, and

---

[20] This survey was funded by the European Monitoring Centre on Racism and Xenophobia. Detailed findings are reported in McGinnity et al. (2006).

included a broad range of non-EU adult migrants from Africa, Asia and Eastern Europe.[21] The questions measure discrimination on the basis of national/ethnic origin as perceived by the respondent.[22] The results presented here are based on usable questionnaires from 624 work-permit holders and 417 asylum seekers, re-weighted to be representative of the relevant population.[23]

Domains of discrimination

Figure 13.7 presents an overall comparison of the different situations where discrimination may have been experienced, grouped into five different domains: 1. Employment; 2. Commercial transactions; 3. Private life and public arenas; 4. Shops and restaurants and 5. Institutions.

Harassment on the street or on public transport was the most common form of racism/discrimination in Ireland, followed closely by harassment at work. Being denied access to employment is the only other form of discrimination experienced by at least 20 per cent of respondents. Fewer respondents generally experience being badly treated by an institution, the one notable exception being poor treatment by the immigration services. The next most common form of racism/discrimination is being badly treated in a restaurant or shop. The pattern of racial discrimination is broadly similar to other European countries, with work-related discrimination and harassment on the street featuring highly in all studies. For example, in the Netherlands, 42 per cent of the sample experienced harassment at work, 28 per cent experienced harassment on the street. In Germany, 27 per cent were refused a job, 26 per cent experienced harassment at work and 27 per cent experienced harassment on the street. In Italy and Greece, the most common form of discrimination was in access to housing (63 per cent in Italy and 66 per cent in Greece). Bad treatment by the police and being denied access to housing is much less common among migrants in Ireland than in most other countries (see EUMC, 2006).

These findings are broadly consistent with previous Irish studies of racism, (Loyal and Mulcahy, 2001; Casey and O'Connell, 2000; Horgan,

---

21 This sampling strategy ensured a reasonably comprehensive coverage of recent migrants to Ireland. Those who fall outside the scope of the study are: EU and American nationals; all illegal immigrants; most refugees; migrants on student visas; migrants on work authorisation visas and dependents of legal residents.

22 The questions thus require a subjective assessment of incidents by the respondent, and the results should be interpreted in light of this.

23 White South/Central Africans are excluded from these results as the group is sufficiently large to affect the findings on reported racism for the regional group, South/Central Africans, but arguably too small to be analysed separately.

Figure 13.7: *Percentage of migrants (work-permit holders and asylum seekers) who experienced discrimination at least 1–2 times in domain specified*

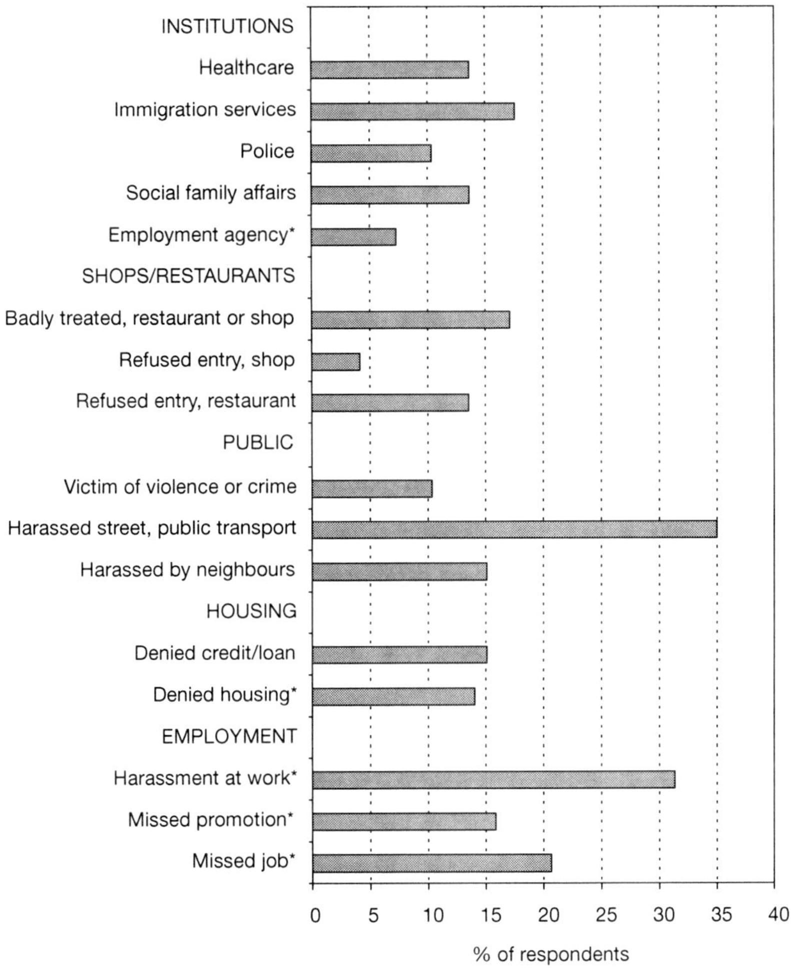

Notes: *Work-related discrimination, access to housing and treatment by the employment service based on work-permit holders only. All other questions relate to those who had contact or experience of the domain in question.

Source: Derived from McGinnity et al., 2006

2000) although none of these are based on representative samples of the population. The CSO included a special module on equality in the QNHS, Quarter 2, 2004 and found that 24 per cent of non-Irish nationals reported having experienced discrimination, compared to less than 12 per cent of Irish nationals (CSO, 2005c). The CSO survey also found that 32 per cent of persons of 'Other Ethnic Backgrounds' reported having experienced discrimination, compared to 12 per cent of those of 'White Ethnic Background'.

How does the experience of discrimination vary between groups of migrants? For most domains studied, Southern/Central Africans, most of whom are Black, experience considerably more racism and discrimination than any of the other groups. South/Central Africans (including, for example, Nigerians and Congolese) experience a particularly high level of racial harassment on the street and on public transport, relative to other migrants. They also experience more discrimination in shops and restaurants and in accessing employment. North Africans and Asians generally experience much lower levels of discrimination than Southern/Central Africans, despite the fact that they too look visibly different from the native Irish population. Non-EU East Europeans also experience relatively low levels of discrimination relative to Southern/Central Africans.

Highly educated migrants are significantly more likely to report experiencing discrimination in all domains. This is consistent with findings from other countries. Migrant women experience discrimination less often in public places and shops/restaurants but experience institutional discrimination more often. Young migrants experience more discrimination than older migrants in all domains except commercial discrimination. This is also true in most other countries. Migrants who have been in Ireland longer tend to have experienced more discrimination in the past year.

Work-permit holders experience significantly less discrimination than asylum seekers. This is true of public racism/harassment, discrimination in shops and restaurants and institutional discrimination. The difference between work-permit holders and asylum seekers is greatest for institutional discrimination, indicating that it is in this domain that differences in legal status are most salient. The overall difference could be due to more favourable attitudes to work-permit holders by the Irish population and authorities, as work-permit holders are seen as 'legitimate', paying taxes and fulfilling a need in the Irish labour market. Asylum seekers are more likely to be seen as illegitimate and a burden on the State (especially as they are not allowed to work). Given the very rapid rise in asylum applications between 1995 and 2000, there was a perception by some people in Ireland that applicants were using the asylum system as a route to economic migration, and that their asylum applications were not genuine. In addition, because of geographical dispersion, asylum seekers tend to be more identifiable, as they live in dedicated accommodation, often in small towns, and they do not work. Work-permit holders are more likely to live in cities and be less distinguishable from the native population.

Racism: Irish policy responses and the extent of racism in Ireland

Ireland has relatively robust legislative provisions around racism and discrimination. As noted above, measures such as the Equality Act, 2004, and the Employment Equality Act, 1998, provide important protections for immigrants in the labour market and in accessing goods and services. The Garda Racial and Intracultural office was set up within the Irish police force to develop and monitor strategies to deal with ethnic and racial diversity, and indeed this may explain why bad treatment by the police was somewhat lower than expected. The National Consultative Committee on Racism and Interculturalism was established in 1998. The publication of the government's National Action Plan on Racism (NAPR) in January 2005 further enhanced protection against racism and discrimination. However, as the ESRI survey found, racism and discrimination is high among Black Africans, relative to other groups, and the recent CSO special module on equality found that 31 per cent of those from other ethnic backgrounds experienced discrimination, which was higher than any of the other subgroups studied (CSO, 2005c).

That said, overall levels of reported racism in Ireland tend to be lower than elsewhere in Europe, particularly Southern European countries. At this point it is uncertain whether racism will increase or decrease as migrant communities become more established and increase as a proportion of the overall population. The Irish experience of migration has coincided with very rapid economic growth and an unprecedented increase in employment and low unemployment. The economic boom may have created an auspicious context for the reception of migrants into Ireland.

Integration of immigrants in Ireland

What type of integration policy is suitable for Ireland and what lessons can be learned from the experience of other more established immigration countries? Detailed analysis of international experiences of integration policy development is beyond the remit of this book. Castles and Miller (2003) identify three different approaches to immigration adopted internationally by immigration countries: differential exclusionary, assimilationist and multicultural. As the authors observe, this somewhat crude distinction neglects the nuances of individual national situations. However, the contrast between the three models hinges on divergent approaches to integration and therefore elucidates this discussion.

It is proposed that former guest-worker countries such as Germany, Switzerland and Austria have pursued a differential exclusionary model of immigration policy development. Immigrants have been encouraged to join the labour market but are excluded from other areas of society. Family reunion is discouraged and secure residence status/naturalisation is more difficult to obtain. France provides an example of a country that has encouraged immigrants to assimilate. The State's role has been viewed as the facilitator of conditions conducive to immigrants becoming indistinguishable from the majority population, for example, by facilitating naturalisation. This assimilationist position was pursued in other former colonial countries, including the UK, but later abandoned in favour of more flexible integration policies.

Countries which are deemed to be 'classical' immigration countries such as the USA, Canada and Australia have adopted a more multicultural (or pluralist) model. This model implies that immigrants should be granted equal rights in all spheres of society and that the diversity of various groups should be respected. Multiculturalism is usually a two-way process with some expectation of conformity on the part of the immigrant to the values of the host society. Multiculturalism is criticised as a threat to the host culture by some, while others view the model as a superficial gesture towards the acceptance of diversity, without the necessary structural change.

Castles and Miller conclude that temporary migrant labour recruitment inevitably leads to some permanent settlement and that the character of the resulting ethnic groups will depend heavily on the policies adopted by the host societies. A multicultural model incorporating access to citizenship is advocated:

> The ethnic groups arising from immigration need their own associations and social networks, as well as their own languages and cultures. Policies which deny legitimacy to these needs lead to isolation and separatism … the best way to prevent marginalisation and social conflicts is to grant permanent immigrants full rights in all social spheres.

The Irish State advisory body – the National Consultative Committee on Racism and Interculturalism (2004) – advocates interculturalism, defined as:

> … interaction between majority and minority cultures to foster understanding and respect. It is about ensuring that cultural diversity is acknowledged and catered for. It is about inclusion for minority ethnic groups by design and planning, not as a default or add-on.

There is therefore a greater emphasis on changing the attitudes and practices of the majority population, as well as those of minorities, rather than simply tolerating diversity. At present Ireland has a specific integration policy for refugees only.[24] However, a new fund has recently been established by the State for projects to assist the integration of all legally resident immigrants. The State's Reception and Integration Agency (RIA) deems integration to be achievable when immigrants, as well as the host community, are able to: speak the host language; gain access to, and delivery of, core services such as education and health; secure jobs commensurate with their abilities; engage in all aspects of civil action; participate fully in the democratic process; and when immigrants are prepared to modify their attitudes and behaviours.[25]

This definition appears to reflect the two-way principle of the multicultural and intercultural approaches. However, recent developments regarding access to citizenship and Ireland's decision to opt out of EU Directives on family reunification[26] and long-term residents[27] imply a more restrictive model. It is anticipated that domestic legislation will address these latter two important issues in the near future through the Immigration and Residence Bill, and future Irish integration policy may therefore begin to take on a clearer shape.

Conclusion

The last decade has ended Ireland's long history of emigration and opened up a new era of immigration. The growth in non-Irish national migrants, both for economic and political reasons, has been very dramatic and has added a substantial non-Irish national population to what formerly was a culturally homogeneous society. Nonetheless, immigration to Ireland has originated primarily from within Europe and so has been less racially, culturally and religiously heterogeneous than that experienced by other immigrant societies.

---

24 Regarding the integration of refugees, a policy document produced by the Department of Justice, Equality and Law Reform (2000) stated: 'Integration is a two-way process that places a real obligation on both society and the individual refugee. From the refugee's perspective, integration requires a willingness to adapt to the lifestyle of Irish society without abandoning or being expected to abandon one's own cultural identity. From the point of view of Irish society, it requires a willingness to accept refugees on the basis of equality and to take action to facilitate access to services, resources and decision-making processes in parity with Irish nationals.'

25 Presentation made by John Haskins, Principal Officer, Reception and Integration Agency; European Network Against Racism seminar on 'Integration and active citizenship', 27 January 2006

26 COM/2002/0225

27 COM/2001/127

We have characterised the evolution of Irish migration in terms of three phases: 1. Substantial outward migration until the early 1990s; 2. A dramatic increase in inward migration from the mid-1990s to 2004, linked to the economic boom; 3. Since 2004, a phase of more secure, stable and perhaps permanent immigration in which the majority of migrants are likely to be entitled to a more comprehensive package of economic and civil rights than in the previous phase.

With this shift towards a greater proportion of long-term immigrants, the expectation that migrants are in Ireland on a temporary basis is increasingly redundant. International experience would suggest that long-term immigration necessitates the development of a comprehensive and coherent long-term strategy to integrate the new Irish.

It should be acknowledged that important developments took place during Phase 2 of the evolution of Irish migration, such as the National Action Plan against Racism and legislation to outlaw discrimination on the grounds of race, ethnicity or national origin. Arguably, however, these constitute piecemeal responses and significant gaps remain, for example, in the education system, in the provision of both public and private services and in enabling migrants to participate actively in civil society.

If current migration trends continue as expected, there is a pressing need for a thorough debate about the framework within which migration policy should evolve. That framework would entail both economic and social components. The economic issues concern the objectives of migration policy and the appropriate balance between skilled and unskilled immigrants. We have discussed the evidence that points to the positive economic impact of migration. Economic imperatives suggest that immigration of skilled labour is essential to a knowledge economy. However, reliance on unskilled immigration raises questions about whether the objective is to increase economic activity (GNP) or standards of living (GNP per capita). It is also necessary to examine whether unskilled immigrant labour is meeting demand for low-skilled low-wage jobs that cannot be met from domestic sources, or to sustain low-wage and low-productivity jobs in declining industries, such as agriculture. Clearly, the skill composition of migration has an impact on living standards and the distribution of earnings. NESC argues that it will be critical to avoid strong migration at the lower end of the market, pushing market wages below the reservation wages of lower-skilled indigenous workers. Important in this respect also is to ensure that migrant workers are not employed in occupations that fall below their skill levels – either because of discrimination or insufficient English language skills. Of course it should be acknowledged that in the long run EU membership entails free movement of labour, irrespective of skill-level. So, relying exclusively on domestic labour supply is not a long-term option. The new employment permits system addresses this tension by combining a very liberal migration regime in relation to nationals of the 25–EU Member States and to highly qualified labour migrants from the rest of the world, with a highly restrictive regime in respect of lower-skilled workers from beyond the borders of the EU–25 states.[28] One of the side effects of a very restrictive non-EU labour migration policy could be to channel would-be migrants towards illegal or irregular entry routes.

The second component is social. It concerns how to integrate the new Irish and their children, and how institutions and organisations can adapt to become open to all residents. This raises controversial issues about socio-cultural assimilation, seen as the attempt at one-way adoption of a host society's social and cultural values, versus multiculturalism, which appears more pluralist but may undermine cohesion of the broader society. Integration can be conceived as a two-way process in which both newcomers and host societies are changed. Papademetriou (2003) argues that 'immigrants thrive best in socially and politically supportive environments that allow them to change most of their social and cultural traditions at their own pace, while learning and adapting to important community practices more quickly'. Such an integration policy is grounded on equity and mutuality, and requires active engagement not only of national government, but also the business sector, trade unions and the range of political, civic, community and voluntary organisations. In this respect it appears that Ireland can learn from other societies that have successfully welcomed and integrated immigrant populations. NESC (2006) argues that successful forward-looking management of migration requires that 'Policies for migrants must be consciously developed that see the whole person and not just the unit of labour, and foster interaction, social learning, and trust between migrant communities and the indigenous population' (p. 143).

It remains to be seen what direction integration policy will take in Ireland. In this respect, the survey findings relating to attitudes in Ireland to immigrants provide grounds for both concern and optimism. Increased immigration appears to have led to increased concerns about the capacity of Irish society to absorb the relatively rapid influx of immigrants. However, notwithstanding these concerns, Irish respondents exhibited substantially greater willingness than many other Europeans to accord civil rights to immigrants, and these attitudes showed no signs of shifting during

[28] At present the more restrictive work permit regime continues to apply to nationals of the new EU accession states, Romania and Bulgaria; however, preference will be given to them over nationals of non-European Economic Area countries.

the period 1997–2003, when immigration increased dramatically. As such, the survey results suggest the importance of developing long-term policies to promote integration, but also that there is a normative foundation for their development. This is not a matter of choice. Laissez-fair migration policies can ultimately sow the seeds of inter-group conflict.

These issues pose considerable challenges for Irish society but need to be addressed to avoid the marginalisation of non-Irish nationals, and ethnic cleavages in Irish society. The challenge for the next decades will be to develop a fair and managed migration policy that will respond to the needs of an increasingly diverse society and that will ensure that Irish institutions are open to all legal residents. It is of course important to recognise that in seeking to assist migrants to settle and incorporate themselves in the economy and the society, we should not lose sight of the interests and priorities of the broader Irish society.

We noted at the outset of this chapter that the new immigration represents a break with a long history of mass emigration. Arguably, migration can be regarded as a gauge of the quality of life: most people emigrate because of lack of economic opportunity or because they cannot achieve sufficient quality of life in their native lands. In this sense the cessation of the long-drawn out exodus from the country itself represents an improvement in the quality of life in that the current generation of young Irish people can choose to live and work in their native land. The influx of immigrants, both returning Irish emigrants as well as non-Irish immigrants, is also a positive measure of the quality of life available in Ireland in the twenty-first century.

14

Crime and its Consequences

Ian O'Donnell

Introduction

This chapter examines the relationships between crime, risk, fear and the politics of punishment. It takes as its frame of reference the period 1990 to 2004. A fundamental change in the way crimes were categorised in 2000, when the focus shifted from 'indictable' to 'headline' crime, makes interpretation problematic, and the limited quality of the data renders international comparisons unreliable. Nonetheless a number of trends are marked and can be summarised as follows:

1. Recorded indictable crime rose steadily between 1990 and 1994.
2. Recorded indictable crime fell sharply between 1995 and 1999.
3. Recorded headline crime fell, surged and then declined between 2000 and 2004.

Narrowing the focus to the most serious type of crime and looking at the public and political response, the following can be said:

1. Homicide accounts for a small fraction of violent deaths. Many more occur at workplaces and on the road.
2. Public anxiety about crime peaked suddenly in 1996, and dealing with lawlessness became a hot topic in the following year's general election. Since then it seems to have oscillated in people's hierarchy of concerns.
3. Victimisation surveys show a doubling in the risk of being assaulted or experiencing theft between 1998 and 2003. Over the same period personal feelings of safety were unchanged.
4. The prison population grew substantially between 1996 and 2001.

The role of the economy varies according to the type of crime in question. There is evidence of an inverse relationship between the level of spending and property crime but a positive correlation with violence (O'Donnell and O'Sullivan, 2001). The crime drop in the latter half of the

T. Fahey et al. (eds.), Quality of Life in Ireland, 245–264.

1990s, which was caused by a reduction in offences against property, can be explained by a decreased motivation to offend when the capacity to acquire goods lawfully was enhanced. Improved health care for heroin users, who can be prolific thieves, played a role also. Another factor – albeit of less significance than is often assumed – was a major expansion in the number of prison places, itself made possible by the country's growing wealth. In addition, a rise in living standards means that security measures can be afforded so that the costs (to the potential offender) of the most prevalent crimes such as burglary, shoplifting and criminal damage are raised by the presence of guards, cameras, alarms and property marking.

The overall fall in crime concealed an increase in offences against the person from around 1995. This can be explained by the tendency for people with greater disposable incomes to spend more time in pubs and clubs, settings where interpersonal confrontations may occur. The rise in street disorder and lethal violence is intertwined with rising levels of alcohol consumption (Institute of Criminology, 2003; O'Donnell, 2005a). In one English study the growth in beer drinking was identified as the single most important factor in explaining the growth in violent crime (Field, 1990).

At the same time as prosperity and the pursuit of profit reduce the motivation for petty theft they broaden the range of opportunities for crimes such as tax evasion and health and safety violations. It would not be surprising if a booming economy were to be accompanied by an increase in workplace deaths and injuries and a flood of money being hidden from the Revenue Commissioners.

The political response to crime can have a powerful impact on public perceptions of risk and feelings of safety. These in turn influence quality of life, regardless of the underlying level of criminal activity.

The experience in other countries is that once the public becomes fearful, it is difficult to nudge them back to confidence. This is true even when crime goes into a downward spiral. In this way the public can remain fretful, uneasy and intolerant, independently of whether their bodily integrity or property is more or less at risk.

There is a tendency for governments to respond with increasingly repressive measures, become preoccupied with imprisonment, and downgrade expert advice in favour of sound bite 'solutions'. Such responses in turn confirm and feed public concerns. These are some of the symptoms of what has been termed a 'culture of control' (Garland, 2001). An attempt will be made in this chapter to investigate whether Ireland has entered the twenty-first century relatively safe but chronically fearful and increasingly punitive.

Trends in recorded crime

The interpretation of crime statistics in every country is fraught with difficulty. The problems are compounded in Ireland because of the over-reliance on police data, the compilation of which is poorly understood. Despite lengthy deliberations, an Expert Group, set up by the Minister for Justice, Equality and Law Reform, remained confused as to how the statistics were assembled and should be interpreted, a minority (including the author) reporting that despite its best efforts it could 'come to no conclusions about the quality, reliability and accuracy of Garda data' (Expert Group on Crime Statistics, 2004, para. 2). This makes it difficult to take the statistics at face value, let alone to compare them with police data from other countries.

There are few alternative sources of information. Although some national and local surveys have been conducted over the years (e.g. O'Connell and Whelan, 1994; Watson, 2000) there remains an excessive dependence on the official picture and when it is unclear, explanation becomes difficult. Matters became more complicated in 2000 when the method of categorising and presenting crime in the Garda annual report changed fundamentally for reasons that were not revealed.

The most significant change for present purposes was the replacement of four categories of 'indictable' crime with ten categories of 'headline' crime. The types of crime covered by each classificatory scheme are broadly similar. In general these are the offences deemed to be most serious. The bulk of them are against property (e.g. burglary and theft), and all serious violence is included (e.g. murder, manslaughter, rape, sexual assault). These changes accompanied the introduction of a new computer system, known as PULSE (Police Using Leading Systems Effectively). It is not possible to map headline offences directly onto their indictable predecessors.

The traditional lack of explanatory text in the annual Garda reports makes it difficult to understand whether changes in offence frequency are due to legislative initiatives, policy developments, new recording practices or real changes in criminal behaviour. This problem is not new. It was highlighted a quarter of a century ago by Rottman (1980) in his pioneering study, *Crime in the Republic of Ireland: Statistical Trends and their Interpretation*, and has been reiterated by more recent commentators. The lack of good quality data has been an impediment to criminological research, although a number of books have managed to build interesting theoretical arguments using the meagre available resources; examples include McCullagh (1996), Brewer, Lockhart and Rodgers (1997), and Kilcommins, O'Donnell, O'Sullivan and Vaughan (2004).

The variation in the number of crimes recorded before and after the introduction of PULSE was substantial. As Table 14.1 shows, a steady and significant downward trend continued briefly before being replaced by a remarkable upward trajectory, an apparent tidal wave of crime. The 20.4 per cent increase in the crime rate in 2002 was one of the greatest on record. In the absence of major social or legislative change, sudden fluctuations in recorded crime levels, in whichever direction, are more likely to be accounted for by changes in data processing than real changes in the level of criminal activity. Changes in the latter are usually more gradual. It seems reasonable to speculate that the drop in 2000 reflected the bedding down of the new system, while the increases in subsequent years are accounted for by the more comprehensive recording required by the new technology. The slowing down of the rate of change in recent years suggests that the system may now be stable.

Table 14.1: *Crimes recorded by An Garda Síochána*

	No. recorded	*Rate per 1,000 population*	*Annual change in rate (per cent)*
Indictable			
1990	87,658	25.0	
1991	94,406	26.8	7.1
1992	95,391	26.8	0.2
1993	98,979	27.7	3.2
1994	101,036	28.2	1.7
1995	102,484	28.5	1.0
1996	100,785	27.8	– 2.3
1997	90,875	24.8	–10.8
1998	85,627	23.1	–6.8
1999	81,274	21.7	–6.1
Headline			
2000	73,276	19.3	
2001	86,633	22.6	16.6
2002	106,415	27.2	20.4
2003	103,360	26.3	–3.0
2004	98,964	24.5	–7.1

Source: O'Donnell, O'Sullivan and Healy, 2005, Tables 1.2 and 1.3; An Garda Síochána, 2005

It is inevitable that technological advances will be introduced from time to time in law enforcement agencies and it would be surprising if crime rates did not rise as a result of the more complete recording that accompanies new data collection methodologies. In this context recorded crime could show an increase even if the underlying rate of victimisation remained stable or fell.

There is an important point to be made about the comprehensiveness of the Garda figures. Most crimes are not included in the indictable/headline categories, although all of the serious ones are. For less serious matters such as road traffic and liquor licensing violations and public order offences (known in Garda parlance as non-indictable or non-headline) we are told only the number that result in proceedings. Thus, while it is possible to count how many offences of all kinds resulted in proceedings, the total amount of recorded crime cannot be ascertained.

Proceedings in non-indictable/non-headline cases have declined greatly over the past decade, from 501,000 in 1994 to 282,000 in 2004 (the total in 1984 was 847,000). This is at odds with the tendency noted above for improved recording systems to lead to improved recording. The explanation for this trend is unclear. It may reflect a reduction in Garda activity, or a change in priorities, as these types of offences usually result from proactive policing rather than victim reports. If these figures are accepted they reflect a substantial change in operational policing, but one which seems to have gone unnoticed, or at least unremarked. It is not possible to say why proceedings were taken in three times as many cases 20 years ago.

The level of crime is often offered as an index of social harmony, with increases seen to flow from fundamental ruptures in the organisation of society. This view was put strongly by a former Garda Commissioner in September 1994, on the cusp of the economic recovery. In a trenchant article published by *The Irish Times*, Patrick Culligan portrayed a society in transition where traditional authorities were being challenged, new social norms were evolving and more opportunities to offend were becoming available. He harked back to a supposed golden age of stability, civility and contentment; a time when life was ordered and predictable, institutions were benign places, and the enforcement of discipline was unproblematic. The scenario outlined by the commissioner suggested a bleak future, with relentlessly escalating crime rates.

In fact, the opposite occurred. Between 1995 and 1999 the number of recorded indictable crimes fell by 21 per cent. This was the sharpest reduction in the European Union. Such a fall is not unprecedented. Between 1983 and 1987, crime dropped by 17 per cent. The number of headline offences recorded in 2000 was 73,276 (19.3 per 1,000 population). This was the biggest fall in the EU between 1999 and 2000, but is likely to have resulted in large part from the new method of compiling and presenting data, which took some time to be fully rolled out. It seems fair to say that the post-1995 decline was reversed but the return to previous levels was not sustained. Since 2002 the rate has begun to dip again.

There are considerable problems associated with comparative analyses. Jurisdictions differ in how crimes are defined, prioritised, recorded and presented for publication. Without a detailed understanding of criminal justice policy and practice at the level of the individual country it is misleading to read too much into international data. While a crude and fallible measure, comparative crime statistics provide the best available rough guide to the extent of a country's response to crime. The most up-to-date figures compiled by the Home Office in London relate to 2001 and these are summarised in Figure 14.1.

Figure 14.1: *Recorded crime in 2001, EU–15*

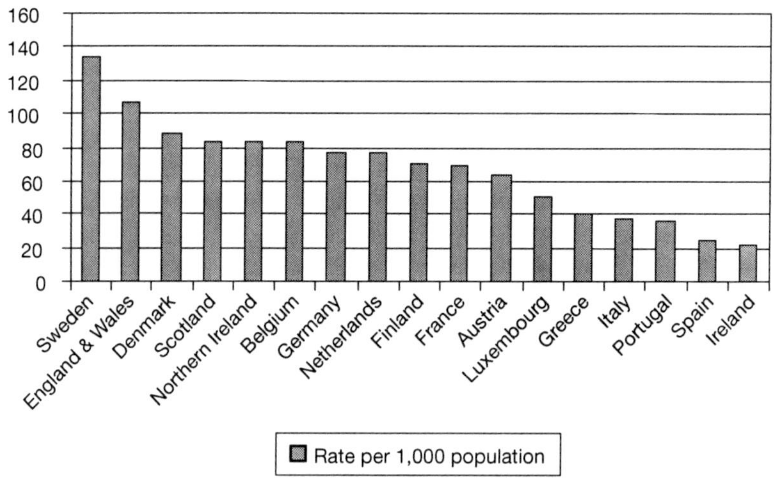

Source: Barclay and Tavares, 2003

Sweden's position at the top of the table probably owes more to Scandinavian thoroughness than to epidemic levels of criminality. For example, the country's most recent available statistics show that in 2004, 71,000 bicycle thefts were recorded as well as 12,000 thefts from libraries and 40,000 incidents of graffiti. Large numbers of minor offences, meticulously recorded, cause the overall total to swell dramatically.

For Ireland, only headline offences are included in the returns made to the Home Office. This is one reason why the rate is so out of line with other European countries where a more comprehensive return is made. In the absence of standardised definitions and crime-specific analyses it is not clear how much comfort can be drawn from such an apparently favourable position at the bottom of the table.

Similar numbers of crimes were recorded in 1994 (indictable) and 2004 (headline) but there was a big change in their geographical spread. Particularly noteworthy are the major falls in two Garda regions: the Dublin Metropolitan area (which includes parts of Wicklow and Kildare) and the South (Cork, Kerry and Limerick). This is driven by big drops in the city areas (Dublin down by 16.9 per cent and Cork by 37.2 per cent).

In overall terms, the amount of crime in the cities (Dublin, Cork, Limerick, Waterford and Galway) fell from 70 per cent of the national total in 1994 to 60 per cent in 2004. There were big rises everywhere else, especially the North and West, albeit from low bases. Even in 2004 the counties that make up the Northern Region – Cavan, Monaghan, Donegal, Sligo and Leitrim – accounted between them for only 100 headline crimes per week. This changing distribution is shown in Table 14.2.

Table 14.2: *Indictable/headline crime recorded by Garda region*

	1994	*2004*	*Per cent change*
Dublin	56,395	46,841	–16.9
East	11,285	15,167	34.4
South East	7,551	9,673	28.1
South	17,212	14,788	–14.1
West	5,239	7,127	36.0
North	3,354	5,368	60.0
All	101,036	98,964	–2.1

Source: An Garda Síochána, annual reports

While the cities no longer carry so much of the national crime burden they still account for most killings. For example, 51.4 per cent of all murders took place in Dublin in 2004 compared to 40 per cent in 1994. In Connaught and the border counties there were fewer murders in 2004 (n = 4) than in 1994 (n = 7). Ireland's trend in homicide is interestingly different from other Western countries where the pattern is for an increase beginning in the 1960s and a decline in the 1990s. In Ireland the increase started a decade later and there is no sign yet of a decline.

Lethal harm

There is value in limiting the focus to crimes where the data quality is most reliable and where definitions change least across national boundaries. Probably the best candidate for such an analysis is homicide. This is not necessarily an appropriate index for the overall level of crime – compare Ireland's position in Figures 14.1 and 14.2 – but it is undoubtedly a type of activity that strongly influences public perceptions of the crime problem and shapes the political response.

Figure 14.2 shows that after Finland, France and Belgium and the three jurisdictions making up the UK, Ireland comes next in the EU league table. The range is narrow, with most countries recording between 10 and 15 homicides per million of the population each year. Despite the staggering drop in homicide in the USA in recent times – from 23,440 victims in 1990 to 16,200 in 2002 – its rate is still far greater (55.9 killings per million of the population) than the most deadly EU country; but far less than South Africa where lives are ended through crime at a rate almost unimaginable anywhere else (488.4 per million, on average, between 2000 and 2002).

Figure 14.2: *Homicides per million population, EU–15 average annual rate, 2000 to 2002*

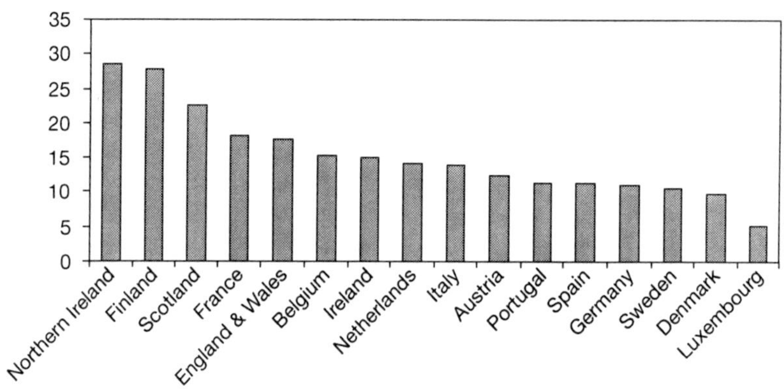

Source: Barclay and Tavares, 2003; Povey, 2005. Greece omitted as homicide data include attempts.

It is clear from Table 14.3 that while the rate of lethal violence in Dublin is not out of line with other European capital cities, it has increased dramatically at a time when the international trend is downward. European cities pale in comparison with the situation in the USA. Between 2000 and 2002, Washington DC clocked up an annual average of 427.8 homicides per million residents, making it one of the most dangerous places in the world (but much safer than in 1991 when the rate stood at 806). Urban areas in Ireland in recent years have seen a significant increase in killings related to gangland activities, often drug-related. These must be taken into account when explaining the upward trend, along with changing patterns of migration and surging alcohol consumption (for a review see O'Donnell, 2005a).

Table 14.3: *Homicides per million population (capital cities, EU–15) average annual rate*

	1990–1992	*2000–2002*	*Per cent change*
Dublin, Ireland	14.7	21.2	44.5
Vienna, Austria	22.1	28.4	28.6
London, England	24.7	26.7	8.2
Edinburgh, Scotland	21.2	16.4	–22.8
Rome, Italy	18.2	13.6	–25.3
Berlin, Germany	29.5	21.7	–26.4
Copenhagen, Denmark	25.3	16.0	–36.8
Stockholm, Sweden	37.7	22.0	–41.6
Paris, France	36.3	18.1	–50.1
Belfast, Northern Ireland	149.9	62.4	–58.4
Helsinki, Finland	48.6	19.2	–60.5
Madrid, Spain	N/a	18.1	–
Lisbon, Portugal	N/a	15.0	–
Amsterdam, Netherlands	N/a	32.3	–
Brussels, Belgium	N/a	30.3	–
Athens and Pireus, Greece	N/a	N/a	–

Source: Barclay and Tavares, 2003; Povey, 2005

Homicides are not the only kind of unlawful deaths that should be the focus of concern. Many road traffic deaths involve flagrant law breaking, such as driving recklessly or at excess speed or under the influence of drugs or alcohol. These are 'accidents' only in the sense that the intention to cause death or serious harm is absent (as indeed it is in many cases of manslaughter). For this reason this category of violent death is included in Table 14.4.

Table 14.4: *Lethal harm (annual averages)*

		1990–1994	*2000–2004*
Homicide	Number	32.0	54.0
	Rate	9.0	13.8
Traffic	Number	434.6	382.2
	Rate	387.1	207.7
Workplace	Number	57.8	63.2
	Rate	49.2	34.6

Note: The national population is used as the denominator when calculating the homicide rate; the number of people in employment is used for the rate of workplace deaths; and the number of vehicles licensed is used for road deaths. All rates are expressed per million.

Sources: An Garda Síochána, National Roads Authority, Health and Safety Authority, Central Statistics Office

There is a dawning realisation that the loss of life on Ireland's roads could be curtailed if drivers changed their behaviour. In its editorial of 22 December 2005, *The Irish Times* declared that 'Drink driving does not happen by chance. It happens by choice.' The newspaper accepted the advice of the National Safety Council that, as driver behaviour contributed to three-quarters of road deaths, describing them as 'accidents' can be inaccurate. It was decided as a matter of policy to substitute the terms 'crash' or 'collision' in future coverage. We have an unusual attitude to the blood spilled by motorists. A bottle thrown recklessly by a drunk person that strikes and kills an innocent passer-by evokes quite a different reaction to a car driven recklessly by a drunk person that has the same consequence. There are many times more deaths on the road (374 in 2004) than homicides (45 in 2004).

Similarly, occupational safety and employee protection fall squarely within the criminal law and many deaths result from ignorance, lax enforcement, deliberate flouting of the regulations and exposure of employees to known (or suspected) hazards. Members of the public can also fall victim to dangerous work practices. Like other violent deaths, these are criminal actions with lethal consequences. However, even among criminologists they are seldom considered as part of the problem of 'crime'. Hillyard et al. (2005) have coined the term zemiology (based on the Greek word, *xemia* meaning harm) to describe the study of all the different types of social harm that impact on people's lives. These include excess winter deaths due to hypothermia, the debilitating consequences of environmental pollution, the poisoning of the food chain through some forms of intensive farming, the adverse financial consequences of duping home owners into buying endowment policies that cost more than they ever realise, and, of course, criminal victimisation.

The point of this perspective is to illustrate that the activities of the State and big business can be more pernicious than those of traditional 'criminals' and we ignore them at our peril.

There are more workplace deaths each year than homicides. In 2004 there were 45 cases of murder and manslaughter, while 49 persons died from injuries sustained at work. It is a sobering fact that Irish citizens are more likely to be lethally harmed at work, sometimes because their employer has broken the law, than they are to be killed by a violent attacker. These deaths are not included in the Garda crime statistics, but are tabulated by the Health and Safety Authority. Indeed, offences of dangerous driving causing serious injury or death and even traffic fatalities that are dealt with as cases of manslaughter are not categorised with offences against the person in the Garda statistics. They appear among a long list of 'other headline offences' somewhere between personation and

Fisheries Act offences. This gives a clear indication of law enforcement priorities and what is considered by the authorities to constitute 'real' crime.

It is difficult to say with any degree of certainty whether the speed at which the economy has grown has led to an increasing disrespect for the law. However, it would be reasonable to hypothesise that the scale and rate of expansion of the construction industry, for example, will have adverse implications for employee protection. Even if standards remained the same or improved, the sheer increase in the number of workers could mean more deaths and injuries, especially with tight deadlines and generous financial rewards on completion. There is the added factor that some of these construction workers will find it difficult to understand written and verbal instructions in English. (The website of the Health and Safety Authority now carries notices in Polish and Turkish.)

It seems plausible therefore to posit a link between workplace deaths and prosperity, but this is not borne out by the figures presented in Table 14.4. While the average number of such deaths each year has risen slightly, the rate per million employees is down by almost one-third. Nor have the increases in traffic volumes, long-distance commuting and car ownership – all symptoms of newfound prosperity – led to a rising death toll on the roads. While the number of road fatalities remains stubbornly high compared to other countries it is less of a problem now than it was a decade ago, especially when the number of vehicles is taken into account. The death rate on the roads (per million licensed vehicles) fell by almost half when the five-year period 2000 to 2004 is compared with 1990 to 1994.

There are other ways that a rich country can be criminogenic but it is difficult to develop any analysis due to a lack of good quality data (or even poor quality data). Garda reports show only a handful of offences that could be considered as white-collar crime (e.g. falsification of accounts, offences against the Companies Act or Stock Exchange Act). This is clearly an underestimate. To give just one example, the financial cost of crimes investigated by the Revenue Commissioners far exceeds that of street crime. The total value of property stolen in robberies, burglaries and thefts in 2004 was €78m (An Garda Síochána, 2005, p. 51). In the same year investigations into tax evasion yielded €698m (Revenue Commissioners, 2004, p. 6).

Not only does the criminal activity not investigated by the Garda cost more to the State than what is traditionally seen as 'crime', but many people are involved in it. For example, the final phase of the investigation into bogus non-resident accounts in January 2004 involved letters being sent to 28,000 individuals who had not come forward under a voluntary disclosure scheme (Revenue Commissioners, 2004, p. 22). The yield from this campaign in 2004 alone was €87.2m, more than the total amount stolen by 'criminals' during the same year. Contrast the single conviction for serious tax evasion obtained in 2004, and highlighted in the Revenue Commissioners' annual report, with a total of 2,098 burglars against whom criminal proceedings were commenced in the same year (An Garda Síochána, 2005, p. 29).

By restricting the focus to police-generated crime figures there is a danger of supporting the stereotypical view which equates the priorities of the criminal justice system with the problem of crime. This ignores the harm and anxiety caused by those against whom police activity is typically not directed, which must surely constitute a large part of the challenge posed by crime to contemporary society.

Victimisation

Because much crime is not reported to the police and because changes in legislation or practice can have such a dramatic impact on the level of recorded crime, victim surveys are used in many countries to provide a more stable measure of people's experiences. The Quarterly National Household Survey administered by the CSO included a module on victimisation in the fourth quarters of 1998 and 2003 (CSO, 1999, 2004b). This provides a valuable point of contrast with the Garda data. The key findings can be summarised as follows:

- In 2003, more than one in twenty (5.2 per cent) persons aged 18 or over indicated that they had been a victim in the previous year of at least one of the following personal crimes: theft with violence; theft without violence; physical assault (excluding domestic violence or sexual assault). This was more than double the comparable rate for 1998 (2.4 per cent).
- The incidence of crimes against property (i.e. burglary; theft of, or from, motor vehicles; bicycle theft; or vandalism) remained relatively unchanged over the five-year period, affecting 11.7 per cent of households surveyed in 2003 compared with 12.1 per cent in 1998.
- While exposure to crimes against property remained highest in the Dublin region (18.7 per cent of households), this represented a slight decrease on the figure recorded five years previously (20.1 per cent). Outside Dublin, exposure to household crime was highest in the Mid-East (12.4 per cent) and Mid-West (11.1 per cent) and lowest in the West (7.2 per cent).

- Of those surveyed in 2003, 80.1 per cent considered that crime was either a 'serious' or 'very serious' problem – compared with 76.7 per cent in 1998. In 1998, 56.1 per cent were worried about becoming victims of crime. This proportion was almost identical in 2003 (56.9 per cent) despite the increase in levels of personal victimisation.
- There was very little change in the public's sense of security as subjectively perceived. Just under three-quarters (74.8 per cent) felt either 'safe' or 'very safe' walking alone in their neighbourhood at night in 2003, virtually no change on the proportion five years previously (73.7 per cent). The vast majority (93.9 per cent in 2003 and 93.2 per cent in 1998) of those surveyed indicated that they felt safe alone in their homes after dark.

While the crime categories, geographical units and reference periods differ, making direct comparison with Garda data impossible, it is important to note that reported personal victimisation increased between 1998 and 2003 for every offence type, age band, geographical region and socio-economic group. However, and crucially, there was little change in the extent to which people thought crime was a problem or felt insecure. Finally, the elderly and women are least at risk of criminal victimisation. But they tend to be most anxious. Thus, people's lives can be destabilised independently of the risk they face.

Has the public reaction to crime changed?

In June 1980, in a survey carried out for *The Irish Times*, members of the public were asked what they thought was the most important problem facing the country. Only 7 per cent put crime at the top of their list. This was at a time when recorded crime was heading for an historic high. The number of indictable offences exceeded 100,000 for the first time in 1983.

Eight years later, a similar question was asked in a survey for *Independent* newspapers. Only 2 per cent were of the view that crime and issues of law and order were the most important problems facing the country. Six years on, in 1994, in a survey conducted for the *Sunday Press*, 3 per cent thought crime was the most important issue facing the country. (In that year 100,000 indictable crimes were recorded for the second time.) Unemployment was ranked highest among those polled, usually followed by inflation, emigration and sometimes the Troubles in Northern Ireland. It seemed that, even in the early 1990s, Ireland remained a nation curiously unconcerned by crime despite recorded crime reaching unprecedented levels (see O'Donnell and O'Sullivan, 2003).

This situation changed suddenly in 1996. In July of that year, when asked what the most critical issue facing the government was, nearly 50 per cent identified crime and law and order. In the same survey, 88 per cent thought the government was losing the fight against crime. Suddenly concern about crime had become a national priority. It was affecting how people saw the world and how safe they felt in it. (At this time recorded crime had begun to fall.)

The reason for the heightened concern is easy to identify. For some time there had been disquiet about the lavish lifestyles enjoyed by many Dublin criminals who had become well known to the public by the nicknames given them by journalists (such as the General, the Monk and the Viper). They had become minor celebrities and appeared to be able to act with impunity. Despite widespread knowledge of their activities the Gardaí seemed unable, or unprepared, to act.

Concern about lawlessness grew in January 1996 due to three rural killings: Patrick Daly's body was found at the bottom of a well; Tommy Casey was killed in his home by intruders; Joyce Quinn was reported missing and found dead two days later. These deaths generated an unusually strong response, including helicopter patrols, national check points and road blocks, because they showed that crime was not just a problem for impoverished urban areas; killing had come to the countryside, the repository of the 'true' Ireland.

On 7 June 1996 Detective Garda Jerry McCabe was shot dead during an attempted robbery of a post office van in Adare, Co. Limerick. Two weeks later the investigative journalist Veronica Guerin was murdered as she sat in her car in Dublin traffic. These killings were defining moments in the debate about law and order in Ireland. They were the catalyst for a hardening in political attitudes. Crime control became a national priority and it was as if a state of national emergency had been declared. The Dáil was recalled for a special debate, and, during the general election campaign which took place in 1997 – as recorded crime continued to fall – public concern seemed to be at an all-time high.

This was a textbook case of what sociologists would call a 'moral panic'. Public anger and anxiety were inflamed and a raft of legal and policy changes was set in motion to clamp down on 'organised' crime. Serious questions were raised about the State's ability to protect its citizens. The calculated killing of a journalist who wrote regularly about Dublin's underworld indicated that crime gangs felt they could operate without fear of consequences. This was a worrying scenario for many people and generated the conditions where a harsh response to perceived lawlessness became acceptable.

These events marked the beginning of a flirtation with Zero Tolerance policing and a more enduring commitment to expand the number of prison places. The decision to punish more was taken despite the fact that recorded crime was falling steeply. It is clear that the public can develop an acute fear of crime due to political hysteria (or cynical calculation) and this can affect quality of life as profoundly as the level of crime.

The fact that the number of prisoners began to rise after the crime rate started to fall is shown in Figure 14.3. Between 1990 and 1996 the number of prisoners fluctuated within a very narrow band, never exceeding 2,200. In 1997 it jumped to more than 2,400 and continued to climb until it achieved a new level of stability at around 3,100. While the prison population has reached a level unprecedented since the foundation of the State, the rate of imprisonment per 100,000 population remains lower than in many EU countries: 81 in 2002 compared with 96 for Germany, 126 for Scotland and 139 for England and Wales.

Figure 14.3: *Daily average number of prisoners*

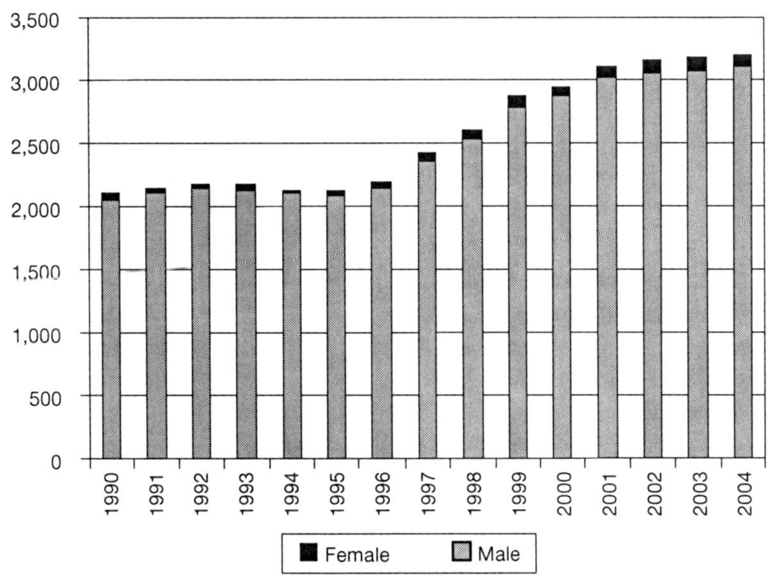

Source: O'Donnell, O'Sullivan and Healy, 2005, Table 3.1; Irish Prison Service, 2005

It is important to note that the prison population rose at a time when the number of committals under sentence fell. The reasons for this contradictory trend are that prisoners are spending a greater proportion of their sentence behind bars than in the past as there is less recourse to temporary release, more people are being denied bail, and a growing number of long sentences is being imposed (see O'Donnell, 2004; O'Donnell, 2005b).

In the late-1990s, public anxieties were inflated out of all proportion to the risk faced by individual citizens, and the business of government became (temporarily) defined by the imperative of crime control. Options and choices were narrowed and shaped by crime-related considerations. The following two sets of opinion poll results illustrate the nature of this change.

1992: What, in your opinion, are the main issues the parties should be addressing in this election campaign?

	Per cent
Unemployment	86
Health service / hospitals, etc.	22
Taxation / PAYE	15
Interest / mortgage interest	11
Social welfare benefits / reform / abuse, etc.	11
Crime / vandalism / law and order	8

MRBI survey for *The Irish Times*, 17–18 November 1992

1997: In your opinion what are the main issues on which the parties should fight the election campaign?

	Per cent
Crime / law and order / justice	41
Unemployment / jobs	40
Drugs	22
Income tax / tax / PRSI	15
Northern Ireland / peace	11
Poor / poverty / lower paid	11

MRBI survey for *The Irish Times*, 26–27 March 1997

In the lead-up to the 2002 general election, despite periodic bouts of anxiety, crime concern seemed to have abated. The perennial worries about unemployment and taxation had also receded. The public was now most concerned about the health service, with house prices making an appearance on the list for the first time. In 2003, with little prospect of an imminent election, concern about the crime problem remained a minority interest. It was higher than in the 1980s but lower than during the late 1990s. These shifts are shown in the following polls.

2001: In the next general election, in your opinion, what are the main issues which will influence the way you vote?

	Per cent
Health	34
Cost of living	29
House prices	21
Unemployment	19
Taxation	17
Crime	14

MRBI survey for *The Irish Times*, 22–23 January 2001

2003: If there was a general election tomorrow, what are the main issues which would influence the way you would vote?

	Per cent
Health / hospitals	66
Cost of living / inflation	31
Jobs / unemployment	26
The economy	24
Education	23
Levels of crime	23

TNS MRBI survey for *The Irish Times*, 16 May 2003

It might be argued that worry about crime is least pressing for societies where economic and national security needs cannot be taken for granted. When families are losing their children through emigration as a result of bleak employment prospects at home, crime is given a lower priority. It would be fair to say that crime was not of major concern to the public before the mid-1990s and that since then it seems to have risen and fallen in significance, at least insofar as it related to perceived priorities for government.

Trends in recorded crime were out of step with trends in public sentiment. When crime was peaking in the early 1980s, the public was relatively unconcerned. When it was falling in the late 1990s, there were strong demands for action. Ireland differs significantly from other countries in that crime has not been used as a 'wedge' issue to set political parties apart. Despite unprecedented funding for prisons and police, the public debate is not soured by law and order policy claims and counter-claims to the same extent as either Britain or the USA, where muscle-flexing by politicians determined to appear 'tough' has had many undesirable consequences. These include simplistic policies, an apparently insatiable desire to introduce more punishment for those who break certain laws and are caught, and a huge burden on the public purse. In this way the politics of punishment directly affect citizens' quality of life. For example, in California, education budgets have been cut to fund prison-building programmes.

The politicisation of law and order, and the anxiety it engenders, is independent of any variation in the crime rate; but it is important. A society that is preoccupied with punishment and exclusion can be a brutish place to live. Public debate is coarse, those on the margins are further excluded, and some law-breakers are not given a second chance. Such developments usually take place in parallel with an enduring disregard for white-collar or corporate wrongdoing. A shift in this direction would have a deleterious effect on the quality of life.

Ireland has not moved as far in this regard as other countries in the Anglophone world. What seems different is the lack of a sustained commitment to the politics of crime control. There has not been the same desire to make a harsh response to crime the issue to unite a political party, or to act as a lightening rod to draw attention away from more urgent, but more potentially problematic, concerns. It would be going too far to say that we are being governed by crime, but it might be reasonable to suggest that public concerns, and the political response to them, have risen from an extraordinarily low baseline. (See Kilcommins et al., 2004, for a review of the extent to which Ireland has developed a 'culture of control' over the past decade.) One factor that distinguishes Ireland is that the lack of information on crime and punishment makes serious debate and rational policy formulation extremely challenging.

Concluding comment

Is it the best of times or the worst of times? Is it the spring of hope or the winter of despair? On balance it seems fair to suggest that Ireland has a modest overall crime problem according to Garda presentations of what is considered serious. Between 1990 and 2004 the number of serious crimes recorded by the police fluctuated somewhat but within a fairly narrow range (Table 14.1). There is no evidence of an escalation in recent times. The crime rate appears low compared with other EU countries (Figure 14.1) but in large measure this is a reflection of recording practice. Closer examination of the national trend reveals a significant reduction of crime in the cities (Table 14.2) and a rising homicide rate (Figure 14.2 and Table 14.3). The latter distinguishes the country from its European neighbours. In other respects trends over the past decade or so are not dramatic.

Two victimisation surveys carried out by the CSO sound a note of caution, showing that levels of crime against the person doubled between 1998 and 2003. But this was not accompanied by growing feelings of insecurity or increased anxiety about becoming a victim of crime. The surveys showed little change in crimes against property over the same period. Combined with an increased ability to protect our belongings with alarms, electronic gates and security guards, the potential harms of crime are reduced. Despite these variations in crime, risk and insecurity, the prison population rose steadily (Figure 14.3).

When drafting this chapter I anticipated that one consequence of the boom would be more people losing their lives as a result of the criminal actions (or inaction) of their employers. There is no evidence of this in terms of workplace fatalities. Similarly, an expected increase in deaths on the road did not materialise and the overall risk of lethal harm remains low (Table 14.4).

It would be reasonable to expect that more middle-class individuals would yield to the wider range of criminal temptations that is an inevitable consequence of rapid economic growth. It is difficult to test this empirically as so few such cases enter the criminal justice system. However, a series of national financial scandals over the past decade has alerted us to the popularity of concealing large amounts of cash offshore, or at home in bogus non-resident accounts, or through undeclared payments into life assurance products. This suggests that variations on this theme may be of increasing significance.

While public concern about crime spiked after 1996 it does not appear to have led to the chronic anxiety and repeated calls for harsh responses that have infected the debate in some other countries. Similarly, the political discourse has not become mired in the search for increasingly 'tough' responses. While reactionary and wrongheaded policies, together with punitive and explosive rhetoric, emerge regularly on the Irish scene, they are not ingrained and have not yet generated sufficient momentum to persist outside of a crisis situation. As the National Crime Forum (1998, p. 10) put it, 'The public is not calling for draconian action.' This helps to insulate us from the worst of times.

Is it possible to divine future trends? In an article published in 1997, based on crime data up to 1996 (O'Donnell, 1997), I speculated that if economic growth continued the following would be observed:

1. In the short term, a drop in the level of property crime, which will be reflected in a reduction in the overall crime rate
2. In the short term, an increase in violence against the person
3. In the long term, a rise in recorded crime

Looking back, with a decade's hindsight, the first two of these predictions proved accurate and time will tell if the same is true of the third. I also opined that if the prevailing law and order policies were pursued there would be:

1. A substantial growth in the size of the prison population
2. An increase in sentence lengths for serious crime together with a growing emphasis on community penalties
3. A concentration of disadvantage and criminal victimisation in a small number of geographically well-defined communities, at the same time as society at large becomes safer and more economically secure
4. A hardening of attitudes in society such that the disadvantaged are blamed for their own misfortune

The first of these predictions has come about. As for the others, the evidence is mixed: sentence lengths seem to have increased somewhat but there has not been a shift of focus to community sanctions; society has become more economically secure but too little is known about the distribution of crime to say whether it has become concentrated in distinct communities; concern about crime has risen but there has not been a universal hardening of attitudes.

What remains constant is the manageable nature of the problem, despite periodic crises.

15

Soaring in the Best of Times?

Robert Erikson

How are we to determine whether a society is developing for the better or worse? This question has occupied philosophers and social scientists for centuries and will presumably do so for centuries to come. The authors of this book approach it with the help of a host of observations from social studies in order to try to determine whether Ireland has become not only a richer but also a better society to live in. Here I will discuss some of the issues that are central to attempts to assess the qualitative aspects of the development of a society, then look at the results in the book from this perspective, and end with a few personal reflections.

Evaluating societal change

To consider whether Irish society has become a nation where people not only earn more but also have better lives, we have to ask in what respect and for whom the term 'better' might apply. To reach the judgement that improvement has taken place it might be argued that no one's conditions should have become worse (this is the well-known 'Pareto principle'). If we adhered strictly to this principle we would never be able to observe improvement, since there will always be someone who will be exposed to change for the worse.

Hence it seems that we have to consider other principles in order to judge societal change. An obvious candidate is to look at *average* change. The question here is whether an increasing average income would indicate a better society even if those with already low incomes got even less. Many would answer no to that question. Suppose, though, that no one's income actually decreased but that income inequality nevertheless increased because those at the bottom received less than others – that is, their relative income position worsened even though their absolute income rose? This actually seems to be what some critics of the Celtic Tiger argue has happened (see Chapters 3 and 6). Despite the absolute improvement involved, many would claim that the change involved here is not for the

T. Fahey et al. (eds.), Quality of Life in Ireland, 265–276.

better. Missing a certain good may become more problematic if the number who have access to it increases, since many aspects of life depend on 'positional goods' (Hirsch, 1976), whose value depends on the extent to which others have access to them. Simple examples are the ownership of a TV or personal computer. It is hardly a problem for a child if such goods do not appear in the family home when only a small number of children can watch TV at home or surf on the Internet. But a child who is among the few who do not have access to these forms of communication may have problems with schoolwork and with social relations.

The absolute value of a positional good depends on its relative position in the distribution of such a good (Brighouse and Swift, 2006). A secondary school certificate is to some extent a positional good. The knowledge and skills acquired certainly have some worth in themselves, but its value in the labour market depends on the number of others who have this much or more schooling. A car makes transportation easier for the owner, but when the number of cars increases, their relative value for the owners decreases, at least in the context of an unchanged infrastructure.

The importance of the number of others who have access to something one lacks oneself and the character of positional goods are the two main reasons why income poverty is mostly defined in relative terms in developed economies, a view held by Adam Smith (1776): 'By necessaries I understand not only the commodities which are indispensably necessary for the support of life, but whatever the custom of the country renders it indecent for creditable people, even of the lowest order, to be without.' The crucial point is that absolute values depend on relative positions (see Sen, 1992).

An increase in average incomes and other material aspects of living standards is thus not sufficient to conclude that a society is developing towards the better if the situation of those worse off is not improving as well. How to judge a development where everyone's situation is improving in absolute terms but those at the bottom of the distribution are worsening in relative terms is a more delicate matter. There must be situations where absolute improvement outweighs relative impairment, as well as the other way around.

Quality of life: what dimensions are important?

So far I have discussed change in one dimension only, that is, income and material conditions. However, it seems obvious that one has to consider more aspects of people's conditions to judge overall improvement. Other important components include health, working conditions, security of life and property, and social relations, but also civil and political rights, housing, knowledge and skills, and time use. These components are generally correlated with economic resources but are far from completely so and need to be considered in their own right. Some of them, notably health, may for most people count as a more important aspect of living circumstances than economic resources.

Furthermore, it does not seem satisfactory just to look at one factor at a time. To judge overall development we ought to consider all relevant aspects simultaneously. The judgement is simple if all factors change in the same direction, but can improvement in one factor compensate for deterioration in another? How should we judge a change where the incomes of all are going up, but where average health becomes worse? Another aspect of multidimensionality is the association between various aspects of welfare. Say that we observe improvements in all aspects for everyone, but that the correlation between aspects increases. This will mean that bad conditions in several respects are more concentrated among the worst off. Suppose that health, housing, income, education, working conditions, and exposure to crime all improve for everyone, but that those who are worst off in these respects increasingly tend to be exposed to all of them simultaneously. Should this increased relative burden of deprivation on a minority be an argument for claiming that society is not becoming better (see Walzer, 1983)?

Subjective well-being and expectations

Which is more important, the actual conditions or the satisfaction with these conditions? It is far from evident that the two move in the same direction. Thus, how should we judge a development where real incomes go up, but where people become less satisfied with these incomes due to an even faster change in aspiration levels? In one sense one could claim that it is most important how people judge their situation. However, it is well known that there is hardly any correlation over time between satisfaction and conditions, which suggests that people adapt their expectations to changing conditions, in which case more weight perhaps should be given to change in factual circumstances. One could claim that a case where factual conditions improve while subjective satisfaction remains stable implies a development for the better. It seems more questionable to regard the development as positive if people become more satisfied with unchanging conditions, a case which seems to imply a disillusioned acceptance of status quo.

A concentration on bad conditions

A common reaction to social reporting relates to its preoccupation with the dismal aspects of life – why not discuss the good life more – as studies of welfare tend to look at bad conditions rather than the extent to which people live the really good life. There are good reasons for this approach, since we may differ greatly in what we regard as the best conditions of life – some would think of creative work, others of exciting leisure or a life in music. We are more likely to be able to agree on unwanted conditions, say, political oppression, poverty, poor health or unsanitary housing. A claim that we are experiencing more of the good life may be disputed by those who do not agree on the account of what is good in life, while everyone may regard a diminishing frequency of experiences of bad conditions as a positive development.

The time experienced in various conditions should also be considered. The same overall level of poverty can arise both if many people are exposed to it for a short time and if a few people experience it more or less permanently. Housing problems, for example, appear to be much less serious for young people who spend a short time in poor housing than for relatively small groups of deprived people for whom poor housing is a long-term condition.

An accurate assessment of the welfare of the population should rely on actual conditions and not on provision of services. An increasing number of hospital beds may indicate better health care, but it may alternatively indicate worsening public health. Similarly, more policemen may indicate a better protection against crime or an increasing level of crime. Rising expenditure on social welfare may indicate that more people are exposed to difficult economic conditions or that difficult economic conditions are being alleviated (if welfare spending is successful in lifting more people out of severe poverty).

This is far from a complete discussion of what could be considered in attempts to gauge the development of a society, but it shows what a difficult task the authors of this book have taken on in their assessment of the recent development of welfare in Ireland. I hope it is a sufficient base for a discussion of whether, through this book, they have painted an accurate picture of how the quality of Irish life has changed in the last decade.

Ireland after the Celtic Tiger – the quality-of-life balance sheet

The foregoing provides a background that allows us to situate our discussion of the assessment of Irish society. Let me first provide a very rough summary of the results in the preceding chapters.

Average national income in Ireland increased considerably, so that it now lies slightly above the OECD average. The level of income inequality remains high in a European context, but there has been little change in this respect, although those with the highest incomes may have increased their share of total income.

Unemployment decreased considerably after the early 1990s. The number of dual-earner families increased while families without anyone in the labour market became fewer. Not surprisingly, average earnings increased. With regard to the occupational structure, the number of positions with relatively advantageous conditions increased, and wage returns to education also grew. The relative share of part-time work increased up to the mid-1990s and has remained unchanged thereafter. Stress at work may have increased although the available information on change in working conditions is inconsistent.

The changing occupational structure has given men and women better chances to find attractive jobs, regardless of their social origins. The association between current position and social origins seems to have decreased as well.

Higher alcohol consumption and more obesity increase the risk of people becoming ill. Death rates are nevertheless decreasing, but are still higher than the EU average. Thus, prolonged life expectancy suggests a healthier Ireland, but people's subjective assessment of their health has not improved.

The situation for pupils in Irish secondary schools has improved in terms of autonomy and possibilities to take a job, but the overall character of schoolwork seems on the whole to be unaltered. Whether education in Ireland generally has become better is a moot point, but the situation for those with little education above compulsory level may have become worse because of decreasing demand for unskilled labour.

Birth rates have declined, but are still high in a European perspective. The number of younger persons living alone has increased considerably since 1990, in spite of an increasing number of marriages during the same period, and is perhaps connected to freer sexual mores. The percentage of separations and divorces has increased, but is still very low compared to other countries in Northern Europe.

Life in the new suburbs does not seem to be as vacuous as some (not living there) believe. Long commuting time in dual-worker families may, however, lead to increased levels of time pressure among those living in the new suburbs.

The number of dual-earner families has increased considerably, related to increasing female labour force participation. As in other European countries this development seems to have had little impact on the division of household work, where women continue to bear the major burden. This is to some extent the cause and consequence of the higher probability of women working part-time, leading to only moderate differences between the sexes in time devoted to various forms of work during weekdays. However, women have more committed time in this sense during weekends.

Victimisation surveys suggest that exposure to crimes against the person, such as theft and assault, doubled from 1998 to 2003, while the incidence of crimes against property remained unchanged in frequency.

During the economic boom Ireland has changed from being a country of emigration to one of immigration. Most of the recent immigrants come to Ireland looking for a job and, in general, are successful in finding one, which may be a major contributor to the fact that Irish people appear to display a rather low level of resistance to the newcomers.

Given this very sparse and most likely partial summary, I will raise six questions:

1 Are there important aspects of Irish welfare development not covered in this book?

2 Were some left behind when average material conditions improved?

3 Did economic improvement coincide with negative developments in other areas, like health and social life?

4 Did adverse conditions become more concentrated within a minority?

5 May structural change have diminished the control-of-life circumstances in Ireland in spite of the increasing material welfare?

6 Were some non-material values lost in the rising tide?

In his famous essay 'Citizenship and Social Class' (1950), T. H. Marshall discussed the importance of civil, political and social rights in the development of a democratic society. The authors of this book can be said to have considered social rights in detail, although they have not considered whether the political rights of any group in Ireland have been jeopardised or whether there are increased problems relating to individual civil rights. These two areas may for good reasons be regarded as unproblematic in mature democracies, but there seems to be at least one group for which this is not self-evident, i.e. immigrants. The revealed preferences of immigrants suggest that they want to be in the new country, but the good society should take care of everyone, including those who, for any reason, are willing to accept adverse conditions. Thus, it would have been of value if the chapter on immigrants had included a more thorough description of immigrant conditions and perhaps particularly with regard to their civil and political rights.[1]

A typical social report provides a multidimensional account of developments and this book clearly falls into this tradition. Thus, we learn about change in income inequality, in employment and quality of work, in health and in several other respects. Are there important aspects of Irish life missing in this account? Answers to this question will differ according to the values of the person who replies, but it seems to me that the most important dimensions are covered.

We learn that there were no great changes in health while death rates declined. This latter development seems, however, not to be related to recent economic change in Ireland, since the decline has been observed for a fairly long period of time and corresponding decreasing rates have been observed in other European nations, although the timing of the decrease differed between countries. The social class differentials in mortality among employed men and women decreased during the 1980s but lack of data made it impossible to find out whether this development continued into the 1990s. While mortality in Ireland in recent years has declined, especially among the working class, the overall impression is that public health in general remained unchanged. It would have been valuable to have learnt somewhat more about the development of some other aspects of health, e.g. mental well-being, but the authors are obviously restricted by the availability of data in this respect.

The general increase in income does not seem to have been matched by a general change in income inequality, except for a possible – but uncertain – increase of the relative share of the very highest incomes. It is, however, noteworthy that income inequality has not *decreased*. The divide between those with employment and those without is generally an important source of income inequality, so the marked increase in employment rates could have been expected to contribute to decreasing income inequality. Furthermore, households where the main earner was unemployed actually caught up slightly because others in these families have increasingly found employment during the economic boom. However, it is possible that countervailing influences were in operation. The number of dual-earner families increased considerably. This increase could well contribute to

1 The authors' remit was to limit the discussion of the legal position of immigrants and to focus on the economic and social conditions faced by immigrants and the impact of immigration. Detailed discussion of legislative developments are contained in other work by authors such as Quinn (2006a, 2006b), Quinn and Hughes (2005).

increasing income inequality if such households were predominantly drawn from those with higher education. Since households where at least one adult was at work and those where all adults were at work both increased in number, the effects on income inequality may have been cancelled out, with the consequence that income inequality overall remained unchanged.

An increase in the highest income earners' relative share of total income probably does not affect social exclusion since it does not cause more people to have difficulties in participating in public life due to relatively low incomes. In the Irish case, therefore, the possible negative effects of increasing income inequality may rather appear as a general dismay and unease with conspicuous consumption and a decreasing sense of solidarity in society due to the behaviour and consumption patterns of the very rich.

The overall degree of income inequality may well remain unchanged while some vulnerable groups improve in relative earnings and others lose out. It seems as if the economic situation of children improved – which may be an effect of their parents earning relatively more or of a decreasing number of families with many children – while that of older people worsened. This change in the relative incomes of older people is probably an effect of the economic boom, since pensions typically do not increase at the same pace as incomes from work. However, even older people with low incomes tend to report significantly lower levels of deprivation than one would expect on the basis of their incomes. This appears to reflect the intervening role of factors such as home ownership, savings and family support systems. Similarly, while older people's relative income position worsened, their relative deprivation levels increased only slightly (Whelan, Nolan and Maître, 2006) and their self-reported health actually improved from 1994 to 2001.

A lack in the book's presentation of the development of Irish society is that we do not get a systematic description of how various groups have fared during the economic boom. We learn much about the relative situations of men and women, but we would have reached a more complete picture of the changing conditions of the Irish population if other groups had been given a more systematic treatment in the text. The reason that a description of change at group level is of value is that it provides a way of avoiding some of the problems associated with distinguishing the effects of choice from those of structural forces. Thus, a person who experiences a decrease in his relative income may opt for a lower consumption level in order not to have to compete in the economic rat race. If, however, we observe decreasing incomes in a population group, it seems more plausible that this is the effect of societal conditions rather than of collectively similar choices.

Change at group level again involves confronting issues relating to the importance to be attached to absolute improvements, reductions in the absolute size of disadvantaged groups and the changing patterns of relativities between groups. Thus, the relative situation of those with low education seems to have become worse with the transformation of the labour market (Whelan, Nolan and Maître, 2006). However, while evidence consequently points to increased returns to education, the significant reduction in long-term unemployment suggests an increase in absolute opportunities. Similarly, Whelan, Nolan and Maître (2006) show that declining trends in vulnerability were observed across the social class spectrum but this was accompanied by some evidence of increased class polarisation in terms of the relative risks of exposure to such vulnerability.

In a similar vein, it would have been of interest to learn more about who were the ones who experienced increasing rates of crime against the person, precisely because, as is mentioned in the chapter on crime, the 'increased ability to protect our property with alarms, electronic gates and security guards' is not common to everyone. It is presumably those with higher incomes who have experienced this increased ability, which makes it possible that the increased exposure to crime is concentrated among those with low incomes.

Another related piece of information that it would have been interesting to have is whether problems of various kinds became interconnected and more concentrated among small groups of people during the boom. It is perfectly possible to observe no change on a number of dimensions that nonetheless became more highly correlated, implying that some groups of people experience a worsening of their situation. On the other hand, if correlations became weaker, multiple deprivation would decline and the outcome would be positive. The available evidence does not permit a precise quantification of such trends over time. Although it is not possible to establish the development in this respect during the most recent years, there is substantial evidence that Irish society after the economic boom is characterised by relatively modest correlation between deprivation dimensions relating to consumption, health, housing and neighbourhood environment.[2] These dimensions certainly are positively correlated. Those exposed to any one of these dimensions are also more likely to experience the others. However, the degree of correlation is a good deal more modest than many may imagine. Absolute levels of multiple deprivation are rather low once one goes beyond a very small number of dimensions. Similarly, objective socio-economic conditions overlap and such multiple disadvantage is associated with increased multiple

---

2 See Chapter 6 and Whelan, Nolan and Maître (2006)

deprivation. However, as the risk of multiple deprivation escalates the numbers involved decline very sharply.[3] Consistent with this finding there is very little tendency towards spatial concentration of poverty and deprivation in Ireland. Distinctively high levels of multiple deprivation are observed among public sector tenants, particularly urban tenants. However, the process that has contributed to this outcome has also involved a substantial reduction in the numbers found in such housing.[4] Thus, while it would be desirable to be able to track these changes more precisely over time, the overall evidence is inconsistent with the emergence of an Irish 'underclass' of any significant magnitude.

Another issue is the duration of bad conditions for those affected. As mentioned above, the same proportion of the population exposed to a bad condition has very different implications depending upon whether a few live in this condition for long periods or most people experience the condition for some short spells. It would thus have been of value to learn more about the length of periods of poverty and deprivation or of health problems.[5] What we do learn is that persistence of class positions over generation is decreasing, which shows that Ireland is becoming a more open society in terms of social class.

The best of times? An outsider's view

The editors invited me to give a personal view on Irish development. To do this with scientific pretensions would demand an encyclopaedic knowledge of Ireland which I certainly do not have, so these comments are observations by an interested outsider and should be taken as no more than that.

The evidence in this volume points to considerable improvements in the absolute welfare of most inhabitants in Ireland. However, as I have emphasised, our own welfare is relative, in that it is affected by how well other people are doing, and so our welfare can be changed by what happens to other people as well as by what happens to ourselves. This is particularly so during an economic boom. The consequence of others'

---

3 See Whelan, Nolan and Maître (2006)

4 See Watson et al. (2005)

5 Editors' note: The available evidence shows that in terms of absolute levels of persistent poverty Ireland is not particularly distinctive. High levels of mobility into and out of poverty are observed while at the same time a minority of individuals experience sustained spells of poverty. In terms of the factors contributing to such persistence, Ireland fits into the liberal welfare regime model, with both social class and labour market status being particularly influential – see Whelan, Layte and Maître (2004), Whelan et al., (2001), Whelan and Maître (2005), Fourage and Layte (2005).

increased prosperity must be obvious to people in the Dublin area every day, when they try get to their jobs through the traffic jam and likewise when they are looking for a place to live. However, the evidence overall does not indicate a general increase in inequality resulting from worsening relative positions for substantial population groups.

An interesting reaction to the change in other persons' behaviour connected to the economic development – or at least assumed to be so connected – is the observation that values and behaviour are changing, as mentioned in the opening pages of the editors' introduction to this volume. Obviously the Ombudsman and Information Commissioner, Emily O'Reilly (2004), finds that people around her behave in a less and less acceptable way, but she is clearly not the only one.[6] She points to 'the rampant, unrestrained drunkenness, the brutal, random violence … the incontinent use of foul language'. Thus, it seems as if her situation has, at least in this respect, become worse as a consequence of the increased affluence that the economic development has afforded to others. From a Swedish perspective it is easy to regard this as an overreaction, but it is worthwhile taking her reaction seriously. O'Reilly and others experience a reduction in their well-being, since they react negatively to some of the ways in which many take advantage of their improved economic conditions.

While negative material consequences of other persons' increased prosperity can be expected to appear among those with low incomes, negative reactions to the improper behaviour of others seem mainly to concern those in the upper part of Irish society. A first question that an empirically oriented sociologist raises is whether the incidence of violence, drinking, bad language and other utterances of improper behaviour really has increased or whether the image of the past is dimmed by protective mechanisms of memory or perhaps whether the acts have become more visible because those exhibiting them now have the economic resources to do so in contexts where the better-off are present. Violence and drinking actually seem to have increased in frequency to judge from the chapters on health and crime, so the Ombudsman's observations seem to be warranted at least in these respects.

Other aspects of her grievances are more questionable. Is the minor increase in divorce rates really a problem to her, as it may be a sign of declining family life in Ireland, or is it perhaps an indication that increased

---

6 Her speech at the Annual Céifin Conference, 2004, can be downloaded at http://www.citsu.ie/publications/backissues/volume6/december2004.pdf

economic independence has made it possible for many women to leave an unsatisfactory and perhaps violent marriage? Likewise, the possibility of Sunday shopping may relieve some of the stress caused by time pressure during weekdays and may give women the possibility of sharing some of the burden of household planning with men.

Change may be rewarding and challenging but also threatening, and this is much more the case if surrounding conditions are changing rapidly as has been the case in Ireland in the last decade. Suddenly, to the despair of some inhabitants, it seems that the Irish way of life is not the same any longer, as an examination of letters to the editors of the main newspapers will confirm. The preceding chapters suggest that the economic boom of recent years has, in terms of material conditions, been to the advantage of nearly everyone in Ireland. That some feel disappointed and disgusted by some of the consequences of rapid economic growth is perhaps its most serious cost. Even so, my guess would be that few would want to go back to the situation in the pre-boom period, and this is presumably particularly true of those in less affluent positions.

The Swedish economist Gösta Rehn regarded the problem of welfare development as one of combining freedom and security, and to achieve it he suggested that we should strive for the security of wings, rather than for the protection of a shell. Are people in Ireland flying more safely after more than a decade of improved economic conditions? My impression is that this is the case, that is, that the economic development has brought both more freedom and more security to the Irish. 'The best of times' would then be a good description of the current living conditions of the population of Ireland.

References

Ahn, N. and Mira, P. (2002), 'A note on the changing relationship between fertility and female employment rates in developed countries', *Journal of Population Economics*, 15, pp. 667–682

Allen, K. (2000), *The Celtic Tiger: The Myth of Social Partnership in Ireland*, Manchester: Manchester University Press

An Garda Síochána (2005), *Annual Report 2004*, Dublin: Stationery Office

Argyle, M. (2001), *The Psychology of Happiness*, New York: Taylor & Francis

Atkinson, A. B. (2001), *Top Incomes in the United Kingdom over the Twentieth Century*, mimeo., Oxford: Nuffield College

Atkinson, A., Marlier, E. and Nolan, B. (2002), *Social Indicators: The European Union and Social Inclusion*, Oxford: Oxford University Press

Bank of Ireland (2004), *Irish Property Review Quarterly Bulletin*

Barclay, G. and Tavares, C. (2003), 'International Comparisons of Criminal Justice Statistics', *Statistical Bulletin 12/03*, London: Home Office

Barrett, A., Bergin, A. and Duffy, D. (2006), 'The Labour Market Characteristics and Labour Market Impact of Immigrants in Ireland', *The Economic and Social Review*, vol. 37, no. 1, pp. 1–26

Barrett, A., Callan, T., Doris, A., O'Neill, D., Russell, H., Sweetman, O. and McBride, J. (2000), *How Unequal? Men and Women in the Irish Labour Market*, Dublin: Oaktree Press and the Economic and Social Research Institute

Barrett, A., Fitz Gerald, J. and Nolan, B. (2000), 'Earnings Inequality, Returns to Education and Low Pay', pp. 127–46, in Nolan, B., O'Connell, P. J. and Whelan, C. T. (eds.), *Bust to Boom? The Irish Experience of Growth and Inequality*, Dublin: Economic and Social Research Institute and the Institute of Public Administration

Barrett, A., Fitz Gerald, J. and Nolan, B. (2002), 'Earnings Inequality, Returns to Education and Immigration into Ireland', *Labour Economics*, vol. 9, no. 5

Barry, F. (ed.) (1999), *Understanding Ireland's Economic Growth*, London: Macmillan

Baumgartner, M. P. (1988), *The Moral Order of the Suburbs*, New York: Oxford University Press

Beggs, J. and Pollock, J. (2006), *Non-national Workers in the Irish Economy*, AIB Global Treasury Economic Research, www.aibeconomicresearch.com

Bennett, K., Johnson, H., Dack, P., Shelley, E. and Feely, J. (2005) 'Changes in Prevalence of and Prescribing for Ischaemic Heart Disease in Ireland 1990–2002', *Irish Journal of Medical Science*, vol. 174, no. 3, pp. 4–8

Bennett, K., Kabir, Z., Unal, B., Shelley, E., Critchley, J., Perry, I., Feely, J., Capewell, S. (2006), 'Explaining The Recent Decrease In Coronary Heart Disease Mortality Rates In Ireland 1985–2000', *Journal of Epidemiology and Community Health*, vol. 60, no. 4., pp. 322–327

Bianchi, S., Milkie, M., Sayer, L. and Robinson, J. (2000), 'Is anyone doing the housework? Trends in the gender division of household labor', *Social Forces*, vol. 79, pp. 191–228

Billari, F. (2005), 'Europe and its fertility. From low to lowest low', *National Institute Economic Review*, 194, pp. 56–73

Bittman, M. and Wajcman, J. (2004), 'The rush hour: the quality of leisure time and gender equity', in Folbre, N. and Bittman, M. (eds.), *Family Time: The Social Organization of Care*, London: Routledge

Blanchard, O. (2002), 'Comments and Discussion', *Brooking Economic Papers*, 2002, 1, pp. 58–66

Blauner, R. (1964), *Alienation and Freedom. The Factory Worker and his Industry*, Chicago: University of Chicago Press

Böhnke, P. (2005), *First European Quality of Life Survey: Life Satisfaction, Happiness and Sense of Belonging*, Dublin: European Foundation for Living and Working Conditions

Bould, S. (2003), 'Caring Neighborhoods: Bringing up the Kids Together', *Journal of Family Issues*, vol. 24, no. 4, pp. 427–47

Brady, D., Beckfield, J. and Seeleib-Kaiser, M. (2005), 'Economic Globalization and the Welfare State in Affluent Democracies, 1975–2001', *American Sociological Review*, vol. 70, pp. 921–948

Braverman, H. (1974), *Labor and Monopoly Capital. The Degradation of Work in the Twentieth Century*, New York: Monthly Review Press

Breen, R. (2004), *Social Mobility in Europe*, Oxford: Oxford University Press

Breen, R. and Goldthorpe, J. H. (1997), 'Explaining Educational Differentials: Towards a Formal Rational Action Theory', *Rationality and Society*, 9, pp. 275–305

Breen, R. and Goldthorpe, J. H. (1999), 'Class Inequality and Meritocracy: A Critique of Saunders and an Alternative Analysis', *The British Journal of Sociology*, 50, pp. 1–27

Breen, R. and Goldthorpe, J. H. (2001), 'Class, Mobility and Merit: The Experience of Two British Birth Cohorts', *European Sociological Review*, 17, pp. 81–101

Breen, R. and Luijkx, R. (2004), 'Social Mobility in Europe Between 1970 and 2000' in Breen, R. (ed.), *Social Mobility in Europe*, Oxford: Oxford University Press

Breen, R. and Whelan. C. T. (1991), 'Life-Course Mobility as an Intergenerational Process; Intra-generational Mobility in Ireland', Economic and Social Research Institute, Working Paper no. 31

Breen, R. and Whelan. C. T. (1992), 'Explaining the Irish Pattern of Social Fluidity: the Role of the Political', in Goldthorpe, J. H. and Whelan, C. T. (eds.), *The Development of Industrial Society in Ireland*, Oxford: Oxford University Press

Breen, R. and Whelan. C. T. (1993), 'From Ascription to Achievement? Origins, Education and Entry to the Labour Force in the Republic of Ireland during the Twentieth Century', *Acta Sociologica*, vol. 36, no. 1, pp. 1–86

Breen, R. and Whelan. C. T. (1994), 'Modelling Trends in Social Fluidity: The Core Model and a Measured Variable Approach Compared', *European Sociological Review*, vol. 10, no. 3, pp. 25–42

Brewer, J., Lockhart, B. and Rodgers, P. (1997), *Crime in Ireland 1945–95: Here Be Dragons*, Oxford: Clarendon Press

Brewster, K. L. and Rindfuss, R. R. (2000), 'Fertility and Women's Employment in

Industrialized Nations', *Annual Review of Sociology*, 26, pp. 271–96
Brighouse, H. and Swift, A. (2006), 'Equality, Priority and Positional Goods', *Ethics 116*, pp. 471–97
Bruni, L. and Porta, P. L. (eds.) (2004), *Economics and Happiness. Framing the Analysis*, Oxford: Oxford University Press
Callan, T., Nolan, B. and Whelan, C. T. (1993), 'Resources, Deprivation and the Measurement of Poverty', *Journal of Social Policy*, vol. 22, no. 2, pp. 141–172
Capelli, P., Bassi, L., Katz, H., Knoke, D., Osterman, P. and Useem, M. (1997), *Change at Work*, Oxford: Oxford University Press
Card, D., Dustmann, C. and Preston, I. (2005), 'Understanding attitudes to immigration: The migration and minority module of the first European Social Survey,' Centre for Research and Analysis of Migration, Discussion Paper Series CDP, no. 03/05
Casey, S. and O'Connell, M. (2000), 'Pain and Prejudice', in MacLachlan, M. and O'Connell, M. (eds.) (2000), *Cultivating Pluralism: Psychological, Social and Cultural Perspectives on a Changing Ireland*, Dublin: Oaktree Press
Castles, F. (2003), 'The World turned Upside Down: Below Replacement Fertility, changing Preferences and Family-Friendly Public Policy in 21 OECD countries' *Journal of European Social Policy*, vol. 13, no. 3, pp. 209–227
Castles, S. and Miller, M. J. (2003), *The Age of Migration*, London: Palgrave Macmillan
Central Statistics Office (1999), *Quarterly National Household Survey: Module on Crime and Victimisation, Fourth Quarter 1998*, Dublin: CSO
Central Statistics Office (2001), *Quarterly National Household Survey: Module on Length and Pattern of Working Time*, Dublin: CSO
Central Statistics Office (2003), *Quarterly National Household Survey, Housing and Households, Third Quarter 2003*, Dublin and Cork: CSO
Central Statistics Office (2004a), *Population and Labour Force Projections, 2006–2036*, Dublin: Stationery Office, Pm. 4017
Central Statistics Office (2004b), *Quarterly National Household Survey: Module on Crime and Victimisation, Fourth Quarter 2003*, Dublin: CSO
Central Statistics Office (2005a), *Women and Men in Ireland*, Dublin: CSO
Central Statistics Office (2005b), *Population and Migration Estimates, April 2005*, Dublin: CSO
Central Statistics Office (2005c), *Quarterly National Household Survey: Special Module on Equality*, Quarter 4, 2004, Dublin: CSO
Central Statistics Office (2006), *National Employment Survey 2003*, Dublin: CSO
Chambers, R. (1989), 'Vulnerability: How the Poor Cope', Editorial, *IDS Bulletin*, 20, 2
Clapson, M. (2000), 'The Suburban Aspiration in England since 1919', *Contemporary British History*, vol. 14, no. 1, pp. 151–74
Clinch, P., Convery, F. and Walsh, B. (2002), *After the Celtic Tiger: Challenges Ahead*, Dublin: O'Brien Press
Coenders, M., Lubbers, M. and Scheepers, P. (2005), 'Majorities' Attitudes to Minorities in European Union Member States: Results from the Euobarometers 1997–2000–2003', Report No 2, European Monitoring Centre on Racism and Xenophobia

Coleman, D. C. (1992), 'The Demographic Transition in Ireland in International Context' in Goldthorpe, J. H. and Whelan, C. T. (eds.), *The Development of Industrial Society in Ireland*, Oxford: Oxford University Press

Coleman, J. (1987), 'Families and schools', *Educational Researcher*, vol. 16, no. 6, pp. 32–38

Collins, J. (2000), 'Are you talking to me? The Need to Respect and Develop a Pupil's Self Image', *Educational Research*, vol. 42, no. 2, pp. 157–166

Comhairle na nOspidéal (2004), *Acute Medical Units*, Dublin: Comhairle na nOspidéal

Connolly, L. (2002), *The Irish Women's Movement: From Revolution to Devolution*, Basingstoke: Palgrave Macmillan

Cooke, M. (2006), *Re-Presenting the Good Society*, Cambridge, MA: The MIT Press

Coolahan, J. (2000), 'School Ethos and Culture within a Changing Education System', in Furlong, C. and Monahan L. (eds.), *School Culture and Ethos*, Dublin: Marino Institute of Education

Coulter, C. (2003), 'The End of Irish History? An Introduction to the Book' in Coulter, C. and Coleman, S. (eds.) *The End of Irish History? Critical Reflections on the Celtic Tiger*, Manchester: Manchester University Press

Courts Service (2004), *Annual Report 2003*, Dublin: Courts Service

Crenson, M. (1978), 'Social Networks and Political Processes in Urban Neigbourhoods', *American Journal of Political Science*, 22, pp. 578–594

Cullen, E. (2004), 'Unprecedented growth – but for whose benefit?', in Douthwaite, R. and Jopling, J. (eds.), *Growth: the Celtic Cancer*, Dublin: Lilliput Press

Curry, P. (2000), '… she never let them in': Popular Reactions to Refugees Arriving in Dublin', Chapter 8 in MacLachlan, M. and O'Connell, M. (eds.) (2000), *Cultivating Pluralism: Psychological, Social and Cultural Perspectives on a Changing Ireland*, Dublin: Oaktree Press

D'Addio, A. C. and d'Ercole, M. M. (2005), 'Trends and Determinants of Fertility Rates', OECD Social, Employment and Migration Working Papers no. 27, Paris: OECD

Daly, A. and Walsh, D. (2004), *Mental Illness in Ireland. Reflections on the Rise and Fall of Institutional Care*, Dublin: Health Research Board

Daly, A. and Walsh, D. with Dunne, Y., Hallissey, D. and Bannon, F. (2006), *Irish Psychiatric Units and Hospitals Census 2006*, Dublin: Health Research Board

Daly, M. and Clavero, S. (2002), *Contemporary Family Policy. A comparative review of Ireland, France, Germany, Sweden and the UK*, Dublin: Institute of Public Administration

Darmody, M. and Smyth, E. (2005), *Gender and Subject Choice: Take-Up of Technological Subjects in Second-Level Education*, Dublin: The Liffey Press/ Economic and Social Research Institute

De Fraine, B., Van Landeghem, G., Van Damme, J. and Onghena, P. (2005), 'An analysis of well-being in secondary school with multilevel growth curve models and multilevel multivariate models', *Quality and Quantity*, vol. 39, pp. 297–316

De Haan (1998), 'Social Exclusion: An Alternative Concept for the Study of Deprivation?', *IDS Bulletin*, vol. 29, no. 1, pp. 10–19

de Róiste, A. and Dinneen, J. (2005), *Young People's Views about Opportunities, Barriers and Supports to Recreation and Leisure*, Dublin: National Children's Office

Delhey, J. (2004), *Life Satisfaction in an Enlarged Europe*, Dublin: European Foundation for Living and Working Conditions

Denny, K., Harmon, C. and Redmond, S. (2000), 'Functional Literacy, Educational Attainment and Earnings: Evidence from the International Adult Literacy Survey', Working Paper 00/09, Institute for Fiscal Studies

Department of Education (1996), *Transition Year Programme 1994–1995: An Evaluation by the Inspectorate of the Department of Education*, Dublin: Department of Education

Department of Education (2004), *Internationalisation of Irish Education Services: Report of Interdepartmental Working Group*, Dublin: Department of Education

Department of Education and Science, (2001) *Report of the National Evaluation of the Leaving Cert Applied Programme*, Dublin: Department of Education and Science

Department of Health and Children (1999), *White Paper on Private Health Insurance*, Dublin: Stationery Office

Department of Health and Children (2001), *National Health Strategy Research*, Dublin: Department of Health and Children

Department of Health and Children (2002), *Health Statistics*, Dublin: Department of Health and Children

Department of Health and Children (2003), *Commission on Financial Management and Control Systems in the Health Service*, Dublin: Stationery Office

Department of Health and Children (undated), 'Report of the Consultative Forum Sub Group on Eligibility', Dublin: Stationery Office

Department of Health and Children (various years), *Health Statistics*, Dublin: Stationery Office

Department of Justice, Equality and Law Reform (2000), *Integration: A two way process*, Dublin: Government Publications

Department of the Environment and Local Government (2002), *National Spatial Strategy for Ireland 2002–2020: People, Places and Potential*, Dublin Stationery Office

Devine, D., Nic Ghiolla Phádraig, M. and Deegan, J. (2004), *Time for Children – Time for Change? Children's Rights and Welfare in Ireland during a Period of Economic Growth*, Report to the COST (European cooperation in the field of scientific and technical research) network

Diener, E. and Seligman, M. E. P. (2004), 'Beyond money. Toward an economy of well-being', *Psychological Science in the Public Interest*, vol. 5, no. 1

Downey, D. (1998), *New Realities in Irish Housing. A Study on Housing Affordability and the Economy*, Dublin: Consultancy and Research Unit for the Built Environment, Dublin Institute of Technology

Downey, D. (2005), 'The challenge of affordability for sustainable access to housing', pp. 44–68 in Norris, M. and Redmond D. (eds.), *Housing Contemporary Ireland: Policy, Society and Shelter*, Dublin: Institute of Public Administration

Doyle, N., Hughes, G. and Wadensjö, E. (2006), *Freedom of Movement for Workers from Central and Eastern Europe: Experiences in Ireland and Sweden*, Stockholm: Swedish Institute for European Policy Studies

Drudy, P. J. and Punch, M. (2005) *Out of Reach: Inequalities in the Irish Housing System*, Dublin: TASC at New Island

Duffy, D. (2002), 'A descriptive analysis of the Irish housing market', *Quarterly Economic Commentary*, summer, Dublin: Economic and Social Research Institute
Duffy, D. (2004), 'A Note on Measuring the Affordability of Homeownership', Policy Discussion Forum, *Quarterly Economic Commentary*, summer, Economic and Social Research Institute
Duffy, D., Fitz Gerald, J. and Kearney, I. (2005), 'Rising House Prices in an Open Labour Market', *Economic and Social Review*, vol. 36, no. 3, winter (www.esr.ie)
Eames, R. (2005), 'Presidential Address. Church of Ireland Synod, 2005', http://synod.ireland.anglican.org/2005/speeches/pdf/tues/presadd.pdf Accessed 21 February 2007
Easterlin, R. A. (2005), 'Building a better theory of well-being', pp. 29–64 in Bruni, L. and Porta, P. L. (eds.) *Economics and Happiness. Framing the Analysis*, Oxford: Oxford University Press
Educational Disadvantage Committee (2003), 'Identifying Disadvantage for the Purpose of Targeting Resources and Other Supports', submission to the Minister for Education and Science
Educational Disadvantage Forum (2003), *Educational Disadvantage Forum: Report of Inaugural Meeting*, Dublin: Educational Disadvantage Committee
Edwards, P. (2005) 'The Puzzle of Work: Insecurity and Stress and Autonomy and Commitment', in Heath et al. (eds.), *Understanding Social Change*, Oxford: Oxford University Press
Erikson, R. and Goldthorpe, J., H. (1992), *The Constant Flux*, Oxford: Oxford University Press
Esping-Andersen, G. (1990), *The Three Worlds of Welfare Capitalism*, Cambridge: Polity Press
Esping-Andersen, G. (1999), *Social Foundations of Post-industrial Economies*, Oxford: Oxford University Press
European Commission (2004), *Joint Report by the Commission and the Council on Social Inclusion*, Brussels: European Commission
European Commission (2005), *Employment in Europe, 2005*, Brussels: European Commission
European Monitoring Centre on Racism and Xenophobia (2006), *Migrants' Experiences of Racism and Xenophobia in 12 EU Member States*, Vienna: EUMC
Eurostat (2004), 'How Europeans Spend their Time. Everyday Life of Women and Men', Data 1998–2002, Luxembourg: Eurostat
Expert Group on Crime Statistics (2004), *Minority Report*, Dublin: Department of Justice, Equality and Law Reform
Fahey, T. (1992), 'Housework, the Household Economy and Economic Development in Ireland since the 1920s', *Irish Journal of Sociology*, vol. 2, pp. 42–69
Fahey, T. (1999), 'Religion and sexual culture in Ireland', pp. 53–70 in Eder, F. X., Hall, L. and Hekma, G. (eds.), *Sexual Cultures in Europe*, National Histories, Manchester: Manchester University Press
Fahey, T. (2001), 'Trends in Irish Fertility Rates in Comparative Perspective', *The Economic and Social Review*, vol. 32, no. 2, pp. 153–180
Fahey, T. (2004), 'Housing affordability: Is the real problem in the private rented sector?' *Quarterly Economic Commentary*, summer, Dublin: Economic and Social Research Institute
Fahey, T. and Lyons, M. (1995), *Marital Breakdown and Family Law in Ireland*, Dublin: Oak Tree Press

Fahey, T. and Smyth, E. (2004), 'Do subjective indicators measure welfare? Evidence from 33 European societies' *European Societies (Journal of the European Sociological Association)*, vol. 6, no. 1

Fahey, T., Hayes, B. and Sinnott, R. (2005), *Conflict and Consensus. A Study of Values and Attitudes in the Republic of Ireland and Northern Ireland*, Dublin: Institute of Public Administration & Leiden: Brill Academic Publishers

Fahey, T., Nolan, B. and Maître, B. (2004), *Housing, Poverty and Wealth in Ireland*, Dublin: Institute of Public Administration and Combat Poverty Agency

Ferrera, M. and Rhodes, M. (2000), 'Recasting European Welfare states: An Introduction', *Western European Politics*, vol. 23, pp. 2–10

Field, S. (1990), *Trends in Crime and Their Interpretation: A Study of Recorded Crime in Post-War England and Wales*, Research Study 119, London, Home Office

Finnegan, R. B. and Wiles, J. L. (2005), *Women and Policy in Ireland: A Documentary History 1922–1997*, Dublin: Irish Academic Press

Fishman, R. (1987), *Bourgeois Utopias: The Rise and Fall of Suburbia*, New York: Basic Books

Fitz Gerald, J. (2000), 'The Story of Ireland's Failure – and Belated Success', in Nolan, B., O'Connell, P. J. and Whelan, C. T. (eds.), *Bust to Boom? The Irish Experience of Growth and Inequality*, Dublin: Economic and Social Research Institute and Institute of Public Administration

Fitz Gerald, J. (2005), 'The Irish housing stock: growth in the number of vacant dwellings', *Quarterly Economic Commentary*, spring

Fitz Gerald, J., Bergin, A., Kearney, I., Barrett, A., Duffy, D., Garrett, S. and McCarthy, Y. (2005), *Medium-Term Review 2005–2012*, no. 10, December, Dublin: Economic and Social Research Institute

Förster, M. F. (2005), 'The European Social Space Revisited: Comparing Poverty in the Enlarged European Union', *Journal of Comparative Policy Analysis*, vol. 7, no. 1, pp. 29–48

Fourage, D. and Layte, R (2005), 'The duration of spells of poverty in Europe', *Journal of Social Policy*, vol. 34, no. 3, pp. 1–20

Frey, B. S. and Stutzer, A. (2002), 'What can economists learn from happiness research?', *Journal of Economic Literature*, 40, pp. 402–435

Friedman, B. M. (2005), *The Moral Consequences of Economic Growth*, New York: Vintage Books

Friel, S., Nic Gabhainn, S. and Kelleher, C. (1999), *The National Health and Lifestyle Surveys*, Dublin: Health Promotion Unit.

Fuller, L. (2004), *Irish Catholicism since 1950. The Undoing of a Culture*, Dublin: Gill & Macmillan

Gallie, D. (forthcoming 2007) 'Task Discretion and Job Quality', in Gallie, D. (ed.), *Employment Systems and the Quality of Working Life*, Oxford: Oxford University Press

Gallie, D., O'Connell, P. J., Tåhlin, M. and Scherer, S. (2004), 'Skills and the Quality of Work: State of the Art Review', prepared for the European CHANGEQUAL network

Gallie, D., White, M., Cheng, Y. and Tomlinson, M. (1998), *Restructuring the Employment Relationship*, Oxford: Clarendon Press

Galligan, Y., Ward, E. and Wilford, R. (eds.) (1999), *Contesting Politics: Women in Ireland, North and South,* Boulder, CO: Westview Press

Gans, H. (1967), *The Levittowners. Ways of Life and Politics in a New Suburban Community*, London: Allen Lane, the Penguin Press

Garland, D. (2001), *The Culture of Control: Crime and Social Order in Contemporary Society*, Oxford: Oxford University Press

Geary, J. (1999), 'The New Workplace: Change at work in Ireland', *International Journal of Human Resource Management*, vol. 10, no. 5, pp. 870–890

Goldberg, D. P. (1972), *The Detection of Psychiatric Illness by Questionnaire*, London: Oxford University Press

Goldthorpe, J. H. (1987), *Social Mobility and Class Structure in Modern Britain*, second edition, Oxford: Clarendon Press

Goode, W. J. (1963), *World Revolution and Family Patterns*, New York: Free Press

Goode, W. J. (1993), *World Changes in Divorce Patterns*, New Haven and London: Yale University Press

Gorby, S., McCoy, S. and Williams, J. (2005), 'Annual School Leavers' Survey: Results of the School Leavers', Survey, 2002/03, Dublin: Economic and Social Research Institute and the Department of Education and Science

Gordon, D., Adelman, L., Ashworth, K., Bradshaw, J., Levitas, R., Middelton, S., Pantazis, C., Patsios, D., Payne, S., Townsend, P. and Williams, J. (2000), *Poverty and Social Exclusion in Britain*, York: Joseph Rowntree Foundation

Gordon, M. (1977), 'Primary-group differentiation in urban Ireland', *Social Forces*, vol. 55, no. 3, pp. 743–752

Gornick, J. C. and Meyers, M. K. (2003), *Families That Work – Policies for Reconciling Parenthood and Employment*, New York: Russell Sage Foundation

Gould, R. V. (1993), 'Collective action and network structure', *American Sociological Review*, vol. 58, no. 2, pp. 182–196

Green, F. and McIntosh, S. (2000), *Working on the Chain Gang? An Examination of Rising Effort Levels in Europe in the 1990s*, London: Centre for Economic Performance

Guinnane, T. W. (1997), *The Vanishing Irish. Households, Migration, and the Rural Economy in Ireland, 1850–1914*, Princeton: Princeton University Press

Halman, L. (2001), *The European Values Study: A Third Wave*, Tilburg: WORC, Tilburg University

Halpin, B. and O'Donoghue, C. (2004), 'Cohabitation in Ireland: evidence from survey data', University of Limerick Department of Sociology Working Paper, no. WP2004-01, http://www.ul.ie/sociology/pubs/

Hannan, D. and Commins, P. (1992), 'The Significance of Small-scale Landholders in Ireland's Socio-economic Transformation', in Goldthorpe, J. H. and Whelan, C. T. (eds.), *The Development of Industrial Society in Ireland*, Oxford, Oxford university Press

Hannan, D. and Ó Riain, S. (1993), *Pathways to Adulthood in Ireland: Causes and Consequences of Success and Failure in Transitions Amongst Irish Youth*, ESRI General Research Series, Paper no. 161

Hannan, D. F., Smyth, E., McCullagh, J., O'Leary, R., McMahon, D. (1996), *Coeducation and Gender Equality: Exam Performance, Stress and Personal Development*, Dublin, Oak Tree Press/Economic and Social Research Institute

Hardiman, N. (2000), 'Social Partnership, Wage Bargaining and Growth', in Nolan, B., O'Connell, P. J. and Whelan, C. T. (eds.), *Bust to Boom? The Irish Experience of Growth and Inequality*, Dublin: Economic and Social Research Institute and Institute of Public Administration

Hardiman, N. (2004), *Which Paths? Domestic Adaptation to Economic Internationalization in Ireland*, ISSC Working Paper, 2004/12

Health Insurance Authority (2003), *Annual Report and Accounts 2003*, Dublin: Health Insurance Authority

Hill, M. (2003), *Women in Ireland: A Century of Change*, Belfast: Blackstaff Press

Hillyard, P., Pantazis, C., Tombs, S., Gordon, D. and Dorling, D. (2005), *Criminal Obsessions: Why Harm Matters more than Crime*, London: Crime and Society Foundation

Hirsch, F. (1976), *Social Limits to Growth*, Cambridge: Harvard University Press

Homeless Agency (2005), *Counted In 2005*, Dublin: Homeless Agency

Honohan, P. and B. Walsh (2002), 'Catching Up With the Leaders: The Irish Hare', *Brookings Papers on Economic Activity*, no. 1, 1–77

Horgan, O. (2000), 'Seeking Refuge', in MacLachlan, M. and O'Connell, M. (eds.) (2000), *Cultivating Pluralism: Psychological, Social and Cultural Perspectives on a Changing Ireland*, Dublin: Oaktree Press

Hug, C. (1999), *The Politics of Sexual Morality in Ireland*, London: Macmillan

Hughes, G. (2002), 'Employment and Occupational Segregation', in *Impact Evaluation of the European Employment Strategy in Ireland*, Department of Enterprise, Trade and Employment

Hughes, G. and Doyle, N. (2006), 'Recent Changes in Migration Movements and Policies: Ireland', in *Trends in International Migration 2005*, Paris: OECD

Hughes, G. and Quinn, E. (2004), *The Impact of Immigration on Irish Society*, European Migration Network, Dublin: ESRI

Humphries, A. J. (1966), *New Dubliners*, London: Routledge and Kegan Paul

Indecon Economic Consultants (2003), *Indecon's Assessment of Restrictions in the Supply of Professional Services*, Dublin: Competition Authority

Inglis, T. F. (1998), *Lessons in Irish Sexuality*, Dublin: UCD Press

Institute of Criminology (2003), *Public Order Offences in Ireland*, Dublin: Stationery Office

Irish Medical Organisation (2004), *Position Paper on Accident and Emergency*, Dublin: Irish Medical Organisation

Irish Prison Service (2005), *Annual Report 2004*, Dublin: Irish Prison Service

Irish Society for Quality and Safety in Healthcare (2001), *National Patient Perception of the Quality of Healthcare Survey 2000*, Dublin: Irish Society for Quality and Safety in Healthcare

Irish Society for Quality and Safety in Healthcare (2003), *National Patient Perception of the Quality of Healthcare Survey 2002*, Dublin: Irish Society for Quality and Safety in Healthcare

Ishii-Kuntz, M. and Seccombe, K. (1989), 'The Impact of Children upon Social Support Networks throughout the Life Course', *Journal of Marriage and the Family*, 51, (August), pp. 777–790

Jacobs, J. (1993), *The Death and Life of Great American Cities*, New York: The Modern Library

Jacobs, J. A. and Gerson, K. (2004), *The Time Divide: Work, Family and Gender Inequality*, Massachusetts: Harvard University Press

Jaumotte, F. (2003), 'Labour Force Participation of Women: Empirical Evidence on the Role of Policy and other Determinants in OECD Countries', *OECD Economic Studies*, no. 37, pp. 51–108

Kahneman, D. (1999), 'Objective happiness', in Kahneman, D., Diener, E. and Scwartz, N. (eds.), *Well-being: The Foundations of Hedonic Psychology*, New York: Russell Sage

Kalleberg, A. L. and Rosenfeld, R. A. (1990), 'Work in the Family and in the Labor Market: A Cross-National, Reciprocal Analysis', *Journal of Marriage and the Family*, vol. 52, pp. 331–346

Kalleberg, A., Reskin, B. and Hudson, K. (2000), 'Bad Jobs in America: Standard and Nonstandard Employment Relations and Job Quality in the United States', *American Sociological Review*, vol. 65, no. 2, pp. 256–278

Keeler, E. (1992), *Effects of Cost Sharing on Use of Medical Services and Health*, Santa Monica: RAND Corporation

Kellaghan, T., McGee, P., Millar, D. and Perkins, R. (2004), *Views of the Irish Public on Education: 2004 Survey*, Dublin: Educational Research Centre

Kennedy, F. (2003), *Cottage to Crèche: Family Change in Ireland*, Dublin: Institute of Public Administration

Keogh, A. F. and Whyte, J. (2005), *Second Level Student Councils in Ireland: A Study of Enablers, Barriers and Supports*, Dublin: Children's Research Centre

Keohane, K. and Kuhling, C. (2006), 'The happiest country in the world?', pp. 29–42 in Corcoran, M. P. and Peillon, M. (eds.), *Uncertain Ireland. A Sociological Chronicle, 2003–2004*, Dublin: Institute of Public Administration

Kilcommins, S., O'Donnell, I., O'Sullivan, E. and Vaughan, B. (2004), *Crime, Punishment and the Search for Order in Ireland*, Dublin: Institute of Public Administration

Kirby, P. (2002), *The Celtic Tiger in Distress: Growth with Inequality in Ireland*, Hampshire: Palgrave

Kirby, P. (2006), *Vulnerability and Violence: The Impact of Globalization*, London: Pluto Press

Kunst, A. E., Cavelaars, A., Groenhof, F., Geurts, J. J. M. and Mackenback, J. P. (1996), 'Socio-Economic Inequalities in Morbidity and Mortality in Europe: A Comparative Study', Department of Public Health, Rotterdam: Erasmus University

Laver, M., Mair, P. and Sinnott, R. (eds.) (1987), *How Ireland Voted: the Irish General Election of 1987*, Dublin: Poolbeg Press

Layard, R. (2005), *Happiness: Lessons from a New Science*, New York: Penguin

Layte, R. and Nolan, B. (2004), 'Equity in the Utilisation of Health Care in Ireland', *Economic and Social Review*, vol. 35, no. 2, pp. 111–34

Layte, R. and Whelan, C. T. (2004), 'Class Transformation and Trends in Social Fluidity in the Republic of Ireland 1973 to 1994', in Breen, R. (ed.), *Social Mobility in Europe*, Oxford: Oxford University Press

Layte, R., McGee, H., Quail, A., Rundle, K., Cousins, G., Donnelly, C., Mulcahy, F. and Conroy, R. (2006), *The Irish Study of Sexual Health and Relationships: Main*

Report, Dublin: Crisis Pregnancy Agency and the Department of Health and Children

Layte, R., Nolan B. and Whelan, C. T. (2000), 'Trends in Poverty', in Nolan, B., O'Connell, P. J. and Whelan, C. T. (eds.), *Bust to Boom? The Irish Experience of Growth and Inequality*, Dublin: Economic and Social Research Institute and Institute of Public Administration

Layte, R., Nolan, B. and Whelan, C. T. (2004), 'Explaining Poverty Trends in Ireland During the Boom', *Irish Banking Review*, summer, pp. 2–13

Leonard, M. (2004), 'Teenage Girls and Housework in Irish Society', *Irish Journal of Sociology*, vol. 13, no. 1, pp. 73–87

Lollivier, S. and Verger, D. (1997), 'Pauverte d'Existence, Monetaire ou Subjective Sont Distinctes', *Economie et Statstique*, nos. 308/309/310, INSEE, Paris, pp. 113–142

Loyal, S. and Mulcahy, A. (2001), *Racism in Ireland – The Views of Black and Ethnic Minorities*, Dublin: Amnesty International

Lück, D. (2005), 'Cross-national Comparison of Gender Role Attitudes and their Impact on Women's Life Courses', Globalife Working Paper, no. 67

Lück, D. and Hofäcker, D. (2003), 'Rejection and Acceptance of the Male Breadwinner Model', Globalife Working Paper no. 60

Lynch, K. (1989), *The Hidden Curriculum: Reproduction in Education, an Appraisal*, London: The Falmer Press

Lynch, K. and Lodge, A. (2002), *Equality and Power in Schools: Redistribution, Recognition and Representation*, London: RoutledgeFalmer

Madden, D., Nolan, A. and Nolan, B. (2005), 'GP Reimbursement and Visiting Behaviour in Ireland', *Health Economics*, vol. 14, pp. 1047–1060

Maître, B., Nolan, B. and Whelan, C. T. (2006), *Reconfiguring the Measurement of Deprivation and Consistent Poverty in Ireland*, Dublin: Economic and Social Research Institute

Maître, B., Whelan, C. T. and Nolan, B. (2003), 'Female Partner's Income Contribution to the Household Income in the European Union', European Panel Analysis Group Working Paper no. 43

Marshall, T. H. (1950), *Citizenship and Social Class and Other Essays*, Cambridge: Cambridge University Press

Mc Kay, S. (2004), 'Poverty or Preference: What Do "Consensual Deprivation Indicators" Really Measure?', *Fiscal Studies*, vol. 25, no. 2, pp. 201–223

Mc Kay, S. and Collard, S. (2003), 'Developing Deprivation Questions for the Family Resources Survey', Department for Work and Pensions Working Paper, no. 13, Corporate Document Series

McAdam, D. and Paulsen, R. (1993), 'Specifying the relationship between social ties and activism', *American Journal of Sociology*, vol. 99, no. 3, pp. 640–667

McAleese, M. (2003), Speech by the President of Ireland, Mary McAleese, at the 'Re-Imagining Ireland' Conference, Charlottesville, Virginia, 7 May 2003, Dublin: Áras an Úachtaráin, http://www.president.ie/

McCoy, D., Duffy, D. and Smyth, D. (2000), *Quarterly Economic Commentary*, September 2000, Dublin: Economic and Social Research Institute

McCoy, S. and Smyth, E. (2003), 'Educational expenditure: implications for equality', in Callan, T., Doris, A. and McCoy, D. (eds.), *Budget Perspectives 2004*, Dublin: Economic and Social Research Institute/Foundation for Fiscal Studies

McCoy, S. and Smyth, E. (2004), *At Work in School: Part-Time Employment among Second-Level Students*, Dublin: Economic and Social Research Institute, in association with the Liffey Press

McCoy, S., Smyth, E., Darmody, M. and Dunne, A. (2006), *Guidance for All? Guidance Provision in Second-Level Schools*, Dublin: Economic and Social Research Institute/Liffey Press

McCullagh, C. (1996), *Crime in Ireland: A Sociological Introduction*, Cork: Cork University Press

McGee, H., O'Hanlon, A., Barker, M., Hickey, A., Garavan, R., Conroy, R., Layte, R., Shelley, E., Horgan, F., Crawford, V., Stout, R. and O'Neill, D. (2005), *One Island – Two Systems: A Comparison of Health Status and Health and Social Service Use by Community-Dwelling Older People in the Republic of Ireland and Northern Ireland*, Institute of Public Health in Ireland, Dublin

McGinnity, F. and Russell, H. (2006), 'Work Rich, Time Poor? Time Use of Men and Women in Ireland', ESRI Seminar Paper, January 2006, Dublin: Economic and Social Research Institute

McGinnity, F., O'Connell, P., Quinn, E. and Williams, J. (2006), *Migrants' Experience of Racism and Discrimination in Ireland*, Dublin: ESRI

McGinnity, F., Russell, H., Williams, J. and Blackwell, S. (2005), *Time Use in Ireland, 2005: Survey Report*, Dublin: Economic and Social Research Institute

McKenna, P. and O'Maolmhuire, C. (2000), *Work Experience as an Education and Training Strategy for the 21st Century*, Dublin: School of Education Studies, Dublin City University

McLoughlin, O. (2004), 'Citizen Child – The Experience of a Student Council in a Primary School', in Deegan, J., Devine, D. and Lodge, A. (eds.), *Primary Voices – Equality, Diversity and Childhood in Irish Primary Schools*, Dublin: Institute of Public Administration

McPherson, M. J. (1981), 'A Dynamic Model of Voluntary Affiliation', *Social Forces*, vol. 59, no. 3, pp. 705–728

McQuinn, K. (2004), 'A model of the Irish housing sector', Research Technical Paper 1/RT/04, Dublin: Central Bank and Financial Services Authority of Ireland

McWilliams, D. (2006), *The Pope's Children. Ireland's New Elite*, Dublin: Gill & Macmillan

Miller, L. J. (1995), 'Family Togetherness and the Suburban Idea', *Sociological Forum*, vol. 10, no. 3, pp. 393–418

Molotch, H., Freudenburg, W. and Paulsen, K. E. (2000), 'History Repeats Itself, but How? City Character, Urban Tradition and the Accomplishment of Place', *American Sociological Review*, vol. 65, pp. 791–823

Murphy, B. (2005), 'Child-Centred Curricula: Insights into some Realties of Practice in Irish Infant Classrooms Thirty Years On', paper to the Educational Studies Association of Ireland Annual Conference

Murray, K. and Norris, M. (2002), *Profile of Households Accommodated by Dublin City Council. Analysis of Socio-Demographic, Income and Spatial Patterns, 2001*, Dublin: The Housing Unit and Dublin City Council

National Anti-Poverty Strategy, (1997) *Sharing in Progress*, Dublin: Stationery Office

National Consultative Committee on Racism and Interculturalism (2004), NCCRI Progress Report 2002–2004 + Strategy Statement 2005–2007, Dublin. NCCRI

National Council for Curriculum and Assessment (2003), *Developing Senior Cycle Education: Directions for Development*, Dublin: NCCA
National Council for Curriculum and Assessment (2005), *Proposals for the Future Development of Senior Cycle Education in Ireland*, Dublin: NCCA
National Crime Forum (1998), *Report*, Dublin: Institute of Public Administration
National Disability Authority (2006), *How Far Towards Equality: Measuring How Equally People with Disabilities are Included in Irish Society*, Dublin: NDA
National Disease Surveillance Centre (2004), *National Disease Surveillance Centre Annual Report 2003*, Dublin: NDSC
National Economic and Social Council (2005), *NESC Strategy 2006: People, Productivity and Purpose*, Dublin: NESC
National Economic and Social Forum (2003), *Labour Market Issues for Older Workers*, Forum Report no. 26, Dublin: NESF
National Economic and Social Forum (2006), *Creating a More Inclusive Labour Market*, Report no. 33, Dublin: NESF
National Suicide Research Foundation (2004), *Young People's Mental Health*, Cork: NSRF
Nolan, A. (2005), 'A Dynamic Analysis of the Utilisation of GP Services', *Working Paper No. 13 of Research Programme on Health Services*, Health Inequalities and Health and Social Gain: Economic and Social Research Institute, UCD and University of Ulster
Nolan, A. and Nolan, B. (2004), 'Ireland's Health Care System: Some Issues and Challenges', in Callan, T. and Doris, A. (eds.), *Budget Perspectives 2005*, Dublin: Economic and Social Research Institute
Nolan, A. and Nolan, B. (2005), 'Eligibility for Free Care, Need and GP Services in Ireland', mimeo., Dublin: Economic and Social Research Institute
Nolan, B. (1991), *The Utilisation and Financing of Health Services in Ireland*, Dublin ESRI
Nolan, B. (2003), 'Income Inequality during Ireland's Boom', *Studies*, vol. 92, no. 366, pp. 132–143
Nolan, B. and T. Smeeding, (2005), 'Ireland's Income Distribution in Comparative Perspective', *Review of Income and Wealth*, vol. 54, no. 4, pp. 537–560
Nolan, B. and Whelan, C. T. (1996), *Resources, Deprivation and Poverty*, Oxford and New York: Oxford University Press, Clarendon Press
Nolan, B. and Whelan, C. T. (2005), 'On the Multidimensionality of Poverty and Social Exclusion', paper presented at European Consortium for Sociological Research Conference on Comparative European Studies: Assessing Ten Years of Sociological Research 1995–2005, Paris: 25–26 November
Nolan, B. and Wiley, M. (2001), 'Private Practice in Irish Public Hospitals', General Research Series no. 175, Dublin: Economic and Social Research Institute
Ó Riain, S. and O'Connell, P. (2000), 'The Role of the State in Growth and Welfare' in Nolan, B., O'Connell, P. and Whelan, C. (eds.), *Bust to Boom? The Irish Experience of Growth and Inequality*, Dublin: Economic and Social Research Institute and Institute for Public Administration
O'Connell, M. and Whelan, A. (1994), 'Crime victimisation in Dublin', *Irish Criminal Law Journal*, vol. 4, no. 1, pp. 85–112

O'Connell, P. J. (2000), 'The Dynamics of the Irish Labour Market in Comparative Perspective', in Nolan, B., O'Connell, P. J. and Whelan, C. T. (eds.), *Bust to Boom: The Irish Experience of Growth and Inequality*, Dublin: Economic and Social Research Institute and the Institute of Public Administration

O'Connell, P. J. (2005), *Data Analysis of In-employment Education and Training in Ireland*, Dublin: Expert Group on Future Skill Needs, Forfás

O'Connell, P. J. and Gash, V. (2003), 'The Effects of Working Time, Segmentation, and Labour Market Mobility on Wages and Pensions in Ireland', *British Journal of Industrial Relations*, vol. 41

O'Connell, P. J. and Russell, H. (2005), *Equality at Work? Workplace Equality Policies: Flexible Working Arrangements and the Quality of Work*, Equality Research Series, Dublin: The Equality Authority

O'Connell, P. J., Clancy, D. and McCoy, S. (2006), *Access to Higher Education in 2004*, Dublin: Higher Education Authority

O'Connell, P. J., McGinnity, F. and Russell, H. (2003), 'Working time flexibility in Ireland', in O'Reilly, J. (ed.), *Time Rules: Regulating Working-time Transition in Europe*, Cheltenham: Edward Elgar

O'Connell, P. J., Russell, H., Williams, J. and Blackwell, S. (2004), *The Changing Workplace: A Survey of Employees' Views and Experiences*, Dublin: Economic and Social Research Institute/NCPP

O'Donnell, I. (1997), 'Crime, punishment and poverty,' *Irish Criminal Law Journal,* vol. 7, no. 2, pp. 134–151

O'Donnell, I. (2004), 'Imprisonment and penal policy in Ireland,' *Howard Journal of Criminal Justice*, vol. 43, no. 3, pp. 253–266

O'Donnell, I. (2005a), 'Violence and Social Change in the Republic of Ireland', *International Journal of the Sociology of Law*, vol. 33, no. 2, pp. 101–117

O'Donnell, I. (2005b), 'Putting prison in its place', *Judicial Studies Institute Journal*, vol. 5, no. 1, pp. 54–68

O'Donnell, I. and O'Sullivan, E. (2001), *Crime Control in Ireland: The Politics of Intolerance*, Cork University Press

O'Donnell, I. and O'Sullivan, E. (2003), 'The Politics of Intolerance – Irish Style,' *British Journal of Criminology*, vol. 43, no. 1, pp. 41–62

O'Donnell, I., O'Sullivan, E. and Healy, D. (2005), *Crime and Punishment in Ireland 1922 to 2003: A Statistical Sourcebook*, Dublin: Institute of Public Administration

O'Hearn, D. (1998), *Inside the Celtic Tiger: The Irish Economy and the Asian Model*, London: Pluto Press

O'Hearn, D. (2000), 'Globalization. "New Tigers" and the End of the Developmental State? The Case of the Celtic Tiger', *Politics and Society*, vol. 28, no. 1, pp. 67–92

O'Hearn, D. (2001), *The Atlantic Economy: Britain, the US and Ireland*, Manchester: University of Manchester Press

O'Reilly, E. (2004), 'Imagining the future – an Irish perspective', in Kennedy, G. and Bohan, H. (eds.), *Imagining the Future*, Dublin: Veritas

O'Reilly, J. and Fagan, C. (eds.) (1998), *Part-time Prospects: An International Comparison of Part-time Work in Europe, North America and The Pacific Rim*, London: Routledge

OECD (2005), *Education at a Glance 2005*, Paris: OECD

OECD (2006), *Education at a Glance 2006,* Paris: OECD

Oliver, P. (1984), '"If you don't do it, nobody else will": active and token contributors to local collective action', *American Sociological Review*, vol. 49, no. 5, pp. 601–10

Oliver, P., Davis, I. and Bentley, I. (1981), *Dunroamin. The Suburban Semi and its Enemies*, London: Pimlico

Papademetriou, D. (2003), 'Policy Considerations for Immigrant Integration', Migration Policy Institute: http://www.migrationinformation.org/feature/print.cfm?ID=171

Parsons, T. and Bales, R. F. (1955), *Family, Socialisation and Interaction Process*, New York: Free Press

Peillon, M., Corcoran, M. and Gray, J. (2006), *Civic Engagement and the Governance of Irish Suburbs*, Dublin: The Policy Institute

Perez-Mayo, J. (2004), 'Consistent Poverty Dynamics in Spain', IRISS, Working papers, no. 2004-09

Permanent tsb/ESRI (2006), *House Price Index 2006* at www.permanenttsb.ie or www.esri.ie

Phillipson, C., Bernard, M., Phillips, J. and Ogg, J. (1999), 'Older People's Experiences of Community Life: Patterns of Neighbouring in Three Urban Areas', *Sociological Review*, vol. 47, no. 4, pp. 715–743

Piketty, T. (2001), *Les hauts revenus en France au 20^{ieme} siecle – Inegalites et redistributions, 1901–1998,* Paris : Editions Grassets

Piketty, T. (2003), 'Income Inequality in France, 1901–1998', *Journal of Political Economy*, vol. 222, no. 5, pp. 1004–1042

Piketty, T. and Saez, E. (2003), 'Income Inequality in the United States, 1913–1998', *Quarterly Journal of Economics*, vol. CXVIII, no. 1, pp. 1–39

Plasman, A., Plasman, R., Rusinek, M. and Rycx, F. (2002), 'Indicators on Gender Pay Equality', *Cahiers Economiques de Bruxelles*, n° 45 (2)

Povey, D. (2005), 'Crime in England and Wales 2003/2004: Supplementary Volume 1: Homicide and Gun Crime', *Statistical Bulletin 02/05*, London: Home Office

Putnam, R. D. (2000), *Bowling Alone: The Collapse and Revival of American Community*, New York: Touchstone Books

Quinn, E. (2006a), *Migration and Asylum in Ireland: Summary of Legislation, Case Law and Policy Measures and Directory of Organisations, Researchers and Research 2005*, European Migration Network

Quinn, E. (2006b), *Policy Analysis Report on Asylum and Migration: Ireland mid-2004 to 2005*, European Migration Network

Quinn, E. and Hughes, G. (2005a), *Illegally Resident Third Country Nationals in Ireland: State Approaches Towards their Situation*, European Migration Network

Quinn, E. and Hughes, G. (2005b), *Policy Analysis Report on Asylum and Migration: Ireland 2003 to mid-2004*, European Migration Network

Revenue Commissioners (2004), *Annual Report*, Dublin: Office of Revenue Commissioners

Rhodes, M. (1998), 'Globalization, Labour Markets and Welfare States: A Future of "Competitive Corporatism"', in Rhodes, M. and Mêny, Y. (eds.), *The Future of European Welfare States: A New Social Contract?*, London: Sage

Roche, M. (2001), 'The rise in House Prices in Dublin: bubble, fad or just fundamentals?', *Economic Modelling*, 18, pp. 281–295

Roche, M. (2003), 'Will there be a Crash in Irish House Prices?', *ESRI Quarterly Economic Commentary*, winter

Roche, W. K. and Geary, J. (1998), *Collaborative Production and the Irish Boom: Work Organization and Direct Involvement in the Irish Workplace*, UCD Graduate School of Business, Working Paper no. 26

Rottman, D. B. (1980), *Crime in the Republic of Ireland: Statistical Trends and their Interpretation*, Paper no. 102, Dublin: Economic and Social Research Institute

Rubery, J. (1998), 'Part-time Work: A Threat to Labour Standards?', pp. 137–155, in O'Reilly, J. and Fagan, C. (eds.) (1998), *Part-time Prospects: An International Comparison of Part-time Work in Europe, North America and The Pacific Rim*, London: Routledge

Ruddle, H. (1999), *Reaching out. Donating and Volunteering in the Republic of Ireland*, Dublin: National College of Ireland

Ruddle, H. and O'Connor, J. (1993), *Reaching out. Charitable giving and volunteering in the Republic of Ireland*, Dublin: National College of Industrial Relations

Rudduck, J., Chaplan, R. and Wallace, G. (eds.) (1996), *School Improvement: What Can Pupils Tell Us?*, London: David Fulton

Ruhs, M. (2005), *Managing the Immigration and Employment of Non-EU nationals in Ireland*, The Policy Institute, Dublin: Trinity College

Rundle, K., Leigh, C., McGee, H. and Layte, R. (2004), *Irish Contraception and Crisis Pregnancy [ICCP] Study: A Survey of the General Population*, Crisis Pregnancy Agency, Dublin

Russell, H. and Gannon, B. (2002), 'The Gender Wage Gap in Ireland' in *Impact Evaluation of the European Employment Strategy in Ireland*, Department of Enterprise, Trade and Employment

Russell, H., Layte, R., Maître, B., O'Connell, P. and Whelan, C. (2004), *Work-Poor Households: The Welfare Implications of Changing Household Employment Patterns*, ESRI Policy Research Series no. 52, Dublin: Economic and Social Research Institute

Russell, H., Smyth, E. and O'Connell, P. J. (2005), *Degrees of Equality: Gender Pay Differentials among Recent Graduates*, Dublin: Economic and Social Research Institute

Russell, H., Smyth, E., Lyons, M. and O'Connell, P. J. (2002), *Getting Out of the House: Women Returning to Employment, Education and Training*, Dublin: Economic and Social Research Institute/Liffey Press

Saez, E. and Veall, M. (2005), 'The Evolution of High Incomes in Northern America: Lessons from Canadian Evidence', *American Economic Review*, vol. 95, no. 3, pp. 831–849

Savage, M., Bagnall, G. and Longhurst, B. (2005), *Globalisation and Belonging*, London: Routledge

Sayer, L. C., Bianchi, S. M. and Robinson, J. P. (2004), 'Are parents investing less time in children? Trends in Mothers' and Fathers' Time with Children', *American Journal of Sociology*, vol. 110, no. 1, pp. 1–43

Scitovsky, T. (1976), *The Joyless Economy: An Inquiry into Human Satisfaction and Consumer Dissatisfaction*, Oxford: Oxford University Press

Scott, J., Braun, M. and Alwin, D. (1998), 'Partner, Parent, Worker: Family and Gender Roles', in Jowell, R., Curtice, J., Park, A., Brook, L., Thomson, K. and Bryson, C. (eds.), *British and European Social Attitudes*, Aldershot: Ashgate

Sen, A. (1992), *Inequality Re-examined*, Cambridge: Harvard University Press

Sennett, R. (1970), *The Uses of Disorder: Personal Identity and City Life*, Harmondsworth: Penguin Books.

Sexton, J. J. (2001), 'Recent Changes in Migration Movements and Policies: Ireland', in *Trends in International Migration 2001*, Paris: OECD

Sexton, J. J., Hughes, G., and Finn, C. (2002), 'Occupational Employment Forecasts 2015', *FÁS/ESRI Manpower Forecasting Studies*, Report no. 10, Dublin: Economic and Social Research Institute

Shelton, B. A. and John, D. (1996), 'The Division of Household Labor', *Annual Review of Sociology*, vol. 22, pp. 299–322

Shiel, G., Cosgrove, J., Sofroniou, N. and Kelly, A. (2001), *Ready for Life? The Literacy Achievements of Irish 15-Year Olds with Comparative International Data*, Dublin: Educational Research Centre

Simon, H. and Russell, H. (2004), 'Firms and the Gender Pay Gap: A Cross-National Comparison', Pay Inequality and Economic Performance Working Paper Series, London School of Economics, http://cep.lse.ac.uk/piep/papers

Simonsen, K. (1997), 'Modernity, Community or a Diversity of Ways of Life: A discussion of Urban Everyday Life', in Kalltorp, O., Elander, I., Ericsson, O. and Frantzen, M. (eds.) *Cities in Transformation: Transformation in Cities*, London: Avebury

Sleebos, J. E. (2003), 'Low Fertility Rates in OECD Countries: Facts and Policy Responses', OECD Social, *Employment and Migration Working Papers* no. 15, Paris: OECD

Smith, A. (1776), *The Wealth of Nations*, quoted from http://www.econlib.org/LIBRARY/Smith/smWN.html [Book V, Chapter II]

Smyth, E. (1999), *Do Schools Differ? Academic and Personal Development among Pupils in the Second-Level Sector*, Dublin: Oak Tree Press/Economic and Social Research Institute

Smyth, E. and Byrne, D. (2004), *The Potential Supply of Mature Students to Higher Education*, Report to the Higher Education Authority

Smyth, E., Byrne, D. and Hannan, C. (2004), *The Transition Year Programme. An Assessment*, Dublin: The Liffey Press/Economic and Social Research Institute

Smyth, E., Dunne, A., McCoy, S. and Darmody, M. (2006), *Pathways through the Junior Cycle*, Dublin: Liffey Press/Economic and Social Research Institute

Smyth, E., McCoy, S. and Darmody, M. (2004), *Moving Up. The Experiences of First-Year Students in Post-Primary Education*, Dublin: The Liffey Press/Economic and Social Research Institute

Swisher, R., Sweet, S. and Moen, P. (2004), 'The Family-friendly community and its life-course fit for dual-earner couples', *Journal of Marriage and the Family*, vol. 66, May, pp. 281–292

Tåhlin, M. (2006), 'Skill Change and Skill Matching in the Labour Market: A Cross National Overview' in Gallie, D. (ed.), *Research Group Employment and the Labour Market (EMPLOY) State of the Art Report*, Equalsoc.

Task Force on Student Behaviour in Second-Level Schools (2006), 'School Matters: Report of the Task Force on Student Behaviour in Second-Level Schools', Dublin: Department of Education and Science

Taub, R., Surgeon, G., Lindholm, S., Betts Otti, P. and Bridges, A. (1977), 'Urban Voluntary Associations: Locality Based and Externally Induced', *American Journal of Sociology*, vol. 83, no. 2, pp. 425–442

United Nations (2003), *Report on the World Social Situation: Social Vulnerability: Sources and Challenges*, New York: United Nations Department of Economic and Social Affairs

Van Doorslaer, E., Wagstaff, A., Van Den Berg, H., Christiansen, T., De Graeve, D., Duchesne, I., Gerdtham, U. G., Gerfin, M., Geurts, J., Gross, L., Häkkinen, U., Leu, R. E., Nolan, B., O'Donnell, O., Propper, C., Puffer, F., Schellhorn, M., Sundberg, G. and Winkelhake, O. (2000), 'Equity in the delivery of health care in Europe and the US', *Journal of Health Economics*, vol. 19, no. 5, pp. 553–583

Veenhoven, R. (1995), 'The cross-national pattern of happiness. Test of predictions implied in three theories of happiness', *Social Indicators Research*, vol. 34, pp. 33–68

Waite, L. and Gallagher, M. (2000), *The Case for Marriage*, New York: Doubleday

Walzer, M. (1983), *Spheres of Justice*, New York: Basic Books

Watson, D. (2000), *Victims of Recorded Crime in Ireland: Results from the 1996 Survey*, General Research Series Paper no. 174, Dublin: Oak Tree Press

Watson, D. and Williams, J. (2001), *Perceptions of the Quality of Healthcare in the Public and Private Sectors in Ireland*, Dublin: Economic and Social Research Institute

Watson, D. and Williams, J. (2003), *The Irish National Survey of Housing Quality, 2001–2002*, Dublin: Economic and Social Research Institute

Watson, D., Whelan, C. T., Williams, J. and Blackwell, S. (2005), *Mapping Poverty: National, Regional and County Patterns*, Dublin: Combat Poverty Agency and Institute of Public Administration

Whelan, C. T and Maître, B. (2007a), 'Levels and Patterns of Multiple Deprivation in Ireland: After the Celtic Tiger', *European Sociological Review*, vol. 23, no. 2

Whelan, C. T and Maître, B. (2007b), 'Measuring Material Deprivation with EU SILC Data: Lessons from the Irish Survey,' *European Societies*, vol. 9, no. 2

Whelan, C. T. and Layte, R. (2002), 'Late Industrialisation and the Increased Merit Selection Hypothesis', *European Sociological Review*, vol. 18, no. 1, pp. 35–50

Whelan, C. T. and Layte, R. (2004), 'Economic Change, Social Mobility and Meritocracy: Reflections on the Irish Experience', special article in *Quarterly Economic Commentary*, autumn 2004, Economic and Social Research Institute, Dublin

Whelan, C. T. and Layte, R. (2006), 'Economic Boom and Social Mobility: The Irish Experience', *Research in Social Stratification and Mobility*, vol. 24, pp. 193–208

Whelan, C. T. and Maître, B. (2005a), 'Economic Vulnerability, Multi-dimensional Deprivation and Social Cohesion in an Enlarged European Union', *International Journal of Comparative Sociology*, vol. 46, no. 3, pp. 215–239

Whelan, C. T. and Maître, B. (2005b), 'Vulnerability and Multiple Deprivation Perspectives on Economic Exclusion in Europe: A Latent Class Analysis', *European Societies*, vol. 7, no. 3, pp. 423–450

Whelan, C. T. and Maître, B. (2006), 'Levels and Patterns of Multiple Deprivation in Ireland', ESRI Working Paper no. 166, Dublin: Economic and Social Research Institute

Whelan, C. T., Hannan, D. F. and Creighton, S. (1991), 'Unemployment, Poverty and Psychological Distress', General Research Series 150, Dublin: Economic and Social Research Institute

Whelan, C. T., Layte, R. and Maître, B. (2004), 'Understanding the Mismatch Between Income Poverty and Deprivation: A Dynamic Comparative Analysis', *European Sociological Review*, vol. 20, no. 4, pp. 287–301

Whelan, C. T., Layte, R., Maître, B., Gannon, B., Nolan, B., Watson, D., Williams, J. (2003), *Monitoring Poverty Trends in Ireland*, Dublin: Economic and Social Research Institute

Whelan, C. T., Layte, R., Maître, B., Nolan, B. (2001), 'Income, Deprivation and Economic Strain: An Analysis of the European Community Household Panel', *European Sociological Review*, vol. 17, no. 4, pp. 357–337, chapter 6

Whelan, C. T., Nolan, B. and Maître, B. (2006), 'Trends in economic vulnerability in the Republic of Ireland', *The Economic and Social Review*, vol. 37, no. 1, pp. 91–119

Wiley, M. (2005), 'The Irish Health System: Developments in Strategy, Structure, Funding and Delivery since 1980', *Health Economics*, 14, S169–S186

Wilkinson, R. G. (1996), *Unhealthy Societies: The Afflictions of Inequality*, Routledge, London

Wilmott, P. and Young, M. (1960), *Family and Class in a London Suburb*, London: Routledge and Kegan Paul

Wirth, L. (1938), 'Urbanism as a Way of Life', *American Journal of Sociology*, vol. 44, no. 1, pp. 1–24

World Bank (2000), *World Development Report 2000–01: Attacking Poverty*, New York: Oxford University Press

Wren, M. A. (2004), 'Health Spending and the Black Hole', *Quarterly Economic Commentary*, autumn 2004, Dublin: Economic and Social Research Institute

Wren, M. A. and Tussing, A. D. (2006), *How Ireland Cares: the Case for Health Care Reform*, Dublin New Island

Young, M. (1958), *The Rise of the Meritocracy*, Harmondsworth: Penguin

Young, M. and Wilmott, P. (1957), *Family and Kinship in East London*, London: Routledge and Kegan Paul

Index

Social Indicators Research Series

1. V. Møller (ed.): *Quality of Life in South Africa.* 1997 ISBN 0-7923-4797-8
2. G. Baechler: *Violence Through Environmental Discrimination.* Causes, Rwanda Arena, and Conflict Model. 1999 ISBN 0-7923-5495-8
3. P. Bowles and L.T. Woods (eds.): *Japan after the Economic Miracle.* In Search of New Directories. 1999 ISBN 0-7923 6031-1
4. E. Diener and D.R. Rahtz (eds.): *Advances in Quality of Life Theory and Research.* Volume I. 1999 ISBN 0-7923-6060-5
5. Kwong-leung Tang (ed.): *Social Development in Asia.* 2000 ISBN 0-7923-6256-X
6. M.M. Beyerlein (ed.): *Work Teams: Past, Present and Future.* 2000 ISBN 0-7923-6699-9
7. A. Ben-Arieh, N.H. Kaufman, A.B. Andrews, R. Goerge, B.J. Lee, J.L. Aber (eds.): *Measuring and Monitoring Children's Well-Being.* 2001 ISBN 0-7923-6789-8
8. M.J. Sirgy: *Handbook of Quality-of-Life Research. An Ethical Marketing Perspective.* 2001 ISBN 1-4020-0172-X
9. G. Preyer and M. Bös (eds.): *Borderlines in a Globalized World.* New Perspectives in a Sociology of the World-System. 2002 ISBN 1-4020-0515-6
10. V. Nikolic-Ristanovic: *Social Change, Gender and Violence: Post-communist and war affected societies.* 2002 ISBN 1-4020-0726-4
11. M.R. Hagerty, J. Vogel and V. Møller: *Assessing Quality of Life and Living Conditions to Guide National Policy.* 2002 ISBN 1-4020-0727-2
12. M.J. Sirgy: *The Psychology of Quality of Life.* 2002 ISBN 1-4020-0800-7
13. S. McBride, L. Dobuzinskis, M. Griffin Cohen and J. Busumtwi-Sam (eds.): *Global Instability.* Uncertainty and new visions in political economy. 2002 ISBN 1-4020-0946-1
14. Doh. Chull Shin, C.P. Rutkowski and Chong-Min Park (eds.): *The Quality of Life in Korea.* Comparative and Dynamic Perspectives. 2003 ISBN 1-4020-0947-X
15. W. Glatzer: *Rich and Poor.* Disparities, Perceptions, Concomitants. 2002 ISBN 1-4020-1012-5
16. E. Gullone and R.A. Cummins (eds.): *The Universality of Subjective Wellbeing Indicators.* A Multi-disciplinary and Multi-national Perspective. 2002 ISBN 1-4020-1044-3
17. B.D. Zumbo (ed.): *Advances in Quality of Life Research 2001.* 2003 ISBN 1-4020-1100-8

18. J. Vogel, T. Theorell, S. Svallfors, H.-H. Noll and B. Christoph: *European Welfare Production.* Institutional Configuration and Distributional Outcome. 2003 ISBN 1-4020-1149-0
19. A.C. Michalos: *Essays on the Quality of Life.* 2003 ISBN 1-4020-1342-6
20. M.J. Sirgy, D. Rahtz and A.C. Samli (eds.): *Advances in Quality-of-Life Theory and Research.* 2003 ISBN 1-4020-1474-0
21. M. Fine-Davis, J. Fagnani, D. Giovannini, L. Højgaard and H. Clarke: *Fathers and Mothers: Dilemmas of the Work-Life Balance.* 2004 ISBN 1-4020-1807-X
22. M.J. Sirgy, D.R. Rahtz and D.J. Lee (eds.): *Community Quality-of-Life Indicators.* Best Cases. 2004 ISBN 1-4020-2201-8
23. A. Dannerbeck, F. Casas, M. Sadurni and G. Coenders (eds.): *Quality-of-Life Research on Children and Adolescents.* 2004 ISBN 1-4020-2311-1
24. W. Glatzer, S. von Below and M. Stoffregen (eds.): *Challenges for Quality of Life in the Contemporary World.* 2004 ISBN 1-4020-2890-3
25. D.T.L. Shek, Y. Chan and P.S.N. Lee (eds.): *Quality of Life Research in Chinese, Western and Global Contexts.* 2005 ISBN 1-4020-3601-9
26. A.C. Michalos (ed.): *Citation Classics from Social Indicators Research.* The Most Cited Articles Edited and Introduced by Alex C. Michalos. 2005 ISBN 1-4020-3722-8
27. A. Ben-Arieh and R.M. Goerge (eds.): *Indicators of Children's Well Being.* Understanding Their Role, Usage and Policy Influence. 2006 ISBN 1-4020-4237-X
28. M.J. Sirgy, D. Rahtz and D. Swain (eds.): *Community Quality-of-Life Indicators.* Best Cases II. 2006 ISBN 1-4020-4624-3
29. R.J. Estes (ed.): *Advancing Quality of Life in a Turbulent World.* 2006 ISBN 1-4020-5099-2
30. D. Kucera (ed.): *Qualitative Indicators of Labour Standards.* Comparative Methods and Applications. 2007 ISBN 1-4020-5200-6
31. H. Mollenkopf and A. Walker (eds.): *Quality of Life in Old Age.* International and Multi-Disciplinary Perspectives. 2007 ISBN 978-1-4020-5681-9
32. T. Fahey, H. Russell and C.T. Whelan (eds.): *Quality of Life in Ireland.* Social Impact of Economic Boom. 2008 ISBN 978-1-4020-6980-2

Printed in the United States
122421LV00002B/261-278/P

9 781402 069802